AAS
Agents and Actions Supplements
Vol. 21

Edited by
K. Brune, Erlangen

Birkhäuser Verlag
Basel · Boston

PAF, Platelets, and Asthma

Edited by

M. Schmitz-Schumann
G. Menz
C.P. Page

1987

Birkhäuser Verlag
Basel · Boston

Volume Editorial Office:

Hochgebirgsklinik, Davos-Wolfgang
CH-7265 Wolfgang/Switzerland

Library of Congress Cataloging in Publication Data

PAF, platelets, and asthma.
(Agents and actions. Supplements ; vol. 21)
Based on a meeting held Sept. 7–9, 1986.
Includes bibliographies and index.
1. Asthma -- Etiology -- Congresses. 2. Platelet activating factor -- Physiological effect -- Congresses. 3. Blood platelets -- Congresses. I. Schmitz-Schumann, M., 1952– . II. Menz, G. III. Page, C. P. IV. Series: Agents and actions supplement ; v. 21. [DNLM: 1. Asthma -- etiology -- congresses. 2. Blood platelets -- congresses. 3. Platelet Activating Factor -- congresses. W1 AG33A v21 / WF 553 P127 1986]
RC591.P336 1987 616.2'38071 87–21863
ISBN 0-8176-1806-6 (U.S.)

CIP-Kurztitelaufnahme der Deutschen Bibliothek

PAF, platelets, and asthma / ed. by M. Schmitz-Schumann ... –
Basel ; Boston : Birkhäuser, 1987.
(Agents and actions : Supplements ; Vol. 21)
ISBN 3-7643-1806-6 (Basel)
ISBN 0-8176-1806-6 (Boston)
NE: Schmitz-Schumann, Michael [Hrsg.];
Agents and actions / Supplements

Printed in Germany
ISBN 3-7643-1806-6
ISBN 0-8176-1806-6

PREFACE

Bronchial asthma is a disease with many unsolved problems and despite an increased availability of anti-asthma drugs, morbidity and mortality from this disease are not improving. It is now recognized that asthma should be considered as a chronic inflammatory disease of the lung resulting in bronchial hyperreactivity and subsequent symptoms.
The mechanisms underlying airways inflammation and bronchial hyperreactivity have now become a focal point of research in the quest for knowledge about how the management of this disease can be improved.

Platelet activating factor (PAF-acether AGEPC) is a naturally occurring ether-linked phospholipid discovered in 1972 associated with IgE mediated allergic responses which has potent effects on platelet activation. PAF is now recognized as a molecule having a diverse range of biological effects relevant to allergic inflammation and asthma including the ability to induce long lasting airway inflammation and associated increases in bronchial reactivity. Certain activities of PAF are known to be secondary to platelets activation raising the possibility that this blood element plays a role in the pathogenesis of asthma.

The involvement of platelets in the physiology and pathophysiology of haemostasis and thrombosis is now well recognized, but there is increasing evidence for the participation of platelets in inflammatory processes inducing asthma. A meeting was held on September 7-9, 1986 to discuss the available experimental and clinical data on the possible involvement of platelets and PAF in the pathogenesis of asthma. It can be seen from the manuscripts that this topic represents a rapidly expanding area of research of considerable relevance to our future understanding of the mechanisms and treatment of bronchial asthma. The increasing availability of drugs that selectively interfere with the actions of PAF will help to unravel the role of this phospholipid in asthma and hopefully the further study of platelets and PAF in the context of asthma will lead to a better understanding and improved therapeutic management of bronchial asthma.

(Prof. Dr. Christian Virchow)

TABLE OF CONTENTS

Platelet Activation in Asthma

Aspirin-Induced Asthma

AAS 21:
PAF, Platelets, and Asthma

PLATELETS: SOME HISTORICAL BACKGROUND

G.V.R. Born

Platelets in haemostasis

When blood vessels are injured so that they bleed, circulating platelets adhere to the damaged vessel walls and aggregate, so diminishing or arresting the haemorrhage. This interaction between platelets and vessel walls therefore has an easily demonstrable physiological function. There is much clinical and experimental evidence that a deficiency or defect in circulating platelets is associated with "spontaneous" haemorrhages from small vessels. This suggests that platelets are somehow essential for the functional integrity of these vessels, but if there is such a mechanism it has still to be established.

Platelets in atherogenesis

The old thrombogenic hypothesis of atherosclerosis (von Rokitansky, 1841; Duguid, 1949) has recently reappeared in modern costume as claims that platelets contribute to atherogenesis in three ways: first, through damaging arterial endothelial cells by releasing injurious agents, presumably where circulating platelets adhere (Mustard et al. 1977a); secondly, through the release in such situations of a factor responsible for smooth muscle proliferation in the arterial wall (Ross & Glomset, 1973); and thirdly through the formation of persistent mural thrombi which are organised into intimal thickenings. Such evidence as there is for these propositions fails to establish any of them as relevant to atherosclerosis in animals or human beings (see Walton, 1975). Underlying all three claims is the assumption that some normal circulating platelets settle on arterial walls for long enough to release some of their contents. There is no observational basis for this assumption in normal arteries, although quantitative observations should now be possible with modern imaging techniques.

We have begun an investigation designed to quantify the adhesion of circulating platelets in different types of blood vessels. (Kortenhaus, Schröer & Born, 1982) So far, the observations were mainly on small veins because the comparative slowness of the blood flow made it easier to develop and control the new methods required.

The experiments provide evidence that there is very little tendency for cirulating platelets to stick to the walls of small veins and arterioles, even under conditions in which the adhesion propensities of both platelets and vessel walls might be expected to be increased by preparative manipulations.

It has also been claimed (Ross, 19) endothelium is continuously subject to "damage" or "injury" of some kind as a precondition for the adherence of platelets. There is no convincing evidence for this generalisation, especially not in human beings. The first lesions of atherosclerosis, the fatty streaks, commonly begin during childhood or adolescence. It seems most improbable that these could be caused by any conceivable "injury". Specifically, the common assertion that damage is produced by shear stresses in the high-pressure blood system is inherently improbable because of functional adaptations in the course of evolution. The only finding that could conceivably apply to human arteries is that guinea pig aorta has a higher replacement rate of endothelium around the openings of branches than elsewhere (Payling-Wright & Born, 1971). This is most simply explained by assuming that endothelial turnover depends, inter alia, on haemodynamic effects over such areas. But this should be thought of more correctly as a quasi-physiological effect and, even there, platelets are rarely if ever seen adhering to the walls. The turnover rate of endothelium is increased in experimental hypertension (Payling-Wright, 1972).

This is compatible with hypertension as a "risk factor" for coronary heart disease. It seems more likely that this is due to an accelerating effect of inter-endothelial gaps on plasma lipoprotein accumulation (Stehbens, 1965; Caro, 1977) than to an increase in the indiscriminate or even selective deposition of platelets on arterial walls.

Platelets in thrombogenesis

There is conclusive evidence that occlusive thrombi in arteries damaged by atherosclerosis contain platelets as a major, if not the main, component (Davies & Thomas, 1981, 1984). What is the mechanism responsible for rapid and extensive platelet aggregation in an artery as an apparently random event in time (see Born, 1979)? Close serial sectioning of obstructed coronary arteries has established that the platelet thrombus responsible is invariably associated with recent haemorrhage into an underlying atherosclerotic plaque (Friedman, 1970; Davies & Thomas, 1981). The haemorrhages occur through fissures or fractures in the plaque; and the sudden appearance of such a fissure or fracture may well be the random, individually unpredictable event affecting coronary arteries that has to be assumed to occur to account for the clinical onset of acute coronary thrombosis (Born, 1979).

How does haemorrhage into a ruptured plaque start off platelet thrombogenesis ? This can be regarded as part of the general question of how platelets are caused to aggregate through haemorrhage, and most effectively through haemorrhage from arteries. The formation of platelet thrombi appears so similar to that of haemostatic plugs of platelets that analysis of the mechanism of the latter is likely to provide an understanding of the former. Until recently the question was commonly answered by assuming that the process depends on the adhesion of platelets to collagen which is exposed where damaged vessel walls are denuded of endothelium. Adhering platelets then release other agents, including thromboxane A_2 *and ADP, which in turn are responsible for the adhesion of more platelets as growing aggregates. This explanation is unlikely to be correct, for the following reasons. First, haemostatic and thrombotic aggregates of platelets grow without delay and very rapidly. For example, when an arteriole 200 um in diameter is cut into laterally, the rate of accession of platelets to the haemostatic plug is of the order of* 10^4*/s (Born & Richardson, 1979). In contrast, although the adhesion of platelets to collagen itself is almost instantaneous, the subsequent aggregation of platelets, even under optimal conditions for their reactivity, begins only after a delay or lag period of several seconds (Wilner et al. 1969). Secondly, platelets tend to aggregate as mural thrombi when anti-coagulated blood flows through the plastic vessels of artificial organs such as oxygenators or dialysers (Richardson et al. 1976) that contain no collagen or anything else capable of activating platelets similarly. This implies* *that there are conditions under which platelets are activated in the blood by something other than collagen or other constituents of the walls of living vessels.*

The plaque on which a thrombus grows has usually narrowed the arterial lumen. At constant blood pressure the flow of blood is faster through the constriction than elsewhere in the artery. Therefore, high flow and wall shear rates are no hindrance to the aggregation of platelets as thrombi (Born, 1977). Indeed, the question arises of whether the activation of platelets which precedes their aggregation depends in some way on such abnormal haemodynamic conditions.

The blood-flow velocities that would be experienced by platelets closest to the vessel wall and therefore with the highest probability of colliding with the sites of damage can be calculated. Human platelets have a major diameter of about 1.5 um. In an arteriole of medium size the flow velocity of plasma and of any cells in it at a distance of 1 um from the wall is of the order of 10-100 um/ms. Therefore, a platelet flowing within a distance no greather than its own diameter would pass an injury site 100 um long in at most 10 ms. In the absence of other influences, this would seem to be the time available for such a platelet to adhere to the damaged wall.

The time just calculated as available to circulating platelets "at risk" for adhering to a wall lesion has to be compared with what is known about the ime required for platelets to be activated into a condition in which their collision with such a lesion would very probably result in adhesion (Born & Richardson, 1980). That a process of <u>activation</u> is an essential prerequisite for adhesion and aggregation is inferred from the non-reactivity of normal circulating platelets. Presumably, activation consists of a sequence of physical and biochemical events analogous to the activation of muscle (Pringle, 1978). The sequence is still being worked out, but several similarities with muscle are already established. Thus, it is known that in platelets an early event is an increased influx of sodium unaccompanied by an equivalent amount of cloride (Feinberg et al., 1977) and that activation is associated with an increase of free calcium in platelets (Käser-Glanzmann et al., 1977; Le Breton, Sandler & Feinberg 1976).

As activation is indicated by adhesiveness, the change must involve one or more constituents of the outer surface of platelets. There is ividence that the essence is the exposure or formation (Maguerie, plow a Edguiton 1979) of surface receptors for fibrinogen, which has long been known to be an essential and specific plasma co-factor for platelet aggregatin (Born & Cross, 1964; Cross, 1964). The activation time of platelets may then be defined as the interval between the encounter of platelets with an activating agent such as ADP and their ability to react with plasma fibrinogen.

That circulating platelets can be activated to adhere in much less time than that required by their gross change in shape where t1/2 = 1-2 s at 37 ° (Born, 1970) is indicated by direct experimental observations. An arteriole can be irradiated by a laser in such a way that damage is limited to a few square micrometres of endothelium (Arfors et al., 1976). The site of damage is covered almost immediately with platelets that must have been activated in small fractions of a second.

Very similar events follow the application of the activating agent ADP by micro-iontophoresis to the outside of an arteriole or venule under conditions in which appropriate controls indicate that there is no evidence of any damage at all to the endothelial layer (Begent & Born, 1970). Platelet aggregates grow in the vessel exactly opposite the tip of the micropipette, while the blood continues to flow rapidly and without noticeable disturbance over the site. This is explained most simply by assuming that sufficient ADP diffuses between the endothelial cells into the blood to reach platelets passing close to the wall and that this ADP activates them within a few nulliseconds.

An extension of this technique has provided a basis for calculating an average activation time for circulating platelets. It was found that the size of platelet aggregates produced by the iontophoretic application of ADP increases exponentially; the rate constant of this increase depended on the mean blood flow velocity, determined in the same vessels at the same time (Begent & Born, 1970). The shape of the experimentally determined curve was simulated closely by a theoretical curve (Richardson, 1973) derived on the single assumption that platelets require an activation time of about 100 - 200 ms. This time is still one to two orders of magnitude greater than that indicated by the earlier theoretical considerations; so either this experimental derivation overestimates the true activation time or the earlier considerations failed to take something into account that would allow flowing platelets more than a few milliseconds for activation. When branching vessels of the microcirculation are observed microscopically, platelets can often be seen trapped in vortices for up to several seconds. Such delays may occur in the immediate vicinity of major vessel wall lesions, whether caused by disease such as the sudden rupture of an atheromatous plaque (Davies & Thomas, 1984) or by traumatic injury such as a puncture or transection. However, there is no evidence of even the smallest disturbances in the flow of blood in a normal vessel in which platelets are caused to adhere by iontophoretically applied ADP. Moreover, it seems most unlikely that any endothelial unevenness produced by laser injury would give rise to flow disturbances large enough to delay the passage of platelets.

The chemical enviromnent of platelets aggregating in vivo has been in doubt until recently. In vitro platelets are activated by various chemical agents, and it was uncertain which if any of these are responsible for the haemostatic aggregation of platelets in living blood vessels.

Recent evidence (Zawilska, Born & Begent, 1982) establishes that ADP is involved in activating platelets in vivo. Novel techniques were developed for the reproducible determination of bleeding times from small arteries of rats and rabbits in the territory supplied by the superior mesenteric artery. One of its main branches was cannulated and infusions were made into the mesenteric circulation of the enzyme which specifically removes ADP. The infusions increased the bleeding times very significantly. It is reasonable to conclude that the observed increases in bleeding time are caused by removal from the blood plasma of ADP, the presence of which makes a major contribution to the haemostatic aggregation of arriving platelets.

A reservation about the conclusion arises out of the presence of nucleotide-dephosphorylating enzymes in normal blood, both in plasma (Haslam & Mills, 1967) and as ectoenzymes on the surface of circulating cells (De Pierre & Karmnovsky, 1973, 1974; Manery & Dryden, 1979). These enzymes hydrolyse the gamma-phosphate of ATP several times more rapidly than the beta-phosphate of ADP. The infused enzyme systems convert ADP to ATP, which the dephosphorylating enzymes presumably reconvert into ADP. It must be assumed, therefore, that the overall balance between the reaction rates in both directions is such as to diminish the concentration of ADP.

Apyrase increases the bleeding time from transected vessels in isolated rabbit mesenteries (Bergqvist & Arfors, 1980) and from punctures or cuts into artificial vessels (Born et al., 1976); this is in vitro and ex vivo evidence for the dependence of the haemostatic aggregation of platelets on free ADP in the blood. The results reported here are the first to provide similar evidence in vivo, as far as the primary physiological function of platelets is concerned.

Our observations increase current interest in the following questions. First, is it possible to demonstrate plasma ADP directly in blood at sites of haemostasis or thrombosis at concentrations required to activate platelets? Secondly, what is the cellular source (or sources) of the ADP? And thirdly, how does this evidence affect therapeutic possibilities for the prevention or reversal of intravascular, particularly arterial thrombosis?

Free ATP has been demonstrated in blood emerging from cuts in small arteries during haemostasis (Born et al., 1981: Kratzer & Born, 1982). On the assumption that this ATP was accompanied by ADP in their normal intracellular proportions, the blood contained enough ADP, at least 10^{-8} *M (Frojmovic, personal communication; see also Milton et al., 1980) to aggregate the platelets.*

The source of the ATP was investigated by perfusing arteries in vivo with physiological saline contraining altumin and heparin. The arteries were punctured and the emerging fluid contained no blood but ATP at about 1.0 x 10^{-7} *M in the first 2 sec, which decreased rapidly thereafter. The results confirm a long-standing proposition (Born, 1962) that at sites of vascular injury enough ADP is rapidly released from damaged cells into the blood to contribute significantly to haemostatic platelet aggregation. Whatever the source of the plasma ADP, its demonstration suggests novel therapeutic possibilities in the prevention of arterial thrombosis (see Born, 1979).*

One such possibility would turn on the feasibility of infusing enzyme systems which remove free ADP from the blood. In spite of immunological and other problems, it is conceivable that an enzyme with this specificity and a sufficiently long half-life in blood could be investigated for this purpose under appropriate clinical conditions.

Acknowledgements

I wish to thank the British Heart Foundation, the Minna-James-Heineman Foundation of Hanover, and the Fritz Thyssen Foundation of Cologne for generous support.

REFERENCES

1. *Arfors, K.E., Cockburn, J.S. and Gross, J.F. (1976) Measurement of growth rate of laser-induced intravascular platelet aggregation, and the influence of blood flow velocity. Microvasc. Res. 11: 79-87.*

2. *Begent, N.A. and Born, G.V.R. (1970) Growth, rate in vivo of platelet thrombi produced by iontophoresis of ADP, as a function of mean blood flow velocity. Nature (Lond) 227: 926-930.*

3. *Bergqvist, D. and Arfors, K.E. (1973) Influence of platelet count on haemostatic plug formation and plug stability. An experimental study in rabbits with graded thrombocytopenia. Thromb. Diath. Haemorrh., 30: 586-596.*

4. *Bergqvist, D. and Arfors, K.E. (1980) Haemostatic platelet plug formation in the isolated rabbit mesenteric preparation - an analysis of red blood cell participation. Thrombosis and Haemostasis, 4: 6-8.*

5. *Born, G.V.R. (1970) Observations on the change in shape of blood platelets brought about by adenosine diphosphate. J. Physiol. 209: 487-511.*

6. *Born, G.V.R. (1962) Nature, 194: 927-929.*

7. *Born, G.V.R. and Richardson, P.D. (1980) Acitvation time of blood platelets. J. Membrane Biol. 57: 87-90.*

8. *Born, G.V.R., Bergqvist, D. and Arfors, K.E. (1976) Evidence for inhibition of platelet activation in blood by drug effect on erythrocytes. Nature, 259: 233-235.*

9. *Born, G.V.R., Görög, P. and Kratzer, M.A.A. (1981) Aggregation of platelets in damaged vessels. Philosophical Transactions of the Royal Society, B, 294: 241-250.*

10. *Born, G.V.R. (1979) Arterial thrombosis and its prevention. Proceedings of VIIIth World Congress of Cardiology (ed. by S. Hayase and S. Murao), pp. 81-91. Excerpta Medica, Amsterdam.*

11. *Born, G.V.R. (1977) Fluid-mechanical and biochemical interactions in haemostasis. Br. Med. Bull. 33: 193-197.*

12. *Born, G.V.R. (1979) Arterial thrombosis and its prevention (Proc. VIII*

World Congr. Cardiol., Tokyo 1978). Excerpta Medica, Amsterdam, ICS 470, p. 81-91.

13. *Born, G.V.R. and Cross, M.J. (1964) Effects of inorganic ions and of plasma proteins on the aggregation of blood platelets by adenosine diphosphate. J. Physiol. (Lond) 170: 394-414*

14. *Born, G.V.R. and Richardson, P.D. (1986) Activation time of blood platelets. Proc. R. Soc. Lond. B Biol. Sci. (submitted)*

15. *Caro, C.G. (1977) Mechanical factors in atherogenesis. In: Cardiovascular flow dynamics and measurement. University Park Press, Baltimore.*

16. *Constantinides, P. (1966) Plaques fissures in human coronary thrombosis. J. Atheroscler. Res. 6: 1-17.*

17. *Cross, M.J. (1964) Effect of fibrinogen on the aggregation of platelets by adenosine diphosphate. Thromb. Diath. Haemorrh. 12: 524-527.*

18. *Davies, M.J. and Thomas, T. (1981) The pathological basis and microanatomy of occlusive thrombus formation in human coronary arteries. Phil. Trans. R. Soc. Lond. B, 294: 225-229.*

19. *Davies, M.J. and Thomas, A. (1984) Thromboiss and acute coronary artery lesions in sudden coronary ischaemic death. New Engl. J. Med. 310: 1137-40.*

20. *De-Pierre, J.W. and Karnovsky, M.L. (1973) Plasma membranes of mammalian cells. A review of methods for their characterisation and isolation. Journal of Cell Biology, 56: 275-303.*

21. *Duguid, J.B. (1949) Pathogenesis of atherosclerosis. Lancet 2: 925.*

22. *Feinberg, H., Sandlter, W.C., Scorer, M., Le Breton, G.C., Grossman, B. and Born, G.V.R. (1977) Movement of sodium into human platelets induced by ADP. Biochem. Biophys. Acta. 470: 317.*

23. *Forster, G., Bernt, E. and Bergmeyer, H.V. (1974) Creatine kinase. Methods of enzymatic analysis (ed. by H.V. Bergmeyer), vol. 2 pp. 784-797.*

24. *Friedman, H. (1970) Pathogenesis of coronary thrombosis, intramural and intraluminal haemorrhage. In: Halonen LA (ed) Thrombosis and coronary heart disease. Karger, Basel, vol. 4:3*

25. *Haslam, R.J. and Mills, D.C.B. (1967) The adenylate kinase of human plasma, erythrocytes and platelets in relation to degradation of adenosine diphosphate in plasma. Biochemical Journal, 103: 773-784.*

26. *Haslam, R.J. (1964) Role of adenosine diphosphate in the aggregation of human platelets by thrombin and by fatty acids. Nature, 202, 765-768.*

27. *Mustard, J.F., Packham, M.A. and Kinlough Rathbone, R.L. (1977b)*

Platelets, thrombosis and atherosclerosis. Adv. Exp. Med. Biol. 104: 127-144.

28. *Mustard, J.F., Perry, D.W., Ardlie, N.G. and Packham, M.A. (1972) Preparation of suspension of washed platelets from humans. British Journal of Haematology, 22: 193-204.*

29. *Payling-Wright, H.P. (1972) Mitosis patterns in aortic endothelium. Atherosclerosis, 15: 93-95.*

30. *Payling-Wright, H.P. and Born, G.V.R. (1971) Possible effect of blood flow on the turnover rate of vascular endothelial cells. In: Hartert, H.H., Coplex, A.L. (eds) Theoretical and clinical haemorheology. Springer-Verlag, Berlin, pp. 220-226.*

31. *Pringle, J.W.S. (1978) Stretch activation of muscle: function and mechanism. The Croomian Lecture 1977. The Royal Society.*

32. *Richardson, P.D. (1973) Effect of blood flow velocity on growth rate of platelet thrombi. Nature (Lond) 245: 103-104.*

33. *Richardson, P.D., Galetti, P. and Born, G.V.R. (1976) Regional administration of drugs to control thrombosis in artificial organs. Trans. Am. Soc. Artif. Intern. Organs. 22: 22-29.*

34. *Izrael, V., Zawilska, K., Jaisson, F., Levy-Toledano, S. and Caen, J. (1974) Effect of fast removal of plasmatic ADP by the creatine-phosphate and creatine phosphokinase system on human platelet function in vivo. Platelets: Production, Function, Transfusion and Storage. (ed. by. M.G. Baldini and S. Ebbe), pp. 187-195. Grune & Stratton. New York.*

35. *Kaser-Glanzmann, R., Jakobova, M., George, J.N. and Luscher, E.F. (1977) Stimulation of calcium uptake in platelet membrane vesicles by adenosine 3',5'-cyclic monophosphate and protein kinase. Biochem. Biophys. Acta 466: 429.*

36. *Kortenhaus, H., Schroer, P., and Born, G.V.R. (1982) Quantification of the adhesion of platelets in hamster venules in vivo. Proc. R. Soc. Lond. B, 215: 135-145.*

37. *Kratzer, M.A.A. and Born, G.V.R. (1981) Free ATP in blood during haemorrhage. Thrombosis and Haemostiasis, 46: 393.*

38. *Le Breton, C.G., Sandler, W.C. and Feinberg, H. (1976) The effect of* D_2O *and chlortetracycline on ADP-induced platelet shape change and aggregation. Thrombos. Res. 8: 477.*

39. *Manery, J.F. and Dryden, E.E. (1979) Ecto-enzymes concerned with nucleotide metabolism. Physiological and Regulatory functions of adenosine and adenine nucleotides (ed. by H.P. Baer and G.I. Drummond), pp. 323-339. Raven Press, New York*

40. *Mustard, J.F., Moore, S., Packham, M.A. and Kinlough Rathbone, R.L.*

(1977a) Platelets, thrombosis and atherosclerosis. Proc. Biochem. Pharmacol. 13: 312-325.

41. *Ross, R. and Glomset, J.A. (1973) Atherosclerosis and the arterial smooth muscle cell. Proliferation of smooth muscle is a key event in the genesis of the lesions of atherosclerosis. Science (Wash. DC) 180: 1332-1339.*

42. *Schmid-Schönbein, H., Rieger, H. and Fischer, T. (1976) Blood vessels: problems arising at the borders of natural and artificial blood vessels. In: Effert, S., Mayer-Erkelenz, J. (eds) Springer, Berlin pp. 57-63.*

43. *Stehbens, W.E. (1965) Endothelial cell mitosis and permeability. J. Exp. Physiol. (Cogn. Med. Sci.) 50: 90-92.*

44. *von Rokitansky (1941-46) Handbuch der pathologischen Anatomie. Braunmüller & Seidel, Vienna.*

45. *Walton, K.W. (1975) Pathogenetic mechanisms in atherosclerosis. Am. J. Cardiol. 35: 542-558.*

46. *Wilner, G.D., Nossel, H.L. and Le Roy, E.D. (1969) Aggregation of platelets by collagen. J. Clin. Invest. 47: 2616-2621.*

47. *Zawilska, K., Izrael, V., Chelloul, N. and Caen, J. (1975) Prévention de la coagulation intravasculaire disseminée au course due Phénomène de Schwartzmann generalisé chez le lapin par un system enzymatique consommant l'ADP plasmatique. Actualitees Hématologiques, 9: 269*

48. *Zawilska, K.M., Born, G.V.R. and Begent, N.A. (1982) Effect of ADP-utilizing enzymes on the arterial bleeding time in rats and rabbits. British Journal of Haematology, 50: 317-325.*

PLATELET ACTIVATION - AN OVERVIEW

J.F. Mustard, R.L. Kinlough-Rathbone and M.A. Packham

*McMaster University, Dept. Pathology, Hamilton, Ontario, Canada
and University of Toronto, Dept. Biochemistry, Toronto, Ontario, Canada*

Introduction

Platelets are important in: 1) maintaining the integrity of vessel walls; 2) haemostasis; 3) arterial thrombosis; 4) some aspects of the development of atherosclerosis; and 5) some inflammatory reactions. The most detailed studies concerning platelets and their response to stimuli have been centered on haemostasis, and on atherosclerosis and its associated thromboembolic complications. In this review we shall examine what is known about the response of platelets to stimuli in relation to haemostasis and thrombosis and then examine some of these platelet responses in terms of the more limited information concerning the role of platelets in inflammatory reactions.

Vessel Wall Integrity and Haemostasis

In severely thrombocytopenic animals or humans, the integrity of the vessels in the microcirculation breaks down and there may be extensive escape of red cells across the endothelial cell barrier and occasionally, fatal haemorrhage (1,2). Little is known about what platelets do to maintain the integrity of the endothelial lining. Platelets do not normally stick to the endothelium (3), but if platelets are given to a thrombocytopenic animal, they adhere to the vessel wall mainly at the junctions between endothelial cells (4).

In addition, individuals with severe thrombocytopenia are at a high risk of bleeding from injured vessels because of their inability to form a haemostatic plug. During haemostasis platelets adhere to connective tissue (particularly to collagen) and are induced to release the contents of their *granules, including adenosine diphosphate (ADP) and serotonin, and to form thromboxane A_2; these materials stimulate platelets in the flowing blood to adhere to platelets already adherent to the connective tissue. This results in the formation of a mass of aggregated platelets. On the surface of platelets that have undergone the release reaction, platelet factor 3 becomes available and accelerates two steps of the intrinsic coagulation pathway leading to thrombin generation. Thrombin can itself cause further aggregation, release of platelet granule contents and activation of the arachidonate pathway as well asconverting fibrinogen to fibrin, which helps to stabilize the mass of aggregated platelets (4,5).*

Arterial Thrombosis

Studies of arterial thrombosis indicate that similar pathways to those observed in haemostasis are involved in the formation of a thrombus at a site of vessel injury. However, in addition to thrombus formation as a consequence of the interaction of platelets with connective tissue, thrombi can form as a result of reinjury of previously injured vessels (6). In the latter case, tissue thromboplastin from the damaged cells of the vessel wall can initiate the extrinsic coagulation pathway leading to the formation of fibrin on the injured surface. During polymerization of fibrin, platelets can adhere to fibrin strands, initiating a platelet-fibrin thrombus which is largely the result of the action of thrombin. The constituents of atherosclerotic plaques which may initiate thrombosis have not been well defined although it is recognized that thrombi frequently occur on ruptured atherosclerotic plaques (7). Probably both the interactions of platelets with connective tissue and thrombin generation on the surface of the ruptured atherosclerotic plaques are involved.

Pathways in Platelet Aggregation and Release

There are a number of agonists that induce platelet aggregation and/or release of the contents of platelet granules. These include adenosine diphosphate, thromboxane A_2, serotonin, thrombin, platelet activating factor (PAF, PAF-acether, 1-0-alkyl-2-acetyl- sn -glycero-3-phosphorylcholine), collagen, microfibrils in the presence of von Willebrand factor, immune complexes, particulate matter, and some viruses, bacteria and parasites (5,8). Epinephrine acts synergistically with these agonists to augment *platelets aggregation (9). The most detailed studies of the pathways in platelet aggregation have been concerned with platelet activation by ADP, thrombin, collagen, PAF and thromboxane A_2 which is formed from arachidonic acid that is freed from platelet phospholipids.*

These agonists fall into two broad classes, a) agonists such as ADP and serotonin that induce aggregation without the release of platelet granule contents and b) those that induce the release reaction (such as thrombin, collagen, PAF, thromboxane A_2). Those that induce the release reaction also stimulate the production of thromboxane A_2.

Although studies with ADP are often reported in which activation of the arachidonate pathway occurs, these studies have almost always been done with human platelets suspended in a medium that contains a low concentration of ionized calcium such as citrated platelet-rich plasma. In a medium such as this that contains only micromolar concentrations of ionized calcium, the close platelet-to-platelet contact induced by ADP leads to activation of the arachidonate pathway and the formation of thromboxane A_2, which causes further platelets aggregation and the release of platelet granule contents (5). However, when human platelets are aggregated by ADP in the presence of physiological concentrations of calcium, the arachidonate pathway is not activated, the release reaction does not occur and the platelets rapidly deaggregate (10). ADP-induced aggregation involves changes in the glycoprotein IIb/IIIa receptors on the surface of platelets that allow fibrinogen binding; fibrinogen binding is required for extensive aggregation in response to ADP and fibrinogen dissociates from the platelets during deaggregation (11,12). The mechanism by which ADP induces these changes is not clear, but may involve stimulation of inositol phospholipid metabolism (13). ADP may interact with receptors that influence the interconversion of phosphatidylinositol 4,5-bisphosphate (PIP_2) and phosphatidylinositol 4-phosphate (PIP) in the platelet membrane; this cycle of phosphatidylinositide metabolism is believed to be involved in sodium:potassium ATPase activity (14) and may be the mechanism that initially triggers the changes in glycoproteins IIb/IIIa so that fibrinogen binding can occur.

In contrast to ADP, thrombin can induce platelet aggregation, release of granule contents and activation of the arachidonate pathway in the presence of physiological concentrations of ionized calcium. The mechanism by which thrombin induces these changes appears to involve *stimulation of phospholipase C which degrades PIP_2 to inositol trisphosphate (IP_3) and to 1,2-diacylglycerol (13,15,16); this leads to the mobilization of calcium and the activation of myosin light chain kinase and protein kinase C which are responsible for the phosphorylation of myosin light chain (a 20 Kd protein) and of a 40 Kd protein (17-19). These reactions lead to changes in the platelet cytoskeleton that are involved in platelet aggregation and the release reaction (19). Calcium mobilization is also involved in the activation of phospholipase A_2 and formation of thromboxane A (20). PAF appears to have similar actions to thrombin. Collagen is a complex agonist since it is the platelets that adhere to the collagen that are initially stimulated to release their granule contents and to form thromboxane A_2 (21). When platelets interact with collagen, their phospholipase C is activated resulting in the conversion of PIP_2 to IP_3 and 1,2-diacylglycerol (22). Platelets not adherent to collagen are stimulated by the released ADP and by the thromboxane A_2 that is formed and aggregate and undergo further release of granule contents and formation of additional thromboxane A_2 (21). ADP and thromboxane A_2 can act synergistically in aggregation so that their combined effects are far more extensive than their effects alone (9). Although epinephrine has been reported to induce platelet aggregation in citrated platelet-rich plasma, it does not do so in the presence of physiological concentrations of ionized calcium (23). However, it does enhance platelet responsiveness to other aggregating agents (9). There are receptors on the platelet surface for many of these agonists and platelets have been reported to have both alpha- and beta-adrenergic receptors (9).*

When platelets are stimulated by release-inducing agents, they lose the contents of their amine storage granules and alpha-granules, but there is little release from the lysosomal granules. The proteins released from the alpha-granules include: fibrinogen, thrombospondin, fibronectin, von Willebrand factor, cationic proteins, platelet-derived growth factor, platelet factor 4, and beta-thromboglobulin (5,24). The relative importance of these substances is not completely understood, but when the release reaction occurs, not only fibrinogen, but also thrombospondin, von Willebrand factor and fibronectin can bind to the platelet surface (25,26). These proteins may play a part in platelet aggregation and contribute to the stability of platelet aggregates. When platelets are aggregated by thrombin, extensive release occurs and the platelets form stable aggregates that do not deaggreagte readily compared with aggregates that form in response to ADP under conditions in which the release reaction does not occur (27).

The changes induced in platelets by ADP, thrombin, or thromboxane A_2 *do not damage the platelets in such a way that they are rapidly cleared from the circulation (6). Thus, platelets that have taken part in the formation of intravascular platelet aggregates and then deaggregated survive in the circulation for a normal length of time. However, if platelets are exposed to enzymes such as plasmin that cause degradation of membrane glycoproteins, the platelets are rapidly cleared from the circulation (6,28). In conditions in which shortened platelet survival has been reported in association with vascular injury, it is likely that the platelets have been exposed to proteolytic enzymes that have modified them sufficiently to reduce platelet survival.*

In addition to converting arachidonic acid to thromboxane A_2 *via the cyclo-oxygenase pathway, platelets also convert this fatty acid to hydroxy eicosatetraenoic acid (12-HETE) via the lipoxygenase pathway (29). However, no role in platelet function has been established for 12-HETE or its hydroperoxy precursor (30). Platelets are not capable of forming leukotrienes, but it has been suggested that platelet-derived arachidonate may serve as a precursor for the neutrophil-derived eicosanoids, leukotriene* B_4 *and 5-HETE (31).*

Platelets in Inflammation

When platelets are stimulated with agents such as thrombin, collagen, or antigen-antibody complexes that induce the release reaction and activate the arachidonate pathway, some of the factors that are released from the platelet granules, or formed by the platelets, cause an acute inflammatory reaction with increased vessel permeability, and white cell accumulation. This has been shown by injection of materials released from stimulated platelets into the skin of experimental animals (32). Furthermore, when platelet aggregates are induced in the microcirculation by infusions of ADP, some of the aggregates persist and an inflammatory reaction develops at the sites where they lodge (33-35). Although almost all the platelet aggregates soon deaggregate because ADP-induced aggregation is a reversible process, in some areas a secondary reaction occurs that may be caused by persistent platelet aggregates. When platelet aggregates lodge in *the microcirculation, an intense accumulation of inflammatory cells including polymorphonuclear leukocytes can be found in the vessel wall and in the platelet aggregates, and in some cases there are substantial alteration of the vessel wall (33). In some studies, platelets have been found in the subendothelial space (33). Although some investigators have not been able to produce vessel wall changes with platelet aggregates induced by the infusion of collagen fibrils (36), others have found that platelet aggregates formed in response to ADP cause substantial changes in the blood vessels of the brain (34). Thus it can be concluded that platelet aggregates can effect the vessel walls in the microcirculation and contribute to inflammatory changes. The substances produced or released by platelets that influence the vessel wall include ADP, thrombxane A_2, postaglandins, other products of arachidonate metabolism such as those formed by the lipoxygenase pathway (in particular 12-HETE), serotonin, and substances released from alpha granules such as platelet-derived growth factor and a cationic protein which increases vessel permeability.*

Platelets have been shown to participate in defense mechanisms, and to interact with components of the immune system (37); platelets can bind to IgG (38,39) and, through a different receptor, IgE (49). When human platelets that have bound IgE are exposed to the appropriate antigen, they form cytocidal factors that can kill parasites (41).

The IgE receptor appears to be associated with the membrane glycoprotein IIb/IIIa complex since IgE does not bind to thrombasthenic platelets (42). One aspect of the interaction of IgE bound to the platelet surface with its appropriate antigen is that although it can induce the formation of a cytotoxic factor, this reaction apparently does not lead to the release of the contents of the platelet granules, or platelet aggregation (40). The cytotoxic effect of the material formed by the platelets can be inhibited by catalase, indicating that the formation of hydrogen peroxide and/or oxygen metabolites is probably responsible for the cytotoxic action (43). Platelets from allergic asthmatics will generate cytotoxic mediators when exposed to the appropriate antigen, and furthermore, monoclonal antibodies to IgE will cause these platelets to form cytotoxic factors, indicating that IgE is bound to the surface of platelets from these patients (44). Thus, it appears that platelets from allergic individuals have an increased amount of IgE bound to their surface. The approximately 10% of asthmatics in whom an attack can be precipitated by the ingestion of non-steroidal anti-inflammatory drugs such as aspirin, have platelets that release cytocidal mediators in response to this class of drugs (41). This does not appear to be an IgE-mediated process although it is analogus to it. A major difference between the aspirin-induced response and the IgE/antigen-induced response is that only the former can be inhibited by inhibitors of the lipoxygenase pathway (45). This implies that under certain circumstances the products of the lipoxygenase pathway may be involved in producing some of the inflammatory response. At one time it was throught that administation of drugs that inhibit cyclo-oxygenase would shunt arachidonate to the lipoxygenase pathway, leading to increased formation of leukotrienes which could cause bronchoconstriction (46). Of course, this does not apply to platelets, which do not form leukotrienes, but, as mentioned earlier, platelets could supply leukotriene precursors to other cells such as leukocytes (31).

The Role of PAF

PAF is another factor that is produced by IgE-stimulation of platelets, although platelets produce less PAF than do stimulated monocytes, leukocytes, basophils and eosinophils (47-49); even endothelial cell have been reported to produce PAF (50). The role of PAF in intravascular responses is complex. Both intravascular injections of PAF, and inhalation of PAF cause bronchoconstriction (51-53). Furthermore, PAF is believed to sensitize the bronchial smooth muscle to other agents such as histamine (54). Substances formed or released by the platelets may take part in a hypersensitive reaction of this sort.

In addition to causing bronchospasm, PAF is a strong platelet aggregating agent and also induces the release of contents of platelet granules (55-57). There are considerable differences in the sensitivities of platelets from various species: human platelets are less sensitive than rabbit platelets whereas rat platelets are practically insensitive to PAF (56,58). Although there are conflicting reports (59), several groups have shown that PAF can induce platelet aggregation that is independent of release ADP or the formation of thromboxane A_2*, although these substances augment the effect of PAF on platelets (55,57,60,60). (There is apparently no evidence about the possibility that PAF may induce the formation of* *cytocidal factors.) If PAF appears in the circulation, it could cause platelet aggregation, release of granule contents, and formation of thromboxane A_2. Thus, PAF could contribute to the involvement of platelets in inflammatory reactions.*

The bronchospasm induced by inhalation or by intravenous infusion of PAF into guinea pigs could be explained by PAF-induced platelet aggregation in the microvascular bed around the airways. The observation that PAF does not induce bronchial spasm in thrombocytopenic animals is compatible with the concept that platelet aggregates disturb blood flow in the vascular bed and release or form factors that cause bronchospasm (51). The observations by Lellouch-Tubiana and associates (62) that extensive platelet aggreation occurs in the microvasculature and that platelets accumulate in the extravascular compartment of the lung upon intravenous injection of PAF, indicate that aggregates in the microcirculation cause vascular changes that lead to oedema and extravasation of platelets. Eosinophils also accumulate (62), but it is not known whether platelets produce factors that influence eosinophil accumulation.

In some species, platelets stimulated with release-inducing agonists can form PAF although there are wide differences among species in the amounts that are formed (56,63). Whether PAF formed by platelets contributes to bronchoconstriction is not clear. Evidence for platelet involvement in human asthmatic attacks is controversial. Demonstration of increased levels of beta-thromboglobulin and platelet factor 4 in the blood of patients during asthma attacks (64,65) has been confirmed by other investigators (66,67). Ind and associates (68) studied the behaviour of autologous platelets labeled with 111-Indium in three young volunteers with atopic asthma and found that an antigen challenge to induce bronchial constriction was not associated with increased accumulation of platelets in the lungs or shortened platelet survival. They concluded that if platelets do play a part in the early phase of antigen-induced bronchial constriction in human asthma, that do so without accumulating in the lung. Morley et al. (69) have argued that platelet activation can occur in asthma without the platelets undergoing the release reaction. If so, one would not expect to find released platelet proteins in the circulation.

Our knowledge concerning the involvement of platelets in inflammatory and immune reactions is incomplete, although some aspects of platelet activation that have been studied intensely in relation to haemostasis and thrombosis are relevant. However, there are some aspects of platelets activation in inflammatory reactions that appear to be different: for example, the evidence that IgE-sensitized platelets can form cytocidal substances without activation of aggregation or the release of granule contents. In addition, the factors from platelets that increase vessel permeability have not received much attention in relation to inflammation. Finally, the mechanism by which platelets can induce vessel injury with extravasation of platelets and red cells is poorly understood.

References

1. Aursnes, I. (1974) Increased permeability of capillaries to protein during thrombocytopenia. An experimental study in the rabbit. Microvasc. Res. 7, 283-295.

2. Kitchens, C.S., Weiss, L. (1975) Ultrastructural changes of endothelium associated with thrombocytopenia. Blood 46, 567-578.

3. Thorgeirsson, G., Robertson, A.L. Jr. (1978) The vascular endothelium - pathobiologic significance. Am. J. Pathol. 93, 803-848.

4. Mustard, J.F., Packham, M.A. (1979) The reaction of the blood to injury. In: Inflammation, Immunity and Hypersensitivity, 2nd edn, ed. Movat, H.Z. (Harper & Row, New York), pp. 61-128.

5. Packham, M.A., Mustard, J.F. (1984) Normal and abnormal platelet activity. In: Blood Platelet Function and Medicinal Chemistry (Elsevier Biomedical, New York), pp.61-128.

6. Kinlough-Rathbone, R.L., Packham, M.A., Mustard, J.F. (1983) Vessel injury, platelet adherence, and platelet survival. Arteriosclerosis 3, 529-546.

7. Davies, M.J., Thomas, A. (1984) Thrombosis and acute coronary-artery lesions in sudden cardiac ischemic death. N. Engl. J. Med. 310, 1137-1140.

8. Mustard, J.F., Packham, M.A., Kinlough-Rathbone, R.L. (1986) Mechanisms in thrombosis. In:Haemostasis and Thrombosis, 2nd edn, eds. Bloom, A.L., Thomas, D.P. (Churchill Livingstone, New York), (In press).

9. Kinlough-Rathbone, R.L., Mustard, J.F. (1986) Synergism of agonists. In:Platelet Responses and Metabolism, Vol.I, Responses, ed. Holmsen, H., (CRC Press, Boca Raton, FL), pp. 193-207.

10. Kinlough-Rathbone, R.L., Mustard, J.F., Packham, M.A., Perry, D.W., Reimers, H.-J., Cazenave, J.-P. (1977) Properties of washed human

platelets Thromb. Haemostas. 37, 291-308.

11. *Mustard, J.F., Packham, M.A., Kinlough-Rathbone, R.L., Perry, D.W., Regoeczi, E. (1978) Fibrinogen and ADP-induced platelet aggregation. Blood 52, 453-466.*

12. *Peerschke, E.I.B. (1985) The platelet fibrinogen receptor. Semin. Hematol. 22, 241-259.*

13. *Vickers, J.D., Mustard, J.F. (1987) Fate of polyphosphoinositides in platelet aggregation and the platelet release reaction. Platelet Responses and Metabolism, Vol. III, ed. Holmsen, H. (CRC Press, Boca Raton,FL), (In press).*

14. *Simmons, D.A., Kern, E.F.O., Winegrad, A.I., Martin, D.B. (1986) Basal phosphatidylinositol turnover controls aortic Na^+/K^+ ATPase activity. J. Clin. Invest. 77, 503-513.*

15. *Berridge, M.J. (1984) Inositol triphosphate and diacylglycerol as second messengers. Biochem. J. 220, 345-360.*

16. *Nishizuka, Y. (1984) Turnover of inositol phospholipids and signal transduction.Science 225, 1365-1370.*

17. *Daniel, J.L., Holmsen, H., Adelstein, R.S. (1977) Thrombin-stimulated myosin phosphorylation in intact platelets and its possible involvement in secretion. Thromb. Haemostas. 38, 984-989.*

18. *Kaibuchi, K., Takai, Y., Sawamura, M., Hoshijima, M., Fujikura, T., Nishizuka, Y. (1983) Synergism functions of protein phosphorylation and calcium mobilization in platelet activation. J. Biol. Chem. 258, 6701-6704.*

19. *Haslam, R.J., Lynham, J.A. (1977) Relationship between phosphorylation of blood platelet proteins and secretion of platelet granule constituents.I. effects of different aggregating agents. Biochem. Biophys. Res. Commun. 77, 714-722.*

20. *Rink, T.J., Hallam, T.J. (1984) What turns platelets on? TIBS 9, 215-219.*

21. *Kinlough-Rathbone, R.L., Cazenave, J.-P., Packham, M.A., Mustard, J.F. (1980) Effects of inhibitors of the arachidonate pathway on the release of granule contents from rabbit platelets adherent to collagen. Lab. Invest. 42, 28-34.*

22. *Rittenhouse, S.E., Allen, C.L. (1982) Synergistic activation by collagen and 15-hydroxy-9 ,11 -peroxidoprosta-5,13-dienoic acid (PGH_2) of phosphatidylinositol metabolism and arachidonic acid release in human platelets. J. Clin. Invest. 70, 1216-1224.*

23. *Lages, B., Weiss, H.J. (1981) Dependence of human platelet functional responses on divalent cations: aggregation and secretion in heparin- and hirudin-anticoagulated platelet-rich plasma and the effects of*

chelating agents. Thromb. Haemostas. 45, 173-179.

4. *Holmsen, H. (1980) Mechanisms of platelet secretion. In: Platelets: Cellular Response Mechanisms and their Biological Significance, eds. Rotman, A., Meyer, F.A., Gitler, C., Silberberg, A. (John Wiley & Son, New York), pp. 249-263.*

25. *Plow, E.F., McEver, R.P., Coller, B.S., Woods, V.L., Marguerie, G.A., Ginsberg, M.H. (1985) Related binding mechanisms for fibrinogen, fibronectin, von Willebrand factor, and thrombospondin on thrombin-stiumulated human platelets. Blood 66, 724-727.*

26. *Silverstein, R.L., Leung, L.L.K., Nachman, R.L. (1986) Thrombospondin: A versatile multifunctional glycoprotein. Arteriosclerosis 6, 245-253.*

27. *Kinlough-Rathbone, R.L., Mustard, J.F., Perry, D.W., Dejana, E., Cazenave, J.-P., Packham, M.A., Harfenist, E.J. (1983) Factors influencing the deaggregation of human and rabbit platelets. Thromb. Haemostas. 49, 162-167.*

28. *Greenberg, J.P., Packham, M.A., Guccione, M.A., Rand, M.L., Reimers, H.-J., Mustard, J.F. (1979) Survival of rabbit platelets treated in vitro with chymotrypsin, plasmin, trypsin or neurominidase. Blood 53, 916-927.*

29. *Smith, J.B. (1980) The prostanoids in hemostasis and thrombosis. Am. J. Pathol. 99, 741-804.*

30. *Brash, A.R. (1985) A review of possible roles of the platelet 12-lipoxygenase. Circulation 72, 702-707.*

31. *Marcus, A.J., Broekman, M.J., Safier, L.B., Ullman, H.L., Islam, N., Serhan, C.N., Rutherford, L.E., Korchak, H.M., Weissmann, G. (1982) Formation of leukotrienes and other hydroxy acids during platelet-neutrophil interactions in vitro. Biochem. Biophys. Res. Commun. 109, 130-137.*

32. *Packham, M.A., Nishizawa, E.E., Mustard, J.F. (1986) Response of platelets to tissue injury. Biochem. Pharmacol. Suppl., 171-184.*

33. *Jorgensen, L., Hovig, T., Roswsell, H.C., Mustard, J.F. (1970) Adenosine diphosphate-induced platelet aggregation and vascular injury in swine and rabbits. Am. J. Pathol. 61, 161-176.*

34. *Fujimoto, T., Suzuki, H., Tanoue, K., Fukushima, Y., Yamazaki, H. (1985) Cerebrovascular injuries induced by activation of platelets in vivo. Stroke 16, 245-250.*

35. *Jorgensen, L., Rowsell, H.C., Hovig, T., Glynn, M.F., Mustard, J.F. (1967) Adenosine diphosphate-induced aggregation and myocardial infarction in swine. Lab. Invest. 17, 616-644.*

36. *Joris, I., Braunstein, P.W., Jr. (1982) Platelets and endothelium: effects of collagen-induced platelet aggregates on pulmonary vessels.*

Exp. Mol. Pathol. 37, 393-405.

37. Henson, P.M., Ginsberg, M.H. (1981) Immunological reactions of platelets. In: Platelets in Biology and Pathology, 2, ed. Gordon, J.L. (Elsevier/North Holland, Oxford), pp. 265-308.

38. Karas, S.P., Rosse, W.F., Kurlander, R.J. (1982) Characterization of the IgG-Fc receptor on human platelets. Blood 60, 1277-1282.

39. Karpatkin, S. (1985) Autoimmune thrombocytopenic purpura. Semin. Hematol. 22, 260-288.

40. Joseph, M., Capron, A., Ameisen, J.-C., Capron, M., Vorng, H., Pancré, V., Kusnierz, J.-P., Auriault, C. (1986) The receptor for IgE on blood platelets. Eur. J. Immunol. 16, 306-312.

41. Joseph, M., Auriault, C., Capron, A., Vorng, H., Viens, P. (1983) A new function for platelets: IgE-dependent killing of schistosomes. Nature (Lond.) 303, 810-812.

42. Capron, A., Ameisen, J.C., Joseph, M., Auriault, C., Tonnel, A.B., Caen, J. (1985) New functions for platelets and their pathological implications. Int. Archs. Allergy Appl. Immunol. 77, 107-114.

43. Joseph, M., Ameisen, J.C., Kusnierz, J.P., Pancré, V., Capron, M., Capron, A. (1984) Participation of the IgE receptor in the toxicity of blood platelets against schistosomes. C.R. Acad. Sci. Paris 298, 55-60.

44. Capron, A., Ameisen, J.C., Joseph, M. (1986) Personal Communication.

45. Ameisen, J.C., Capron, A., Joseph, M., Maclouf, J., Vorng, H., Pancré, V., Fournier, E., Wallaert, B., Tonnel, A.B. (1985) Aspirin-sensitive asthma: Abnormal platelet responses to drugs inducing asthmatic attacks. Int. Archs. Allergy Appl. Immunol. 78, 438-448.

46. Hamberg, M., Samuelsson, B. (1974) Prostaglandin endoperoxides. Novel transformation of arachidonic acid in human platelets. Proc. Natl. Acad. Sci. USA 71, 3400-3404.

47. Benveniste, J., Jouvin, E., Pirotzky, E., Arnoux, B., Mencia-Huerta, J.M., Roubin, R., Vagaftig, B.B. (1981) Platelet-activating factor (PAF-acether): Molecular aspects of its release and pharmacological actions. Int. Archs. Allergy Appl. Immunol. 66, (Suppl. 1), 121-126.

48. Camussi, G., Aglietta, M., Coda, R., Bussolino, F., Piacibello, W., Tetta, C. (1981) Release of platelet activating factor (PAF) and histamine. II. The cellular origin of human PAF: monocytes, polymorphonuclear neutrophils and basophils. Immunology 42, 191-199.

49. Benveniste, J., Chignard, M. (1985) A role for PAF-acether (platelet -activating factor) in platelet-dependent vacular diseases? Circulation 72, 713-717.

50. Zimmerman, G.A., McIntyre, T.M., Prescott, S.M. (1985) Production of

platelet-activating factor by human vascular endothelial cells: evidence for a requirement for specific agonists and modulation by prostacyclin. Circulation 72, 718-727.

51. *Vargaftig, B.B., Lefort, J., Chignard, M., Benveniste, J. (1980) Platelet-activating factor induces a platelet-dependent bronchoconstriction unrelated to the formation of prostaglandin derivatives. Eur. J. Pharmacol. 65, 185-192.*

52. *Pinckard, R.N., McManus, L.M., Halonen, M., Hanahan, D.J. (1984) Immunopharmacology of acetyl glyceryl ether phosphorylcholine (AGEPC). In:Immunopharmacology of the Lung, ed. Newball, H.H. (Marcel Dekker, New York), pp. 73-103.*

53. *Cuss, F.M., Dixon, C.M.S., Barnes, P.J. (1986) Effects of inhaled platelet activating factor on pulmonary function and bronchial responsiveness in man. Lancet II, 189-192.*

54. *Mazzoni, L., Morley, J., Page, C.P., Sanjar, S. (1985) Induction of airway hyper-reactivity by platelet activating factor in the guinea-pig. J. Physiol. 365, 107P.*

55. *Cazenave, J.-P., Benveniste, J., Mustard, J.F. (1979) Aggreagation of rabbit platelets by platelet activating factor is dependent of the release reaction and the arachidonate pathway and inhibted by membrane-active drugs. Lab. Invest. 41, 275-285.*

56. *Marcus, A.J., Safier, L.B., Ullman, H.L., Wong, K.T.H., Broekman, M.J., Weksler, B.B., Kaplan, K.L. (1981) Effects of acetyl glyceryl ether phosphorylcholine on human platelet function in vitro. Blood 58, 1027-1031.*

57. *McManus, L.M., Hanahan, D.J., Pinckard, R.N. (1981) Human platelet stimulation by acetyl glyceryl ether phosphorylcholine. J. Clin. Invest. 67, 903-906.*

58. *Namm, D.H., Tadepalli, A.S., High, J.A. (1982) Species specificity of the platelet responses to 1-O-alkyl-2-acetyl- sn - glycero-3-phosphocholine. Thromb. Res. 25, 341-350.*

59. *Rao, A.K., Willis, J., Hassel, B., Dangelmaier, C., Holmsen, H., Smith, J.B. (1984) Platelet-activating factor is a weak platelet agonist: Evidence from normal human platelets and platelets with congenital secretion defects. Am. J. Hematol. 17, 153-165.*

60. *Chignard, M., Le Couedic, J.P., Tence, M., Vargaftig, B.B., Benveniste, J. (1979) The role of platelet-activating factor in platelet aggregation. Nature (Lond.) 279, 799-800.*

61. *Sturk, A., Asyee, G.M., Schaap, M.C.L., van Maanen, M., ten Cate, J.W. (1985) Synergistic effects of platelet-activating factor and other platelet agonists in human platelet aggregation and release: The role of ADP and products of the cyclooxygenase pathway. Thromb. Res. 40, 359-372.*

62. *Lellouch-Tubiana, A., Lefort, J., Pirotzky, E., Vargaftig, B.B., Pfister, A. (1985) Ultrastructural evidence for extravascular platelet recruitment in the lung upon intravenous injection of platelet-activating factor (PAF-acether) to guinea pigs. Br. J. Exp. Pathol., 66,345 - 355*

63. *Chignard, M., Le Couedic, J.P., Vargaftig, B.B., Benveniste, L. (1980) Platelet-activating factor (PAF-acether) secretion from platelets: effect of aggregating agents. Br. J. Haematol. 46, 455-464.*

64. *Knauer, K.A., Lichtenstein, L.M., Adkinson, N.F., Fish, J.E. (1981) Platelet activation during antigen-induced airway reactions in asthmatic subjects. N. Engl. J. Med. 304, 1404-1407.*

65. *Gresele, P., Todisco, T., Merante, F., Nenci, G.C. (1982) Platelet activation and allergic asthma. N. Eng. J. Med. 306, 549.*

66. *Durham, S.R., Dawes, J., Kay, A.B. (1985) Platelets in asthma Lancet II, 36.*

67. *Greer, I.A., Winter, J.H., Gaffney, D., McLoughlin, K., Belch, J.J.F., Boyd, G., Forbes, C.D. (1985) Platelet activation in allergic asthma. Thromb. Haemostas. 53, 438.*

68. *Ind, P.W., Peters, A.M., Malik, F., Lavender, J.P., Dollery, C.T. (1985) Pulmonary platelet kinetics in asthma. Thorax 40, 412-417.*

69. *Morley, J., Page, C.P., Sanjar, S. (1985) Platelets in asthma. Lancet II, 726-727.*

Dr. J.F. Mustard, Department of Pathology, McMaster University, 1200 Main Street West, Hamilton, Ontario, L8N 3Z5, Canada

PLATELET PRODUCTION IN THE LUNGS

John F. Martin+, David N. Slater, E. Anthony Trowbridge.

The Faculty of Medicine, University of Sheffield, Royal Hallamshire Hospital, Sheffield, U.K. & +Department of Medicine, King's College Hospital School of Medicine, London, U.K.

Introduction

The origin of the asthmatic tendency and of the immediate events leading to an attack of asthma are understood only partially. The complexity of possible cellular and biochemical events seen in asthmatic patients or animal models may reflect the complexity of a single disease or several diseases with different pathological mechanisms but one clinical appearance. Recently haemostasis and asthma have been linked in a study that showed prolonged bleeding time in asthmatics and changes in platelet variables including PAF-acether sensitivity of the platelets (34). Although the causes of such changes may be secondary to asthma or associated with an asthma-predisposing factor, it is possible that such changes are related to changes in platelet production in asthma.

One way in which asthma and platelet production may be linked is via pulmonary platelet production which has been suggested as a cause of pulmonary disease (40).

Platelets are involved in repair of the vascular wall and haemostasis. The most studied abnormality of platelets is thrombosis, but since platelets have biochemical and physical potential that appears to be far greater than the haemostatic needs of man under physiological conditions, other functions may remain still to be discovered. Platelets vary in reactivity, volume and density, both within an individual and between individuals. Changes in these variables may be a cause of disease. Although it was thought that difference in platelet volumes, density and reactivity were the consequences of the aging of cells in the circulation (11) (20), there is now much evidence that under normal conditions platelet heterogeneity arises at thrombopoesis, (5) (15) (16) (35): changes in platelets can be caused by changes in megakaryocytes.

In an animal model, changes in platelet volume and reactivity were related to megakaryocyte changes (28). In myocardial infarction and sudden cardiac death, platelets are larger and denser than controls (14) (17) (19) (37) and these changes are related to changes in bleeding time (4). In myocardial infarction megakaryocytes associated with these platelet changes are bigger than controls (42). The animal model referred to showed large megakaryocytes with large nuclei, containing increased amounts of DNA associated with large reactive platelets. Platelets contain no DNA and therefore have very limited ability for protein production. Their nature is primarily determined in the megakaryocyte. If platelet changes are involved in asthma then these changes may arise in the megakaryocyte. If platelets are produced in the lungs then there may be a mechanism by which megakaryocytes themselves may exert an effect on bronchial smooth muscle.

Platelets are produced by a unique mechanism which is probably common to all mammals and found in no other class of life. All other cells in the body are produced by mitosis, one cell with a 2N complement of DNA producing two similar daughter cells. Megakaryocytes, when mature, have nuclear contents of DNA that vary from 4N to 64N, with a modal value in man of 32N. Each megakaryocyte produces between 1-2 thousand platelets depending on the size of the megakaryocyte (24). Abnormalities of such a unique process may give rise to pathology peculiar to itself.

The Debate

Two major issues of platelet production which are still debated are the site of thrombocytopoiesis and its mechanism. Although it is not possible to present any single experiment as unequivocal proof of pulmonary platelet production by a process of physical fragmentation, there are now many pieces of evidence that make it a reasonable hypothesis. In evaluating the evidence it should be remembered that quantitative results are usually superior to subjective impression and that experimental animal models frequently provide stronger evidence than 'in vitro' or culture studies especially since platelet production is likely to be similar in all mammals.

Two key facts that have been quoted as support for platelet production in the bone marrow are the presence of megakaryocyte naked nuclei at this site and a cinematographic study of bone marrow thrombocytopoiesis (13). The naked nuclei certainly imply that the megakaryocyte cytoplasm must be lost in the marrow but not necessarily that platelets are produced there. The film was made through a glass window inserted in the femur of a rabbit, without the knowledge that megakaryocytes can spread on glass. Hence what was interpreted as platelet production may have been an artefact of the experiment. Moreover the same film did show entire megakaryocytes being carried away in the venous blood.

Howell and Donahue (1937) first suggested pulmonary platelet production but they also thought megakaryocytes were produced there. Kaufman et al (1965) demonstrated the error in this latter conclusion by showing that the number of pulmonary megakaryocytes depends on the volume of venous blood flowing to a lung. Tingaard Pedersen (1978) has shown that megakaryocytes entering the pulmonary circulation generally possess copious cytoplasm whilst those leaving the lungs are predominantly naked nuclei. Furthermore a number of studies have shown that if there is a demand for increased platelet production then the number of pulmonary megakaryocytes is increased. (1) (3) (7) (9) (29).

There are probably four theories attempting to explain the mechanisms of platelet production. The first follows the proposal of Wright (1910) that platelets are produced by the budding of megakaryocyte cytoplasm. The second relies on pre-determination of platelets by the megakaryocyte demarcation membrane system (26). The third proposes that long filamentous processes extending from megakaryocytes produce platelets. (27). The fourth is the physical fragmentation theory of platelet production (39). The evidence which forms the basis for the first three theories is subjective and depends upon the impression of the observer. In contrast there is both qualitative and quantitative evidence to support the physical fragmentation theory.

The Site of Platelet Production

Increased platelet production occurs in response to platelet destruction (21). Rabbits were made thrombocytopenic by daily antiplatelet serum injections for six consecutive days. This process was designed to increase platelet production and therefore allowed the observation of megakaryocyte response under the stimulus of increased demand. Ultra-structural examination of the bone marrow demonstrated both sinusoidal and extra-sinusoidal megakaryocytes (32). Fig. 1 shows a megakaryocyte and its cytoplasm within the bone marrow. Cytoplasm is only attached over a small portion of the nuclear periphery and a subjective interpretation might suggest that this cytoplasm is moving away from the nucleus.

Fig. 2. shows two megakaryocytes, one on each side of the parasinusoidal membrane: one is in the bone marrow, one is in a venous sinusoid. The one in the marrow has small protrusions that enter the venous sinusoid through the fenestrations in the parasinusoidal membrane. Wright (1910) might have interpreted these as cytoplasmic processes that would bud off to form platelets. An equally valid interpretation is that they are associated with the movement of the megakaryocyte into the venous sinusoid. It is of significance to note that there are few granules within the processes. Fig. 3 shows, on light microscopy, a megakaryocyte in a sinusoidal space.

Tinggaard Pedersen has observed large megakaryocyte cytoplasmic fragments circulating without nuclei in peripheral venous blood (personal communication). (These were not included in his quantitative studies of circulating megakaryocytes). Thus the observation of naked nuclei within the bone marrow does not necessarily mean that the cytoplasm associated with those nuclei had produced platelets at that site. It is possible that the whole cytoplasm without nucleus enters the venous circulation.

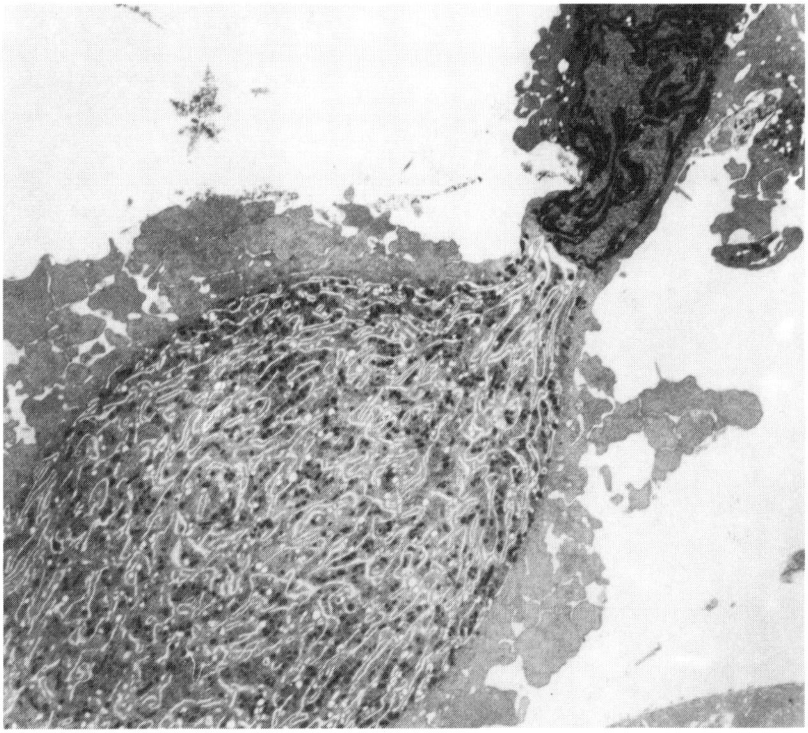

Fig. 1. Amoeboid extra-sinusoidal megakaryocyte. Transmission electron micrograph x3000. (Reproduced by permission of Thrombosis Research).

Quantitative evaluation of the lungs of the rabbits studied by Slater et al (1983) showed that megakaryocyte nuclei were difficult to find in control animals but in the animals with increased thrombopoiesis significantly more pulmonary megakaryocytes were observed. This is probably due to increased pulmonary trapping of the larger megakaryocyte nuclei associated with sustained thrombocytopenia. Fig. 4 shows a megakaryocyte naked nucleus with a minimal rim of cytoplasm trapped in a small pulmonary vessel. In an adjacent vessel there is a megakaryocyte cytoplasmic fragment and two platelets. Fig. 5 shows a mature megakaryocyte wedged in capillaries in the pulmonary circulation.

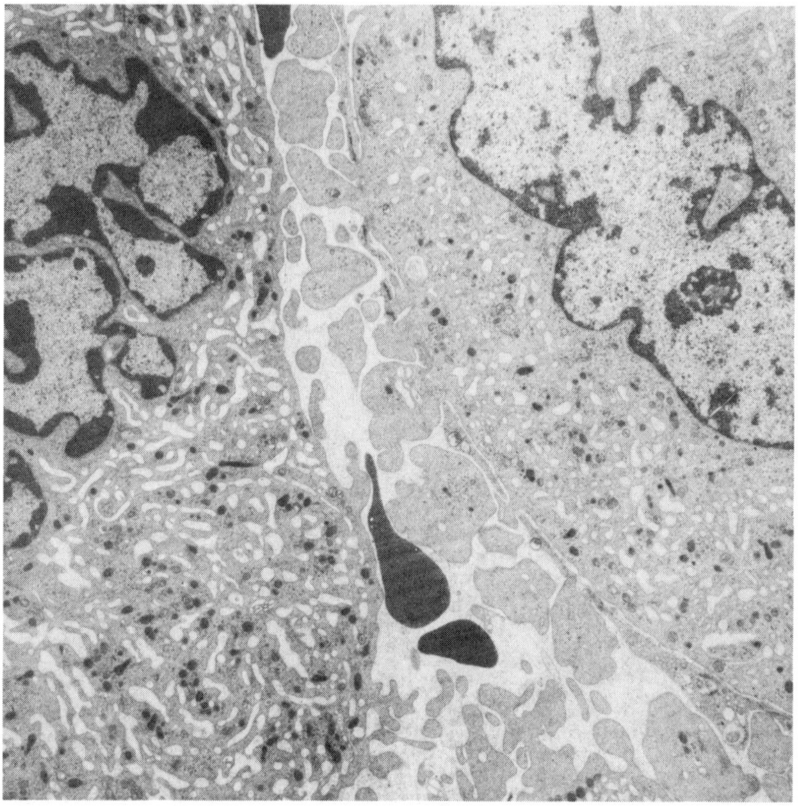

Fig. 2. Bone marrow, rabbit. A mature megakaryocyte is shown with processes protruding between sinusoidal cells. The processes within the sinusoidal spaces could be interpreted as platelets budding off. However, they are more likely to represent early passage of megakaryocytes into sinus spaces. This is supported by the presence of a mature megakaryocyte within the sinusoidal space. Transmission electron microscopy x5000.

This evidence demonstrates that whole megakaryocytes or cytoplasmic fragments unequivocally exist in the bloodstream and that the number of naked nuclei present in the lungs increases during times of

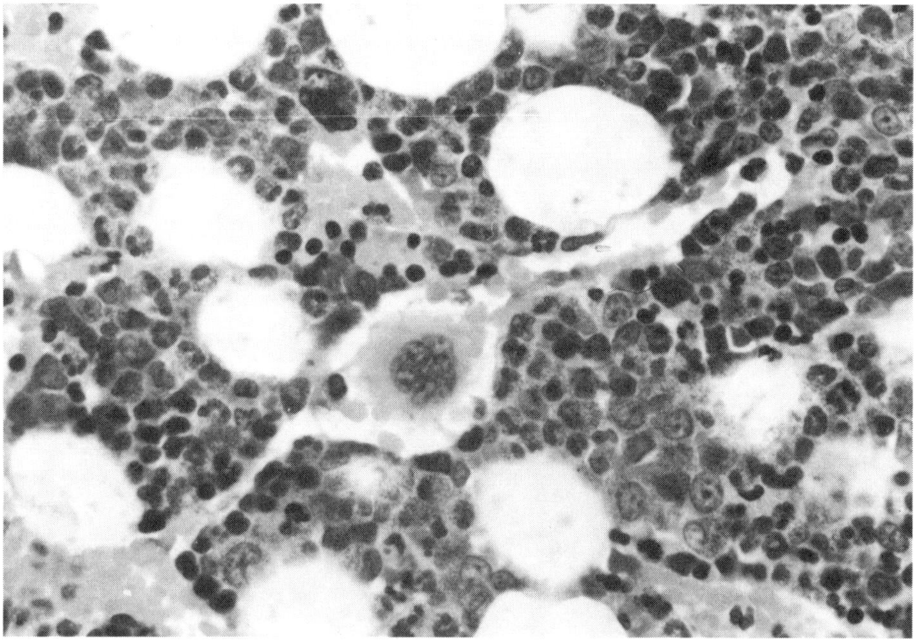

Fig. 3. Bone marrow H/E x720. Rabbit. A mature megakaryocyte is present within one of the sinusoidal spaces.

increased platelet production. However, it is not clear from this evidence what percentage of platelet production occurs in the lungs. In an attempt to answer this point, Table I shows that an estimate may be made of how many megakaryocytes per ml of blood would have to be converted to platelets in the pulmonary circulation to maintain the normal platelet count seen in man and rat. Tinggaard Pedersen (1978) measured the number of megakaryocytes in inferior vena caval blood in man and found on average 12 megakaryocytes per ml of blood, mainly possessing copious cytoplasm. This is of the same order of magnitude as that estimated for man in Table 1. The theoretical estimate may be higher than the experimental finding for two reasons. Firstly only megakaryocytes with nuclei were included in Tinggaard Pedersen's experimental study and secondly the experimental filtration technique may have removed the cytoplasm from some of the

TABLE 1

Data used to calculate the number of megakaryocytes per ml of blood entering the pulmonary artery to maintain a normal platelet count (32). (Reproduced from Clin. Phys. Physiol. Meas. by permission of the Institute of Physics).

Body weight Range	Man 70kg (n=51) (54-94)kg†	Rat 215g (n=9) (100-500)g†
Blood volume (6% body weight)	4.21	12.9ml
Effective platelet blood volume	6.31	19.4ml
Platelet count (platelets l^{-1} of blood)	2.32×10^{11}	10.26×10^{11}
Circulating platelet number	14.6×10^{11}	0.20×10^{11}
Platelet population destroyed per day	0.138‡	0.288§
Number of platelets destroyed per day	2.01×10^{11}	5.8×10^{9}
Number of platelets produced per day	2.01×10^{11}	5.8×10^{9}
Number of platelets produced per megakaryocyte	1088	2129
Number of megakaryocytes released per day	1.85×10^{8}	2.72×10^{6}
Number of megakaryocytes released per minute	1.28×10^{5}	1.89×10^{3}
Cardiac output ($l\ min^{-1}$)	5.6	2.23×10^{-2} (0.015-0.079)
Megakaryocytes per ml of blood entering the pulmonary artery	23	58

† Date from Mitruka and Rawnsley (1977)

‡ Trowbridge and Martin (1983)

§ Evaluated from the experimental data of Jackson and Edwards (1977) by the method described in Trowbridge and Martin (1983).

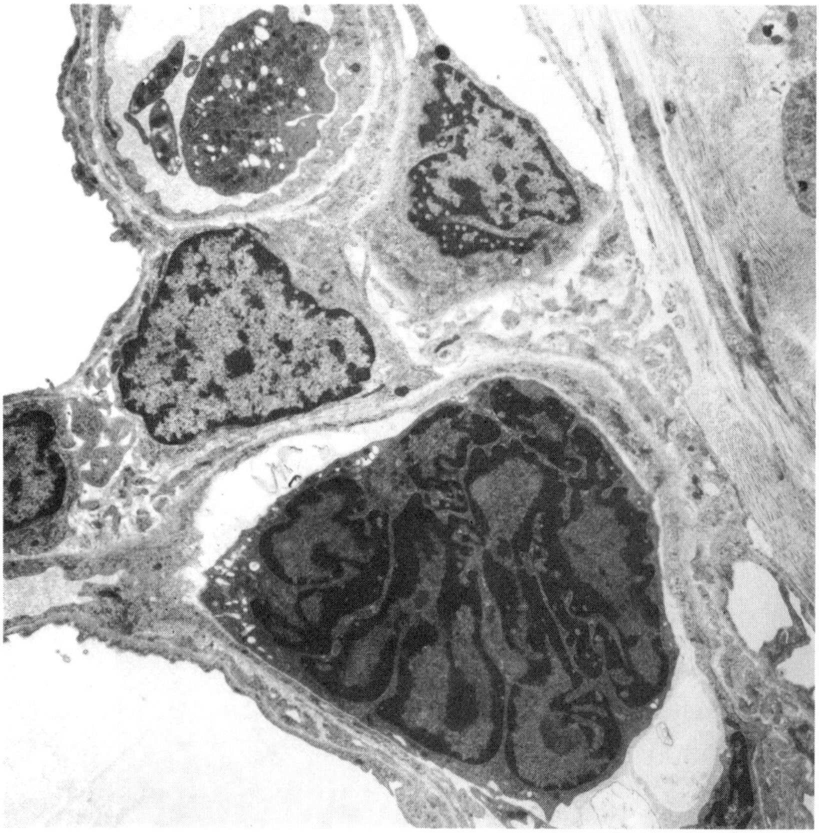

Fig. 4 Naked nucleus in pulmonary circulation. Also pulmonary capillary displaying cytoplasmic fragments from a megakaryocyte and mature platelets. Rabbit. Transmission electron microscopy x 5000.

megakaryocytes. Cytoplasmic particles were excluded from the experimental study although they were found on the filter. Therefore it is possible that sufficient megakaryocytes enter the pulmonary circulation and shed their cytoplasm at that site to account for total platelet production. Experimenters searching for megakaryocytes in the lungs should be aware of the extremely low numbers of pulmonary megakaryocytes predicted from the data in Table 1 to account for total platelet production in the lungs.

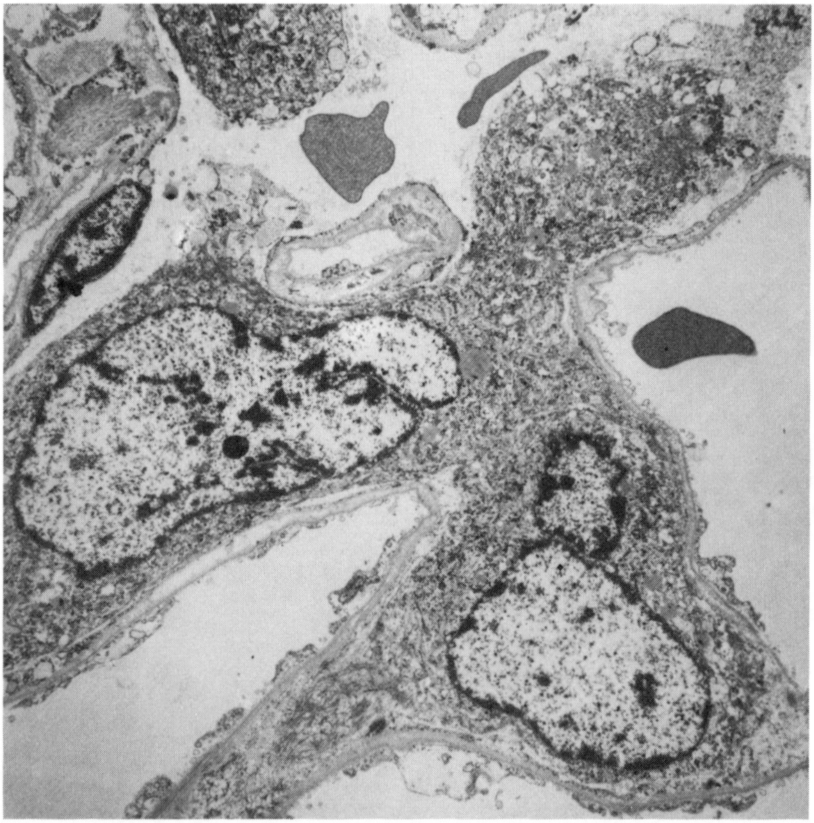

Fig. 5 Mature megakaryocyte wedged in capillaries of pulmonary circulation. Rabbit. Transmission electron microscopy x 3000.

Recently the platelet count was measured at various sites in the circulation from a group of 13 patients undergoing angioplasty for coronary artery atheroma (unpublished data). The platelet count in the pulmonary artery was 200 $\pm$ 21 and 212 $\pm$ 22 in the pulmonary veins. Using a one-tailed paired t-test this increase approached statistical significance ($p<0.06$). In these patients the femoral artery platelet count was 221 $\pm$ 16 and the femoral vein count was 195 $\pm$ 26; a significant decrease ($p<0.04$). It is tempting to attribute this significant increase in platelet count across the pulmonary circulation, which was been described previously by other authors (30), as evidence of pulmonary platelet production. However, it can be calculated that in normal pulmonary platelet production a difference of only 0.01% in platelet count across the pulmonary circulation would be produced, if all platelets were produced in the lungs. Such a difference would not be measurable by present platelet counting techniques. This suggests that sampling bias, or other artefacts may account for the apparent platelet count differences across the pulmonary circulation.

The Mechanism of Platelet Production

Megakaryocytes that circulate in central venous blood must enter the pulmonary arterial circulation. The enormous size of the megakaryocyte means that it cannot pass the pulmonary capilliary bed, (Fig. 4. shows a megakaryocyte nucleus filling a pulmonary capillary). The physical relationships thus generated may then give rise to the platelets' unique volume distribution.

Cellular volume distributions produced through mitosis tend to follow a Gaussian distribution. The platelet volume distribution is unique in that it is positively skewed towards higher volumetric values. This asymmetry has been characterised by assuming a Gaussian model for the logarithms of platelet volumes (25). The logarithmic transformation is attractive since it reduces the asymmetry and allows the log volume platelet population to be estimated from two statistical parameters: the sample mean and variance of the platelet log volumes. Platelets are not produced by mitosis and therefore their mode of production may be reflected in their unique volume distribution.

Methods by which log Gaussian curves are produced have been well reviewed (2). For example, such a curve is produced in industrial processes by a physical fragmentation process. If a number of particles with an arbitrary volume distribution are fragmented physically, the particles produced will tend towards a long Guassian volume distribution as the number of fragmentation steps is increased. A specific fragmentation process has been proposed to explain the production of platelets from megakaryocyte cytoplasm (41). The megakaryocytes are too large to pass through the pulmonary circulation without deforming or fragmenting. The absence of cytoplasm on the megakaryocytes found in the pulmonary vein suggests that cytoplasmic deformation is unlikely. It has been suggested that the megakaryocyte divides into two when it reaches a pulmonary bifurcation, the daughter vessels of which are too small to allow passage of the megakaryocyte without some breakage. The two cytoplasmic particles produced would have a random volume distribution around 0.5 of the cytoplasmic volume that underwent binary division (41). By repeating this process sequentially a number of times, a volume distribution of cytoplasmic particles will be generated. If this theory is correct then this will be the platelet volume distribution.

This hypothesis has been tested. If bone marrow megakaryocyte planimetric areas are measured on histological sections taken from an animal's bone marrow then an estimate can be made of the concomitant volume distribution by stereological methods (37). The individual megakaryocyte cytoplasmic volumes have been derived by the method described above using a Prime computer to produce a volume distribution of particles. By introducing the concept that larger megakaryocytes are more likely to undergo more random binary sequential divisions than smaller megakaryocytes the computer simulation generates particle volume distributions that are in close agreement with the measured platelet volumes found in the blood of the same animal. The computer model accurately predicted the circulating platelet volume distribution for megakaryocyte volumes in man, rat and rabbit (41). Although there are differences between species in certain platelet parameters, platelet production is likely to be similar in principle. All mammals possess platelets, lower orders do not. All mammals possess megakaryocytes which can undergo polyploid change that can give rise to many platelets. In all mammals the platelet volume distribution tends towards the log Gaussian.

The ability of a theory to take actual megakaryocyte volumes and predict the circulating platelet volume distribution in the animal from which the megakaryocytes were taken means that the theory must be a good contender for the actual theory of platelet production.

Application of this theory allows platelet volumes to be related to megakaryocyte cytoplasmic volumes in steady state thrombopoiesis. It has been shown that a larger than normal mean megakaryocyte volume is associated with a larger than normal mean platelet volume after acute myocardial infarction in man (40), during chronic hypoxia in rat (22), as well as in the Kasabach-Merrit syndrome in man. In contrast, in lymphoma larger than normal megakaryocytes produced platelets with a normal mean volume. However, in this pathology microcytic megakaryocytes with a smaller than normal mean cytoplasmic volume also produce platelets with a normal mean volume (unpublished observation). A further study (18), in which rabbits were fed a high cholesterol diet, produced megakaryocytes with larger than normal mean cytoplasmic volumes that gave rise to platelets with a mean volume which was smaller than controls. All of these cases could be explained by small alterations in the average number of fragmentation steps in the process of pulmonary platelet production. An exception is the May-Hegglin syndrome in which normal sized megakaryocytes are observed in the bone marrow (unpublished observation) and which give rise to large platelets. Significant changes in the fragmentation process must be made before the observed megakaryocyte cytoplasmic volumes can be converted into the platelet sizes associated with this condition. The reason for this may lie in the bizarre megakaryocyte cytoplasm ultrastructure found in this syndrome (6).

Recently this laboratory has produced experimental evidence to support the theory of pulmonary platelet production. A rat heart/lung preparation was established so that perfusion fluid, driven by a gravitational pressure head, ran into the catheterised pulmonary artery of the rat and was collected from the pulmonary veins via the catheterised left atrium. To maintain a physiological osmotic pressure a dextran solution was perfused through the lungs of the ventilated animal until the particle count in the fluid sampled from the pulmonary veins was the same as that in the pulmonary artery. Firstly, to act as a control, rat promegakaryoblasts from an eternal line culture were introduced into the pressure head reservoir and allowed to flow into the pulmonary artery and the particle count was observed in the fluid collected from the pulmonary veins. There was no change in particle count in the pulmonary veins but there was a marked decrease in flow, presumably as the promegakaryoblasts occluded the smaller vessels of the pulmonary circulation. Next, mature rat megakaryocytes were separated from rat bone marrow by Percoll velocity gradient and countercurrent flow elutriation. These cells were then

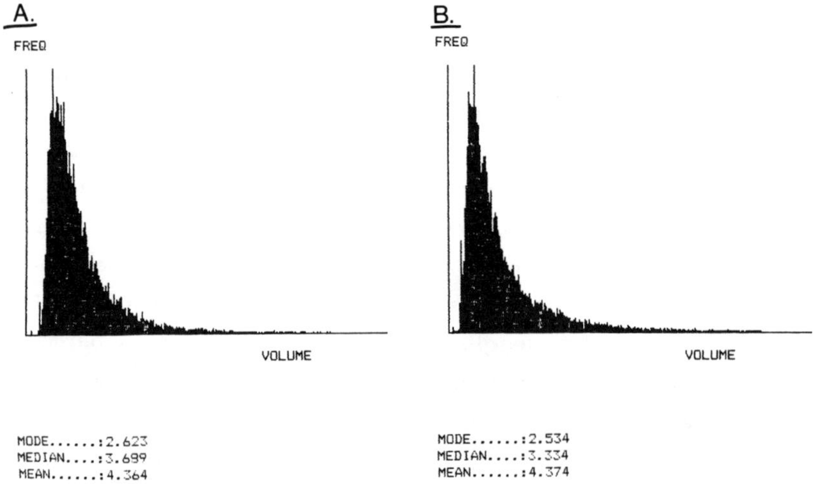

Fig. 6 Volume distributions of rat platelets (A) and particles produced from megakaryocytes in a rat heart/lung preparation (B).

introduced into the pulmonary circulation as before and the particle count and volume distribution observed in the fluid collected from the left atrium. The particle count rose soon after the megakaryocytes had started to enter the lungs and there was no significant reduction in flow. The volume distribution of the particles collected resembled very closely the volume distribution of rat platelets. Fifty-five per cent of the rat platelets and the particles produced from the megakaryocytes lay between 2 and 4 fl. The rat mean platelet volume and that of the particles collected from the heart/lung preparation were both 4.4 fl. (Fig. 6).

Asthma

Abnormalities due to the presence of megakaryocytes may give rise to pulmonary pathology. For example, it has been suggested that platelet derived growth factor (PDGF) from megakaryocytes may be the cause of bone marrow fibrosis in myelofibrosis (33). If that is so then there may be circumstances in which pulmonary fibrosis may be due to PDGF liberated from megakaryocytes in the pulmonary circulation.

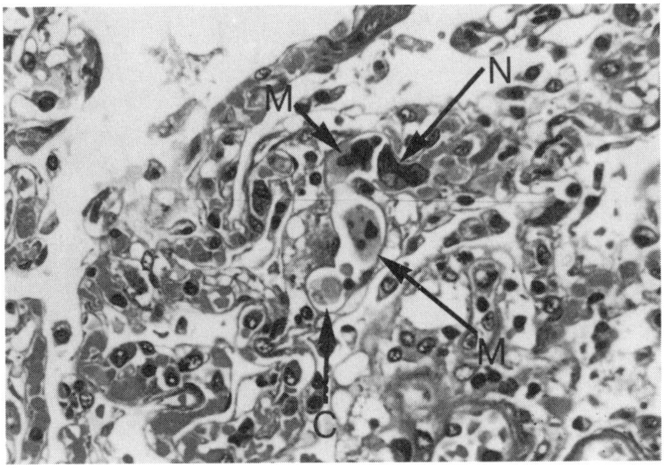

Fig. 7 Lung from 38 year old female dying in status asthmaticus. H/E x320.
M = mature megakaryocyte, N = naked nucleus, C = cytoplasmic fragment.

It has been reported (31) that at autopsy the lungs of three patients dying from status asthmaticus contained large numbers of megakaryocytes (Figs. 7, 8), whereas control lungs contained only rare megakaryocytes. These patients give rare insight into the possible state of lungs during acute asthmatic attack. The relationship of the megakaryocytes to asthma is only speculative, but the presence of the megakaryocyte in these patients is probably significant. They could be either associated with the cause of asthma or be an effect. However, if

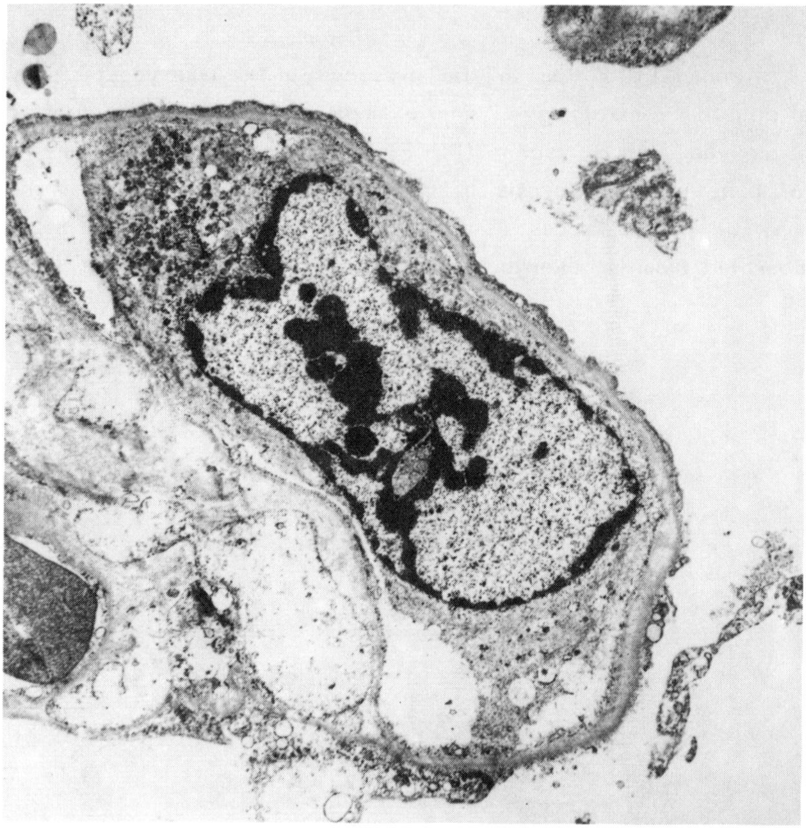

Fig. 8. Lung from 38 year old female dying from status asthmaticus. Mature megakaryocyte in pulmonary capillaries. Formalin fixed. Transmission electron microscopy x5000.

platelets can produce substances that are asthmagenic then megakaryocytes, that are larger and younger than platelets, would be more asthmagenic than platelets. Furthermore, if platelets are produced in the lungs, abnormalities of such production may cause or enhance an asthmatic attack. The answer to why megakaryocytes are found in the lungs of these patients must await further understanding of the normal physiology and pathology of the megakaryocyte.

Conclusions

1. Megakaryocytes can circulate.
2. They are found in sufficient numbers in central venous blood that platelet production from circulating megakaryocytes alone could explain total platelet production.
3. Megakaryocytes are too large to pass through the pulmonary circulation.
4. It is proposed that they fragment in the pulmonary circulation to produce platelets.
5. Abnormalities of this process may produce pulmonary disease.

Acknowledgements

We thank Dr. David Cumberland and Dr. Y.T. Kishk for their assistance in obtaining blood from patients undergoing angioplasty. We are grateful for the skilled assistance of Mr. C. Warren, Mrs. A.M. Stewart and Mr. B. Metcalf in these studies. We are also grateful to Drs. Ciccoria and Hempling for kindly supplying the promegakaryoblast culture. The assistance of Mr. David Crinall in the preparation of and Mrs. Barbara Walton for the typing of the manuscript is also acknowledged.

References

1. Aabo, K.; Hansen, K.B. (1978) Megakaryocytes in pulmonary blood vessels. I. Incidence at autopsy, clinicopathiological relations especially to disseminated intravascular coagulation. Acta Pathol.Microbiol.Scand. Section A, 86, 285-291.
2. Aitchison, J.; Brown, J.A.C. (1957) The lognormal distribution. Cambridge: C.U.P.
3. Breslow, A.; Kaufman, R.M.; Lawsky, A.R. (1968) The effect of surgery on the concentration of circulatory megakaryocytes and platelets. Blood. 32, 382-401.

4. Cameron, H.A.; Phillips, R.; Ibbotson, R.M.; Carson, P.H.M. (1983) Platelet size in myocardial infarction. BMJ. 287, 449-451.

5. Corash, L.; Shafer, B.; Perlow, M. (1978) Heterogeneity of human whole blood platelet subpopulations. II. Use of a subhuman primate model to analyse the relationship between density and platelet age. Blood. 52 726-734.

6. Godwin, H.A.; Ginsburg, A.D. (1974) May-Hegglin anomaly: A defect in megakaryocyte fragmentation. Brit.J.Haemat. 26, 117-128.

7. Hasen, K.D.; Aabo, K. (1978) Megakaryocytes in pulmonary blood vessels. Relations to malignant haematological diseases especially leukaemia. Acta Path.Microbiol.Scand. Section A. 86, 293-295.

8. Howell, W.H.; Donahue, D.P. (1937) The production of blood platelets in the lung. J.Exp. Med. 65, 177-204.

9. Hume, R.; West, J.T.; Malmgren, R.A.; Chu, E.A. (1964) Quantitative observation of circulating megakaryocytes in the blood of patients with cancer. N.Engl.J.Med. 270, 111-117.

10. Jackson, C.W.; Edwards, C.C. (1977) Biphasic thrombopoietic response to severe hypobaric hypoxia. Brit.J.Haematol. 35, 233-244.

11. Karpatkin, S. (1969) Heterogeneity of human platelets. II. Functional evidence suggestive of young and old platelets. J.Clin.Invest. 48, 1083-1087.

12. Kaufman, R.M.; Airo, R.; Pollack, S.; Crosby, W.H.; Doberneck, R. (1965) Origin of pulmonary megakaryocytes. Blood 25, 767-775.

13. Kinosita, R.; Ohno, S. (1961) Biodynamics of thrombopoiesis. In: Blood platelets. Eds. Johnson, S.A.; Monto, R.W.; Rebuck, J.W.; Horn, R.C. Boston: Little, Brown. 611-616.

14. Kishk, Y.T.; Trowbridge, E.A.; Martin, J.F. (1985) Platelet volume subpopulations in myocardial infarction: an investigation of their homogeneity for smoking infarct size and site. Clin.Sci. 68, 419-425.

15. Martin, J.F.; Penington, D.G. (1983) The relationship between the age and density of circulating ^{51}Cr-labelled platelets in the sub-human primate. Thromb. Res. 30, 157-164.

16. Martin, J.F.; Plumb, J.; Kilbey, R.S.; Kishk, Y.T. (1983) Changes in platelet volume and density in myocardial infarction. BMJ. 287, 456-459.

17. Martin, J.F.; Shaw. T.; Heggie, J.; Penington, D.G. (1983) Measurement of the density of human platelets and its relationship to volume. Br.J.Haemat. 54, 337-352.
18. Martin, J.F.; Slater, D.N.; Kishk, Y.T.; Trowbridge, A.E. (1985) Platelet and megakaryocyte changes in cholesterol-induced experimental atherosclerosis. Arteriosclerosis. 5, 604-612.
19. Martin, J.F.; Slater, D.N.; Trowbridge, E.A. (1983) Abnormal intrapulmonary platelet production: a possible cause of vascular and lung disease. Lancet i, 793-796.
20. Martin, J.F.; Trowbridge, E.A.; Salmon, G.F.; Plumb, J. (1983) The biological significance of platelet volume: its relationship to bleeding time, platelet thromboxane-B_2 production and megakaryocyte nuclear concentration. Thromb.Res. 32, 443-460.
21. Martin, J.F.; Trowbridge, E.A.; Salmon, G.L.; Slater, D.N.; (1982) The relationship between platelet and megakaryocyte volumes. Thromb.Res. 28, 447-459.
22. Metcalfe, B.C.; Warren, C.W.; Slater, D.N.; Trowbridge, A.E.; Martin, J.F.; Barer, G.R. (1984) Changes in platelets and megakaryocytes in simulated high attitude. Clin.Sci. 67, 76P.
23. Mitruka, B.M.; Rawnsley, H.M. (1977) Clinical, biochemical and haematological reference values in normal experimental animals.
24. Milner, P.C.; Martin, J.F. (1985) Shortened bleeding time in acute myocardial infarction and its relation to platelet mass. BMJ. 290. 1767-1770.
25. Paulus, J.M. (1975) Platelet size in man. Blood. 46, 321-336
26. Paulus, J.M.; Bury, J.; Grosdent, J.C.; (1979) Control of platelet territory development in megakaryocytes. Blood Cells. 5, 59-88.
27. Radley, J.M.; Scurfield, G. (1980) The mechanism of platelet release. Blood. 56, 996-999.
28. Savage, B.; McFadden, P.R.; Hanson, S.R.; Harker, L.A. (1986) The relation of platelet density to platelet age. Survival of low and high density ^{111}Indium-labelled platelets in baboons. Blood. 68, 386-393.
29. Sharnoff, J.G. (1959) Increased pulmonary megakaryocytes - probable role in postoperative thromboembolism. JAMA 169, 688-691.

30. Sharnoff, J.G.; Scardino, V. (1960) Platelet count differences in blood of the rabbit right and left heart ventricles. Nature (Lond.) 187, 334-335.

31. Slater, D.N.; Martin, J.F.; Trowbridge, E.A. (1985) The platelet in asthma. Lancet. i, 110.

32. Slater, D.N.; Trowbridge, E.A.; Martin, J.F. (1983) The megakaryocyte in thrombocytopenia: A light and electronmicroscope study supporting the theory that all platelets are produced in the lungs. Thromb. Res. 31, 163-176.

33. Sultan, C.; Sigau, F.; Lambert, M.; Reyes, F. (1981) Acute myelodysplasia with myelofibrosis; a report of eight cases. Br.J.Haematol. 49, 11-16.

34. Szczeklik, A.; Milner, P.C.; Birch, J.; Watkins, J.; Martin, J.F. (1986) Prolonged bleeding time, reduced platelet aggregation, altered PAF-acether sensitivity and increased platelet mass are a trait of asthma and hay fever. Thromb.Haemostas. 56 (3), 283-287.

35. Thompson, C.B.; Jakubowski, J.A.; Quinn, P.G.; Deykin, D.; Valeri, C.R. (1984) Platelet size and age determine platelet function independently. Blood 63, 1372-1375.

36. Tinggaard Pedersen, N. (1978) Occurrence of megakaryocytes in various vessels and their retention in the pulmonary capillaries in man. Scand.J.Haematol. 21, 369-375.

37. Trowbridge, E.A.; Harley, P.J. (1984) A computer model of the random binary sequential division of megakaryocyte cytoplasm to produce platelets. Phys.Med.Biol. 29, 1447-1487.

38. Trowbridge, A.E.; Martin, J.F. (1983) A biological approach to the platelet survival curve with criticism of previous interpretations. Phys.Med.Biol. 28, 1349-1368.

39. Trowbridge, E.A.; Martin, J.F.; Slater, D.N. (1982). Evidence for a theory of physical fragmentation of megakaryocytes, implying that all platelets are produced in the pulmonary circulation. Thromb.Res. 28, 461-475.

40. Trowbridge, E.A.; Martin, J.F.; Slater, D.N.; Kishk, Y.T.; Harley, P.J.; Warren, C.W.; Woodcock, B. (1984) The origin of platelet count and volume. Clin.Phys.Physiol.Meas. 5, 145-170.

41. Trowbridge, E.A.; Martin, J.F.; Slater, D.N.; Kishk, Y.T.; Warren, C.W.; (1983) Platelet production: a computer based biological interpretation. Thromb.Res. 31, 329-350.

42. Trowbridge, E.A.; Slater, D.N.; Kishk, Y.T.; Woodcock, B.W.; Martin J.F. (1984) Platelet production in myocardial infarction and sudden cardiac death. Thromb.Haemostas. 52, 167-171.

43. Wright, J.H. (1910) The histogenesis of the blood platelets. J.Morphol. 21, 263-278.

METABOLIC ORIGIN AND FATE OF PLATELET-ACTIVATING FACTOR

JT O'Flaherty[+] and RL Wykle[++]
Wake Forest University Medical Center, Departments of Medicine[+] and Biochemistry[++], Winston-Salem, NC USA.

Introduction

Platelet-activating factor (PAF) is a glycerophosphocholine (GPC) containing a long chain alkyl ether at carbon-1 and an acetyl ester at carbon-2. Polymorphonuclear neutrophils (PMN), monocytes, platelets, macrophages, and endothelial cells, when excited, rapidly produce PAF. These same cells, as well as other cell types (e.g., smooth muscle), are activated by the phospholipid. Furthermore, the compound is implicated in a variety of allergic, inflammatory, and toxic reactions *in vivo*. Thus, experimentally induced endotoxic shock in rats is associated with the release of PAF into the blood stream; kadsurenone, a selective PAF competitive inhibitor, protects animals from the lethal effects of endotoxin (1). Many investigative groups, therefore, are currently studying diverse aspects of this fascinating cellular product. Our work has concentrated on PAF synthesis, degradation, and cellular activation mechanisms using the human PMN as a relevant model cell type. Platelets (2-4), macrophages (5-7), and endothelial cells (8-10), to the extent examined, appear quite similar to PMN in their methods of metabolizing and responding to the compound. Findings with PMN, therefore, may have general application.

2. PAF Synthesis

The total phospholipid pool in PMN contains ∿41% GPC; ∿44% of this is 1-O-alkyl ether GPC. Carbon-2 residues of these ethers are comprised of long chain fatty acid esters, including ∿10% arachidonic acid (11). When PMN are stimulated, they release the carbon-2 fatty acid from 1-O-alkyl-(as well as 1-O-acyl-)GPC's and acetylate the lyso intermediate to form PAF (12-17). Calcium-activated phospholipase A_2 and membrane-associated, kinase-activatable acetyltransferase accomplish this 2-step synthesis (12,15,16). Furthermore, the deacylation reaction releases arachidonic acid, which is then free to be metabolized further into 5-hydroxyicosatetraenoate (5-HETE), leukotriene B_4, prostaglandins, and other bioactive derivatives (13,14,18). Consequently, PAF production is frequently associated with the concurrent formation of several other bioactive compounds. These products may promote function individually or in synergistic combinations. 5-HETE, for instance, increases the PMN degranulating activity of PAF by >100-fold (19).

3. PAF Receptors

The PAF which is produced by stimulated cells appears to accumulate within the parent cell's plasma membrane (20); frequently, only a small fraction of the total product will find its way to the extracellular media. Indeed, in selected cell types, e.g., endothelial cells, synthesized PAF may not leave the cell (10). Nevertheless, this synthesized, membrane-associated PAF appears available for activating other cells. Cultured endothelium, when stimulated with thrombin, form, but do not detectable release, PAF. These thrombin-treated cells, however, can activate nearby PMN through a PAF-specific mechanism (10). PAF, then, may be transmembraneously shuttled between adherent cells. In this regard, PAF activates target cells by a specific, receptor-mediated mechanism. In PMN, these receptors are located in cell surface membranes and appear to be of two affinity types: high (K_d = 0.2 nM, 1100/cell) and low (K_d = 0.2 uM, 2000,000/cell) (21). Transcellular communication, therefore, could also involve an interaction of receptors from one cell with the PAF confined to membranes of a second cell.

4. Receptor-linked Activation Mechanisms

PAF receptors appear to trigger function through several mechanisms. One of these involves rises in subcellular calcium (22,23). A second mechanism (which may act in synergy with stimulated increases in cytosolic calcium [24]) involves the activation of protein kinase C (PKC). During the stimulation of many excitable cells types, PKC moves from cytosol to plasmalemma where it forms a tightly bound complex with intramembraneous diacylglycerol. (The diacylglycerol is produced from phosphotidylinositol during cell stimulation.) Product diacylglycerol remains membrane bound, binds to a specific receptor site on cytosolic PKC, and thereby initiates the construction of a membrane-PKC macrocomplex that is active in phosphorylating critical effector proteins (25). We find that PAF produces a similar cytosol-to-membrane mobilization of PKC in PMN. Thus, at > 0.2 nM, the phospholipid causes a rapid decrease in cytosolic PKC and an associated but quantitatively smaller rise in plasmalemmal PKC. PAF acts reversibly: within 15-30 min, PKC begins to reappear in cytosol. Several findings indicated that this effect of PAF is not due to a diacylglycerol-like direct interaction with PKC. First, PAF acted only on PMN primed with cytochalasin B, an agent which enhances responses to PAF but by itself has no effect on PKC location. Second, PAF did not influence PKC in disrupted PMN or activate PKC in a cell-free system. Direct PKC activators like phorbol myristate acetate (PMA) and diacylglycerol, contrastingly, stimulate cytosol-to-membrane movement of the enzyme independently of cytochalasin B in intact or disrupted cells and are potent activators of the kinase in cell-free systems. Finally, the bioinactive structural analogue, lyso-PAF, did not effect PKC in cytochalasin B-pretreated PMN and the homocholine analogue of PAF was about 80-fold weaker in stimulating PMN degranulation or in mobilizing the cell's kinase C. We conclude, therefore, that PAF activates PKC by an indirect, receptor-mediated mechanism. The PAF-induced mobilization of PKC preceded the cytochalasin-B dependent degranulation response: respective times for inducing half maximal PKC mobilization and release of granule bound B-glucuronidase in PMN treated with 200 nM PAF were < 7 and 40 sec, respectively. Furthermore, polymyxin B, a selective blocker of PKC (26), partially inhibited the PMN degranulation response to PAF and the direct PKC activator, PMA (Table I). Finally, 5-HETE dramatically increased the PKC mobilizing actions of PAF: its synegistic effects on PKC paralleled its influences on the PMN degranulation response. These data suggest that a portion of the cytochalasin B-dependent actions of PAF are mediated by the

Table I. Effect of polymyxin B on PMN degranulation[1]

	polymyxin B (ug/ml)			
stimulus (nM)	0	100	200	400
PAF (200)	20 ± 2[2]	17* ± 2	16* ± 2	14* ± 2
PAF (20)	18 ± 2	15* ± 2	13* ± 2	12* ± 3
PAF (2)	14 ± 2	13 ± 2	11* ± 2	10* ± 3
PMA (1)	38 ± 4	32* ± 4	30* ± 4	27* ± 2
PMA (0.3)	28 ± 4	26 ± 1	22* ± 3	19* ± 2
PMA (0.1)	9 ± 2	6 ± 1	4* ± 2	2* ± 1

1 PMA (2.6 million/ml) were incubated with the indicated concentration of polymyxin B for 20 min at 37°C, treated with 5 ug/ml cytochalasin B for 2-4 min, and challenged for 5 min (PAF) or 20 min (PMA).

2 Net release of granule bound vitamin B-12 binding protein for 5 experiments, ± SEM.

* indicates values significantly lower than those found in the absence of polymyxin B based upon student's paired t-tests.

protein phosphorylating actions of PKC.

5. PAF Degradation

PMN inactivate PAF by enzymatic reactions that take place while the compound resides in the cells' plasma membrane. Following addition of [^{3}H]PAF to PMN, intact radioactive ligand is localized exclusively in plasmalemma (21). At this site, it is deacetylated by a cytosolic acetylhydrolase and acylated by a membrane-bound, activatable transacylase (15,16,18). In human PMN, greater than 80% of the acylated product contains arachidonic acid at the sn-2 position (13,18,27). Both deacetylation and acylation proceed with amazing rapidity: 10 million PMN almost completely metabolize more than 10 pmol PAF in 5-10 min (20). The final acylated compound is then gradually transported to intracellular granules over the ensuing 50 min (21). The 1-O-alkyl-2-acyl-GPC product, like resident alkyl ether GPC, can be converted to PAF during subsequent cell stimulation (18,26,28).

6. Conclusions

These studies suggest the following working hypotheses. Cell stimulation activates phospholipase A_2 and acetyltransferases which convert resident alkyl ether GPC to PAF. Arachidonate is concurrently released and converted to metabolites, e.g., 5-HETE. PAF accumulates in plasmalemma where it may, perhaps in conjunction with 5-HETE, activate its parent cell. The intramembraneous compound may also move directly to the membrane of cells adherent to the parent cell or, alternatively, move to the surrounding aqueous media to activate nearby and more remotely located cells. In any case, cellular activation proceeds through specific membrane-associated receptors which are coupled to intracellular calcium and PKC. Presumably, cellular function is triggered by: a) rises in cytosolic calcium, b) mobilization and activation of PKC, and/or c) initiation of other transduction mechanisms such as the metabolism of arachidonate (29). The receptor bound, intramembraneous ligand is then deacetylated, acylated (principally with arachidonate), and transported to the cell interior where it accumulates in lysosomal granules and may be readily recycled back to bioactive products when recruited by the stimulated cell.

Joseph T. O'Flaherty, M.D., Associate Professor of Medicine, Department of Medicine, Division of Infectious Diseases, Bowman Gray School of Medicine of Wake Forest University, 300 South Hawthorne Road, Winston-Salem, North Carolina 27103, U.S.A.

References

1. Doebber, T.W., Wu, M.S., Robbins, J.C., Choy, B.M., Chang, M.N., Shen, T.Y. (1985) Platelet activating factor (PAF) involvement in endotoxin-induced hypotension in rats. Studies with PAF-receptor antagonist kadsurenone. Biochem. Biophys. Res. Commun. 127, 799-808
2. Kramer, R.M., Patton, G.M., Pritzker, C.R., Deykin, D. (1984) Metabolism of platelet-activating factor in human platelets. Transacylase-mediated synthesis of 1-O-alkyl-2-arachidonoyl-sn-glycerol-3-phosphocholine. J. Biol. Chem. 259, 13316-13320
3. Malone, B., Lee, T-c, Snyder, F (1985) Inactivation of platelet activating factor by rabbit platelets. Lyso-platelet activating factor as a key intermediate with phosphatidylcholine as the source of arachidonic acid in its conversion to a tetraenoic acylated product. J. Biol. Chem. 260, 1531-1534
4. Purdon, A.D., Smith, J.B. (1985) Turnover of arachidonic acid in the major diacyl and ether phospholipids of human platelets. J. Biol. Chem. 260, 12700-12704
5. Albert, D.H., Snyder, F. (1983) Biosynthesis of 1-alkyl-2-acetyl-sn-glycero-3-phosphocholine (platelet-activating factor) from 1-alkyl-2-sn-glycero-3-phosphocholine by rat alveolar macrophages. Phospholipase A_2 and acetyltransferase activities during phagocytosis and ionophore stimulation. J. Biol. Chem. 258, 97-102
6. Jouvin-Marche, E., Ninio, E., Beaurain, G., Tence, M., Niaudet, P., Benveniste, J. (1984) Biosynthesis of PAF-acether (platelet-activating factor). VII. Precursors of Paf-acether and acetyl-transferase activity in human leukocytes. J. Immunol. 133, 892-898
7. Ninio, E., Mencia-Huerta, J.M., Heymans, F., Benveniste, J. (1982) Biosynthesis of platelet-activating factor. I. Evidence for an acetyl-transferase activity in murine macrophages. Biochim. Biophys. Acta 710, 23-31
8. Camussi, G., Aglietta, M., Malavasi, F., Tetta, C., Piacibello, W., Sanavio, F., Bussolino, F. (1983) The release of platelet-activating factor from human endothelial cells in culture. J. Immunol. 131, 2397-2403
9. Prescott, S.M., Zimmerman, G.A., McIntyre, T.M. (1984) Human endothelial cells in culture produce platelet-activating factor (1-alkyl-2-acetyl-sn-glycero-3-phosphocholine) when stimulated with thrombin. Proc. Natl. Acad. Sci. USA 81, 3534-3538
10. Zimmerman, G.A., McIntyre, T.M., Prescott, S.M. (1985) Thrombin stimulates the adherence of neutrophils to human endothelial cells in vitro. J. Clin. Invest. 76, 2235-2246
11. Mueller, H.W., O'Flaherty, J.T., Greene, D.G., Samuel, M.P., Wykle, R.L. (1984) 1-O-alkyl-linked glycerophospholipids of human neutrophils: distribution of arachidonate and other acyl residues in the ether-linked and diacyl species. J. Lipid Res. 25, 383-388
12. Mueller, H.W., O'Flaherty, J.T., Wykle, R.L. (1983) Biosynthesis of platelet activating factor in rabbit polymorphonuclear neutrophils. J. Biol. Chem. 258, 6213-6218
13. Chilton, F.H., O'Flaherty, J.T., Ellis, J.M., Swendsen, C.L., Wykle, R.L. (1983) Metabolic fate of platelet-activating factor in neutrophils. J. Biol. Chem. 258, 6357-6361

14. Swendsen, C.L., Ellis, J.M., Chilton, III, F.H., O'Flaherty, J.T., Wykle, R.L. (1983) 1-O-alkyl-2-acyl-sn-glycero-3-phosphocholine: A novel source of arachidonic acid in neutrophils stimulated by the calcium ionophore A23187. Biochem. Biophys. Res. Commun. 113, 72-79
15. Wykle, R.L., Olson, S.C., O'Flaherty, J.T. (1986) Biochemical pathways of platelet activating factor synthesis and breakdown. Adv. Inflam. Res. 11, 71-81
16. Synder, F. (1985) Chemical and biochemical aspects of platelet activating factor: A novel class of acetylated ether-linked choline-phospholipids. Med. Res. Rev. 5, 107-140
17. Mueller, H.W., O'Flaherty, J.T., Wykle, R.L. (1984) The molecular species distribution of platelet-activating factor synthesized by rabbit and human neutrophils. J. Biol. Chem. 259, 14554-14559
18. Chilton, F.H., Ellis, J.M., Olson, S.C., Wykle, R.L. (1984) 1-O-alkyl-2-arachidonoyl-sn-glycero-3-phosphocholine. A common source of platelet-activating factor and arachidonate in human polymorphonuclear leukocytes. J. Biol. Chem. 259, 12014-12019
19. O'Flaherty, J.T., Wykle, R.L., Redman, J., Samuel, M., Thomas, M. Metabolism of 5-hydroxyeicosatetraenoate by human neutrophils: Production of a novel ω-oxidized derivative. In press
20. Ribbes, G., Ninio, E., Fontan, P., Record, M., Chap, H., Benveniste, J., Douste-Blazy, L. (1985) Evidence that biosynthesis of platelet-activating factor (paf-acether) by human neutrophils occurs in an intracellular membrane. FEBS Lett. 191, 195-199
21. O'Flaherty, J.T., Surles, J.R., Redman, J., Jacobson, D., Piantadosi, C., Wykle, R.L. (1986) Binding and metabolism of platelet-activating factor by human neutrophils. J. Clin. Invest. 78, 381-388
22. O'Flaherty, J.T., Swendsen, C.L., Lees, C.J., McCall, C.E. (1981) Role of extracellular calcium in neutrophil degranulation responses to 1-O-alkyl-2-O-acetyl-sn-glycero-3-phosphocholine. Am. J. Pathol. 105, 107-113
23. Hallam, T.J., Rink, T.J. (1985) Agonists stimulate divalent cation channels in the plasma membrane of human platelets. FEBS Lett. 186, 175-179
24. Melloni, E., Pontremoli, S., Michetti, M., Sacco, O., Sparatore, B., Salamino, F., Horecker, B.L. (1985) Binding of protein kinase C to neutrophil membranes in the presence of Ca^{2+} and its activation by a Ca^{2+}-requiring proteinase. Proc. Natl. Acad. Sci. USA 82, 6435-6439
25. Nishizuka, Y. (1986) Studies and perspectives of protein kinase C. Science 233, 305-312
26. Wise, B.C., Glass, D.B., Chou, C.-H.J., Raynor, R.L., Katoh, N., Schatzman, R.C., Turner, R.S., Kibler, R.F., Kuo, J.F. (1982) Phospholipid-sensitive Ca^{2+}-dependent protein kinase from heart. II. Substrate specificity and inhibition by various agents. J. Biol. Chem. 257, 8489-8495
27. Chilton, F.H., Murphy, R.C. (1986) Remodeling of arachidonate-containing phosphoglycerides within the human neutrophil. J. Biol. Chem. 261, 7771-7777
28. Ramesha, C.S., Pickett, W.C. (1986) Platelet-activating factor and leukotriene biosynthesis is inhibited in polymorphonuclear leukcoytes depleted of arachidonic acid. J. Biol. Chem. 261, 7592-7595
29. Chilton, F.H., O'Flaherty, J.T., Walsh, C.E., Thomas, M.J., Wykle, R.L., DeChatelet, L.R., Waite, B.M. (1982) Platelet activating

factor. Stimulation of the lipoxygenase pathway in polymorphonuclear leukocytes by 1-O-alkyl-2-O-acetyl-sn-glycero-3-phosphocholine. J. Biol. Chem. 257, 5402-5407

PROPERTIES OF PAF RELEVANT TO ASTHMA

C.P. Page and D.N. Robertson
Dept. of Pharmacology
King's College, Chelsea Campus,
Manresa Road, London SW3.

Introduction

Bronchial asthma has recently been described as 'chronic desquamating eosinophilic bronchitis' (1), a concise description reflecting the underlying histopathology (2). This type of clinical definition reflects the change in thinking in our understanding of the pathogenesis of asthma and the therapeutics of this disease toward asthma being considered as a chronic inflammatory disease rather than a reversible disease of airway smooth muscle constriction. The central underlying feature of all asthmatics is a non-specific airways hyperreactivity which seems to be related to inflammatory events in the lung and in particular the recruitment of eosinophils (1,3). Eosinophils are capable of releasing a range of toxic materials from the human lung that result in the loss of airway epithelium (3), a process known to elicit increased airway smooth muscle reactivity (4,5) and a breakdown of the mucociliary escalator (with subsequent formation of mucous plugs).

Many of the experimental and clinical studies investigating the pathophysiological mechanisms contributing to asthma have concentrated on the identification of materials eliciting smooth muscle constriction. However, since asthmatics are non-specifically hyperreactive to a wide range of stimuli including agents as innocuous as distilled water, this approach appears futile and has certainly not led to the development of any novel therapeutic agents. If non-specific bronchial hyperreactivity is a result of airways inflammation, then this would appear to be a better approach to investigate, particularly those factors contributing to eosinophil infiltration. Thus the observations that eosinophils are exquisitely sensitive to the ether-linked phospholipid, platelet activating factor (PAF) and that eosinophils obtained from asthmatics are a good source of PAF in comparison with eosinophils from normals provides a reasonable basis for considering PAF as a mediator of asthma (6,7,8).

PAF has the structure 1-o-alkyl-2-acetyl-sn-glyceryl-3-phosphory-choline (Fig 1) and has a variety of synonyms (Paf-acether, APRL,AGEPC). PAF was first described as a product released by IgE sensitised basophils in the rabbit capable of inducing platelet activation (9). PAF is now recognised as a product of a variety of human inflammatory cell types implicated in the pathogenesis of asthma with the notable exception of the pulmonary mast cell (8), although PAF has been observed to be a product of mastocytes in certain animal species (10).

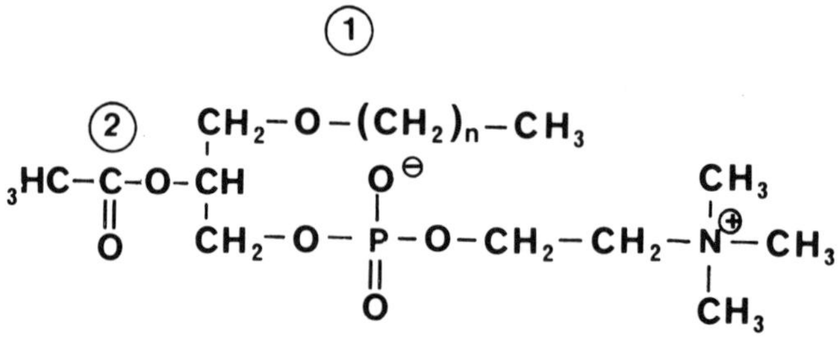

Fig. 1. Structure of PAF

In particular, PAF is released in substantial amounts from alveolar macrophages obtained by bronchoalveolar lavage of sensitised asthmatic subjects and subsequently challenged in vitro with the sensitising antigen (11). Additionally to basophils and eosinophils discussed already, human neutrophils, endothelial cells and platelets are all capable of releasing PAF in response to a variety of inflammatory stimuli (8).

The biosynthesis of PAF is the result of a two step enzymatic pathway involving the initial cleavage of the biologically active precursor lyso-PAF from ether-linked phospholipids (plasmalogens) and the subsequent acetylation of lyso-PAF by a rate-limiting cytosolic acetyl-transferase (12). In eosinophils from asthmatics, the rate-limiting acetyl-transferase enzyme appears to be abnormally activated in comparison with the enzyme activity in eosinophils obtained from normal individuals (12), which provides a plausible explanation for the increased PAFproduction observed in eosinophils obtained from asthmatics (6).

Bronchonstriction

PAF is now recognised as one of the most potent endogenous spasmogens described being active in certain animal species at concentrations as low as 10ng/kg (13). In normal volunteers, PAF administered by inhalation is also the most potent spasmogen yet described being some 30 times more potent than methacholine (14,15). In experimental animals, acute bronchoconstriction induced by PAF is secondary to some aspect of platelet activation since prior depletion of circulating platelets by means of an anti--serum directed against platelets essentially abrogates PAF-induced bronchoconstriction (16,17). The precise mechanism underlying PAF-induced bronchoconstriction is not known, but PAF is not a spasmogen of airway smooth muscle in vitro from either experimental animals or man (18), unless platelets are present (19). The release of spasmogens from activated platelets would seem the most likely explanation for the platelet dependent bronchoconstriction induced by PAF, although which spasmogen is responsible remains unknown (13).

Airways Inflammation

One of the most prominent features of PAF is the ability of this molecule to elicit both acute and more prolonged inflammatory responses in both experimental animals and man. Instillation of PAF into the airways of experimental animals induces a long lasting inflammatory response still evident after 1 month in some animals (20). The first three hours following direct administration of PAF into the lungs is accompanied by a progressive fall in lung function (21) reminiscent of antigen-induced late reactions observed in sensitised rabbits (22) or indeed following antigen challenge of sensitised asthmatics (23). Ultrastructually, such inflammatory changes are characterised by a pulmonary accumulation of a number of inflammatory cells including neutrophils, macrophages, platelets and eosinophils plus dramatic effects on the integrity of both epithelial and endothelial cell layers (20,24, 25). Additional to inflammatory cell recruitment, PAF administration will also elicit oedema formation both in the pulmonary and bronchial circulation of experimental animals (26,27,28). In primates, instillation of PAF directly into the lung results in a selective accumulation of eosinophils which can be observed in bronchoavelor lavage fluid (29). None of these inflammatory changes are found following administration of the PAF precursor, lyso-PAF suggesting a specific effect of PAF rather than non-specific injury resulting from the surfactant properties of this class of molecules. PAF-induced effects on the human lung have yet to be investigated but it is of considerable interest that the local administration of PAF into the skin of healthy human volunteers results in both an acute and more protracted inflammatory response (30,31,32). Intradermal injection of PAF as low as 10ng/site will induce an acute weal and flare response in normal volunteers (30) which from studies in experimental animals probably reflects a direct effect of PAF on the microvasculature leading to increased vascular permeability and blood flow (33,34). Such acute inflammatory changes are dose-dependent and resolve within 30 minutes to 1 hour. Following the administration of higher doses of PAF erythema is observed some 3-6 hours later reminiscent of the antigen induced late response in the skin of sensitised asthmatics (35,36), although of a lesser magnitude. In normal volunteers, biopsy of skin sites at various times after local PAF administration reveals evidence of inflammatory changes. In particular, extensive cellular infiltration is evident with neutrophils predominating at 4 hours and being succeded by a mixed cellular infiltrate comprising of lymphocytes and histiocytes additional to remaining neutrophils 24 hours after administration (31). Additionally, there was evidence of endothelial cell necrosis. Such changes are very similar to those reported by a number of investigators following local administration of PAF in experimental animals (20,37,38).

In atopic volunteers, PAF produces an acute weal and flare response not disimiliar to that observed in healthy volunteers (32). However, in contrast to normal volunteers the succeeding cellular infiltrate is composed almost exclusively of eosinophils (32). The magnitude of eosinophil infiltration being very similar to that observed in these atopics following a local administration of antigen at a concentration sufficent to induce a comparable weal and flare response to that induced by PAF (32). Such clinical studies not only confirm the experimental studies indicating that PAF is a highly potent mediator of acute and more persistant inflammatory responses, but also suggests that atopics and in particular eosinophils from atopics respond in a qualitatively different way to PAF. This difference in the responses of eosinophils to PAF in atopics coupled with the fact that eosinophils from asthmatics generate large quantities of PAF in comparison with eosinophils from normals suggests that PAF may be an important component of the eosinophilia observed in asthma.

Another feature of asthma is increased mucus production and reduced mucociliary clearance. It is therefore of interest that PAF is able to elicit an increase in the secretion of mucous glycoproteins into the airway lumen of experimental animals (39).

Airway Hyperreactivity

The prominent feature of all asthmatics is airway hyperreactivity which in many experimental models appears related to the induction of an inflammatory response in the lung (3,40). Certainly in clinical situations involving exacerbations of airway reactivity, there is an associated inflammatory response in the lung, notably a pulmonary eosinophilia (41). In view of the potency of PAF as a mediator of airways inflammation and the ability of PAF to induce eosinophil recruitment, PAF has been postulated as having a central role in the induction and maintenance of bronchial hyperreactivity in asthma (8). In support of this hypothesis, it has now been demonstrated that PAF will induce a long lasting and non-specific increase in bronchial reactivity in both experimental animals and man analogous to that following antigen exposure in sensitised asthmatics (15,42,43).

In healthy volunteers, inhalation of PAF induces an increased airway reactivity to methacholine that persists for up to 14 days, a property not shared by the PAF precursor, lyso PAF (15). In experimental animals, PAF has been observed to induce bronchial hyperreactivity to a range of spasmogens (42,43). In the guinea-pig, PAF-induced bronchial hyperreactivity is susceptible to inhibition by the four classes of clinically useful prophylactic anti-asthma drugs (namely disodium cromoglycate ketotifen glucocorticosteriods and methylxanthines), whilst being insensitive to non--prophylactic drugs such as beta-adrenceptor agonists, anti-histamines and non-steroidal anti-inflammatory drugs. (44). In this respect, PAF-induced bronchial hyperreactivity would appear to have a pharmacological sensitivity reminiscent of antigen-induced bronchial hyperreactivity in sensitive asthmatics.

The mechanisms underlying PAF-induced bronchial hyperreactivity are not yet understood but it seems likely that such changes in airway reactivity are related to associated inflammatory events in the lung. In the guinea-pig, PAF-induced bronchial hyperreactivity is dependent upon some aspect of platelet activation as prior depletion of circulating platelets by means of a selective anti-serum directed against platelets effectively abolishes the increase in airway reactivity (42). Furthermore, PAF induces an accumulation of platelets into the lung associated with changes in airway reactivity. The platelet recruitment is poorly reversible which may reflect the ability of PAF to induce an extravascular recruitment of platelets with subsequent apposition of platelets to airway smooth muscle (24). Whether extravasated platelets are necessary for the induction of airway reactivity remains to be seen but since platelets are known to release powerful smooth muscle mitogens

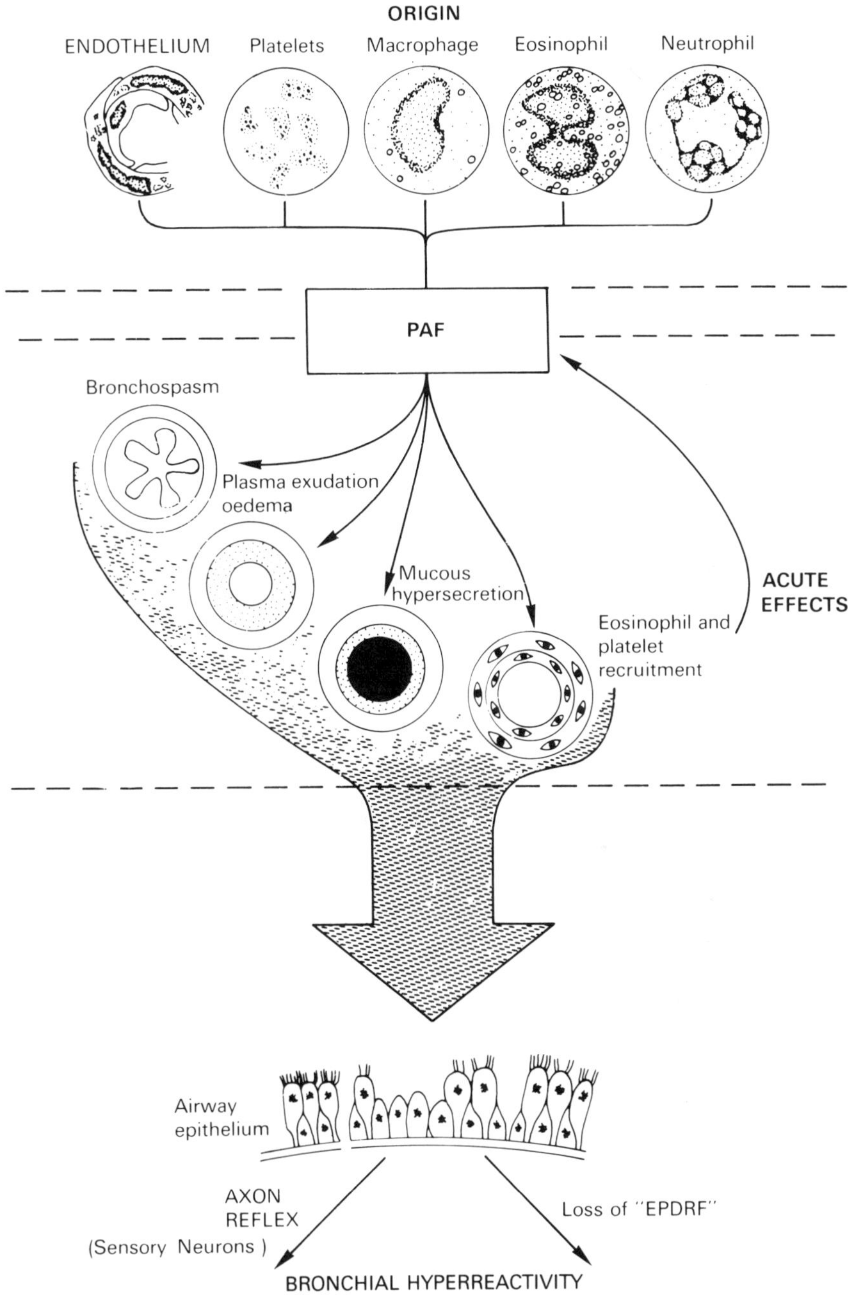

Fig. 2. Schematic representation of the possible relationship between PAF release by inflammatory cells in the lungs and the pathological features of asthma

the possibility remains that PAF-induced platelet extravasation contributes to the smooth muscle hyperplasia that characterises the asthmatic lung and which may well underly irreversible changes in airways reactivity. In the dog (43) and sheep (45), it has been suggested that neutrophils play a role in PAF-induced bronchial hyperreactivity and that PAF-induced bronchial hyperreactivity may be secondary to release of TXB2. However, the dog and sheep would appear not to be predictive models for pharmacological analysis of responses in asthmatics, since the pharmacological sensitivity of antigen--induced hyperreactivity in these species is not the same as observed in allergic asthmatics (46).

PAF-antagonists

A number of selective PAF antagonists have now been described of both synthetic and natural origin (47,48). The structures appear at first sight to be diverse and include phopholipid analogues of PAF (e.g. CV-3988, RO19-370, and SRI-63072), lignans (e.g. kadsurenone), terpenes (ginkgolides -B-BN 52021), triazolobenzodiazapines (e.g. alprazolam) and some type II and III calcium channel blockes.

All the PAF-antagonists seem to inhibit the array of pathological changes produced by PAF both in-vitro and in-vivo (47). In the context of asthma, it is of interest that BN 52021 and alprazolam have been observed to inhibit antigen induced bronchoconstriction in sensitised guinea-pigs (49,50). No formal clinical trials have been performed as yet with any of the PAF antagonists but ginkgolide extracts and plants containing kadsurenone like compounds have been utilised in traditional Chinese medicine for the treatment of asthma and inflammation (51). Furthermore, prelimary clinical data has revealed that treatment of asthmatic children with a ginkgolide preparation for several weeks is able to reduce the necessity for concommitant glucocorticoid therapy (52) and the same prepartion has been shown to inhibit allergen--induced bronchonstriction in sensitised asthmatics (52).

Conclusions

It is now apparent that PAF can mimic the pathological features of bronchial asthma more closely than any other mediator discovered. In particular, the ability of PAF to evoke eosinophil recruitment and a non-selective increase in bronchial hyperreactivity are impressive. A schematic representation depicting the possible relationship between PAF release and the features of asthma is shown in Fig 2. The similarity between the pharmacological sensitivity of PAF-induced bronchial hyperreactivty and antigen-induced bronchial hyperreactivity in asthmatics is also of interest because such a model system may lead to a better understanding of current anti-asthma drugs. It is hoped that the further investigation of the actions of PAF, will help to elucidate the mechanisms underlying bronchial asthma and lead to new treatments for this disease.

Correspondence to: C.P. Page
Dept. of Pharmacology
King's College, Chelsea Campus,
Manresa Road, London SW3.

References

1. Reed, C.E. (1986) New therapeutic approaches in asthma. J. Allergy Clin. Immunol. 77, 537-543.

2. Dunhill, M.S. (1978) The pathology of asthma. In 'Allergy : principles and practice, 1st Edition, Eds. Middleton,E., Reed, C.E., and Ellis, E.F., C.V. Mosby Co. 679-686.

3. Frigas, E., Gleich, G.J. (1986) The eosinophil and the pathophysiology of asthma. J. Allergy Clin. Immunol. 77, 527-537.

4. Barnes, P.J., Cuss, F.M., Palmer, J.B. (1985) The effect of airway epithelium on smooth muscle contraction in bovine trachea. Br. J. Pharmacol. 86, 685-692.

5. Goldie, R.G., Papadimitrium, J.M., Paterson, J.W., Rigby, P.J., Self, H.M., Spina, D. (1986) Influence of the epithelium on responsiveness of guinea-pig isolated trachea to contractile and relaxant agonists. Br. J. Pharmacol. 87, 5-14.

6. Lee, T.C., Leniham, D.J., Malone, B., Roddy, L.L., Wasserman, S.I. (1984) Increased biosynthesis of platelet activating factor in activated human eosinophils. J. Biol. Chem. 259, 5526-5530.

7. Wardlaw, A.J., Kay, A.B. (1986) Paf-acether is a potent chemotactic factor for human eosinophils. J. Allergy. Clin. Immunol. 77, 236.

8. Morley, J., Sanjar, S., Page, C.P. (1984) The platelet in asthma. Lancet ii, 1142-1144.

9. Benveniste, J., Henson, P.M. Cochrane, C.G. (1972) Leucocyte dependant histamine release from rabbit platelets: The role of IgE, basophils and a platelet activating factor. J. Exp. Med. 136, 1356-1377.

10. Mencia-Huerta, J.M., Lewis, R.A., Razin, E., Austen, K.F. (1983) Antigen induced release of platelet activating factor (Paf-acether) from mouse bone-marrow derived mast cells sensitised with monoclonal IgE. J. Immunol. 131, 2958-2964.

11. Arnoux, B., Grimfeld, A., Duroux, P., Denjean, A. (1983) Alveolar macrophages Paf-acether. A new association in the pathogenesis of human asthma. In 'Platelet Activating Factor', INSERM symposium No.23, Eds, Benveniste,J., Arnoux, B. Elsevier Science Publications B.V. pp 335-341.

12. Snyder, F. Chemical and biochemical aspects of platelet activating factor: A novel class of acetylated ether-linked choline phospholipids. (1985) Med. Res. Rev. 5, 107-140.

13. Morley, J., Page, C.P., Sanjar, S. (1985) Pulmonary responses to platelet activating factor. Prog. Resp. Res. 19, 117-123.

14. Patterson, R., Bernstein, P.R., Harris, K.E., Krell, R.D. (1984) Airway responses to sequential challenges with platelet activating factor and leukotriene D of rhesus monkeys. J. Lab. Clin. Med. 104, 340-345.

15. Cuss, F.M., Dixon, C.M., Barnes, P.J. (1986) Inhaled platelet activating factor in man: effects on pulmonary function and bronchial responsiveness. Lancet. 2 189.

16. Vargafig, B.B., Lefort, J., Chignard, M., Benveniste, J. (1982) Platelet activating factor induces a platelet -dependent bronchoconstriction unrelated to the formation of postaglandin derivatives. Eur. J. Pharmacol. 65, 185-192.

17. Halonen, M., Palmer, J.D., Lohman, I.C., McManus, L.M., Pinckard, R.N. (1981) Differential effects of platelet depletion on the physiologic alteration of IgE anaphylaxis and acetyl glyceryl ether phosphorylcholine infusions in the rabbit. Am. Rev. Resp. Dis. 124, 416-421.

18. Cerrina, J., Raffenstin, B., Labat, C., Bayol, A., Boullet, C., Gateau, O., Brink, C. (1983) Absence d'effect in-vitro du Paf-acether sur le muscle lisse pulmonaire de rat, cobaye et homme. J. Pharmacol (Paris) 14, 23.

19. Schellenberg, R.R., Walker, B., Snyder, F. (1983) Platelet-dependent contractions of human bronchus by platelet activating factor. J. Allergy. Clin. Immunol. 71, 145.

20. Cammussi, G., Pawlowski, I., Tetta, C., Roffirello, C., Alberton, M., Brentjens, J., Andres, G. (1983) Acute lung inflammation induced in the rabbit by local instillation of 1-o-octadecyl-2-acetyl-sn-glyceryl-3-phosphorylcholine or of native platelet activating factor. Am. J. Pathol. 112, 78-88.

21. Page, C.P., Guerreiro, D., Sanjar, S., Morley, J. (1985) Platelet activating factor (Paf-acether) may account for late-onset reactions to allergen inhalation. Agents Actions. 16, 30-32.

22. Shampian, M.P., Behrens, B.L., Larsen, G.L., Henson, P.M. (1982) An animal model of late pulmonary responses to Alternaria challenge. Am. Rev. Resp. Dis. 126, 493-498.

23. Cockcroft, D.W., Ruffin, R.E., Dolovich, J., Hargreave, F.E. (1977) Allergen-induced increase in non-allergic bronchial reactivity. Clin. Allergy 7, 503-513.

24. Lellouch-Tubiana, A., Lefort, J., Pirotzky, E., Vargafitg, B.B., Pfister A. (1985) Ultrastructural evidence for extravascular platelet recruitment in the lung upon intravenous injection of platelet activating factor (Paf-acether) to guinea pigs. Br. J. Exp. Path. 66, 345-356.

25. Lewis, J.C., O'Flaherty, J.T., McCall, C.E., Wykle, R.L., Bond, M.G. (1983) Platelet Activating Factor effects on pulmonary ultrastructure in rabbits. Exp. Mol. Pathol. 38, 100-108.

26. Mojarad, M., Hamasaki, Y., Said, S.I. (1983) Platelet activating factor increases pulmonary microvascular permeability and induces pulmonary oedema.

Bull. Europ. Physiopath. Resp. 19, 253-257.

27. O'Donnell, S.R., Ganendran, J.G. (in press) PAF-acether in conscious guinea pigs is a potent mediator of bronchial oedema. Clin. Exp. Pharmacol. Physiol.

28. Evans, T.J., Chung, K.F., Barnes, P.J. Platelet activating factor increases vascular permeability in guinea pig airways. Clin. Sci. (in press).

29. Aronux, B., Denjean, A., Page, C.P., Morley, J., Benveniste, J.(1985) Pulmonary effects of platelet activating factor in a primate are inhibited by ketotifen. Am. Res. Resp. Dis. 131, A2.

30. Archer, C.B., Page, C.P., Paul, W., Morley, J., MacDonald, D.M. (1985) Inflammatory characteristics of Paf-acether in the skin of experimental animals and man. Int. J. Tiss. Reac. 7, 363-365.

31. Archer, C. B., Page, C.P., Paul, W., Morley, J., MacDonald, D.M. (1985) Inflammatory cell accumulation in response to intracutaneous Paf--acether: a mediator of acute and persistent inflammation. Br. J. Dermatol. 113, (suppl 28), 133-135.

32. Henocq, E., Vargaftig, B.B. (1986) Accumulation of eosinophils in response to intracutaneous Paf-acether and allergens in man. Lancet ii, 1378-1379.

33. Humphrey, D.M., McManus, L.M., Satouchi, K., Hanahan, D.J., Pinckard, R.N. (1982) Vasoactive properties of acetyl glyceryl ether phosphorylcholine and analogues. Lab. Invest. 46, 422-427.

34. Morley, J., Page, C.P., Sanjar, S. (1985) Pharmacology of the late response to allergen and its relevance to asthma prophylaxis. Int. Archs. Allergy appl. Immun. 77, 73-78.

35. Basran, G.S., Page, C.P., Paul, W., Morley, J. (1984) Platelet activating factor: A possible mediator of the dual response to allergen. Clin. Allergy. 14, 75-79.

36. Solley, G.O., Gleich, C.J., Jordan, R.E., Schroeter, A.L. (1976) The late phase of the immediate wheal and flare skin reaction. Its dependence upon IgE antibodies. J. of Allergy and Clinical Immunology. 58, 408.

37. Dewar, A., Archer, C.B., Paul, W., Page, C.P., MacDonald, D.M., Morley, J. (1984) Cutaneous and pulmonary histopathological responses to platelet activating factor (Paf-acether) in the guinea pig. J. Path. 144, 25-34

38. Humphrey, D.M., Hanahan, D.J., Pinckard, R.N. (1982) Induction of leukocytic infiltrates in rabbit skin by acetyl glycerly ether phosphorylcholine. Lab. Invest. 47, 227-234.

39. Hahn, H. L., Purnamo, I., Lang, M., Sannwald, V. (1985) Effects of platelet activating factor on tracheal mucus secretion in live ferrets. Respiration (in press).

40. Fabbri, L.M. (1985) Airway inflammation and asthma. Progess in Biochemical Pharmacology, 20, 18-27.

41. De Monchey, S.E.R., Kauffman, H.F., Venge, P., Koeter, G.H., Jansen, H.R., Sluiter, H.J., de Vries, K. (1985) Broncho-alveolar eosinophila during allergen-induced late asthmatic reactions. Am. Rev. Resp. Dis. 131, 373-377.

42. Mazzoni, L., Morley, J., Page, C.P., Sanjar, S. (1985) Inductions of airway hyperreactivity by platelet activating factor in the guinea pig. J. Physiol. 365, 107P.

43. Chung, K., Aizawa, H., Leikauf, G., Veki, I.F., Evans, T.W., Nadel, J.A. (1986) Airway hyper-responsiveness induced by platelet activating factor: role of thromboxane generation. J. Pharm. Exp. Ther. 236, 580-584.

44. Mazzoni, L., Morley, J., Page, C.P., Sanjar, S. (1986) Prophylactic anti-asthma drugs impair the airway hyperreactivity that follows exposure to platelet activating factor (PAF). Br. J. Pharmacol. 86, 571P.

45. Christman, B.W., Portes, D.K., King, G.A., Lefferts, P.L., Snapper, J.R. (1986) Synthetic platelet activating factor alters pulmonary haemodynamics, lung mechanics, and lung fluid/solute exchange in awake sheep: Role of platelets and granulocytes and effects of synthetic platelet activating factor on airway reactivity. Am. Rev. Resp. Dis. 133, A174.

46. Morley, J., Hanson, J.M., Page, C.P. Platelet activation and airway hyperreactivity in asthma. Asthma Review (in press).

47. Braquet, P., Godfroid, J.J. PAF-acether specific binding sites: 2. design of specific antagonists. Trends in Pharmacol. Sci (in press).

48. Kornecki, E., Ehrlich, Y.E., Lenox, R.H. (1984) Platelet activating factor-induced aggregation of human platelets specifically inhibited by triazolobenzodiazepines. Science 226, 1454-1456.

49. Touvay, C., Etienne, A., Braquet, P. (1985) Inhibition of antigen--induced lung anaphylaxis in the guinea pig by BN 52021 a new specific Paf--acether receptor antagonist isolated from Ginkgo biloba. Agents and Actions (in-press).

50. Darius, H., Lefer, D.J., Smith, J.B., Lefer, A.M. (1986) Role of platelet activating factor - acether in mediating guinea pig anaphylaxis. Science. 232, 58-60.

51. Chinese Pharmacopea (Peking, China) (1977).

52. Braquet, P. Proofs of involvement of Paf-acether in various immune disorders using BN 52021 (Ginkgolide B): A powerful Paf-acether antagonist isolated from Ginkgo biloba L. In 'Prostaglandins in Health and Disease', U. Zof(Ed). Raven Press (in press).

EFFECT OF PLATELET ACTIVATING FACTOR ON HISTAMINE RELEASE FROM RAT MAST CELLS

M. Kurosawa

First Department of Internal Medicine, Gunma University School of Medicine, Maebashi 371, Japan

Introduction

PAF is a newly discovered mediator of anaphylaxis released by various inflammatory cells such as platelets (1), macrophages (2), eosinophils (3), neutrophils (4), and basophils (5). It was reported (6) that it was also released from mast cells in some species, but recent evidence (7) indicated that mast cells do not release PAF in situations where they release histamine in response to the calcium ionophore A23187 or compound 48/80. However the interaction between mast cells and PAF has received very little attention and in the present study the effect of PAF on histamine release and protein kinase C and PI kinase activation has been studied in rat mast cells.

Materials and methods

Reagents and their sources were as follows: C_{16}-and C_{18}-PAF (Nova Biochem, Laufelfingen, Switzerland), goat anti-rat IgE (epsilon specific) (Bethyl Laboratories, Montgomery, U.S.A), (gamma ^{32}P) ATP (4500 µ Ci/mmol) (ICN Pharmaceuticals, Irvine, U.S.A.), silica gel plate (20 x 20 cm, 250 um layer) (Brinkmann, Westbury, U.S.A.), Percoll, compound 48/80, calcium ionophore A23187, diacylglycerol, diphosphoinositide (DPI), phosphatidylinositol (PI) and the other phospholipids, bovine serum albumin (BSA), lysine-rich histone, phenylmethylsulfonyl fluoride (PMSF), ethylene glycol bis (beta-aminoethyl ether)-NNN'N'-tetraacetic acid (EGTA), Tris/HCl

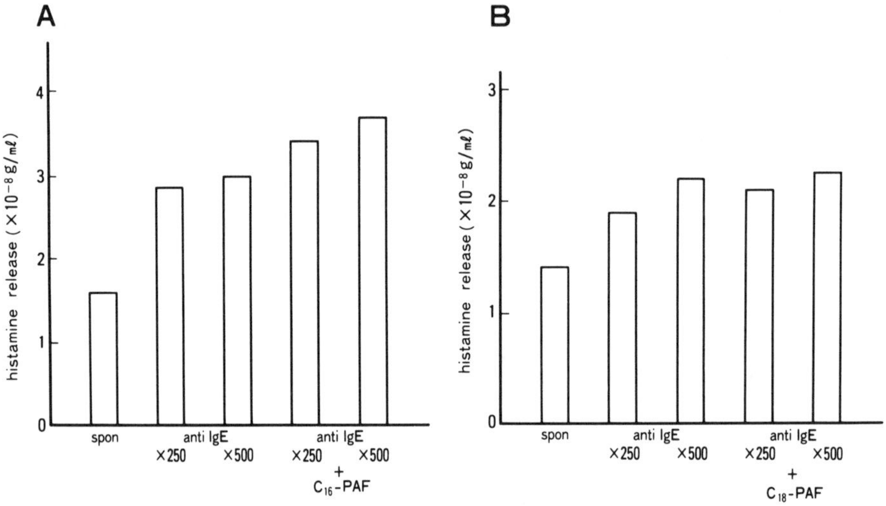

Fig.1.: Effect of PAF on anti-IgE-induced histamine release from rat mast cells. Anti-IgE was diluted to 1/250 and 1/500. A, C_{16}-PAF; B, C_{18}-PAF.

(Sigma Chemical, St. Louis, U.S.A.), oxalic acid, sodium pyrophosphate and the other reagents (Fisher Scientific, Fair Lawn, U.S.A.).

Rat mast cell preparations: Rat mast cells mixed with leukocytes and serosal cells were obtained by peritoneal and pleural lavage of male Sprague-Dawley rats weighing from 250 to 300 g. The lavage medium was a heparinized (10 U/ml) balanced salt solution (BSS) (4.0 mM Na_2HPO_4, 2.7 mM KH_2PO_4, 150 mM NaCl, 2.7 mM KCl, 0.9 mM $CaCl_2$ pH 7.2) containing 0.046 % (w/v) BSA. The mast cells in this mixture were purified on a Percoll gradient (9) and were more than 90 % pure by a toluidine blue dye staining reaction.

Isolation of rat mast cell granules: Granules were isolated from sonicated rat mast cells on a Percoll gradient by the method of Kruger et al. (13). As described by them, the granules distribute in two distinct bands in the gradient: the upper band close to the top and the lower band close to the bottom of the gradient. Electron microscopy and ruthenium red staining (13) revealed that the upper band consisted largely (more than 90 %) of swollen granules lacking membranes and the lower band largely (more than 95 %) of granules with intact membranes. Intact membrane granules washed twice with BSS after recovery from the gradient were used in the experiments below.

Cell incubation conditions: Mast cells (1.2-1.7 x 10^6) were incubated with 100 ng/ml PAF for 1 min at 37° C and then were stimulated by mast cell activating agents for the indicated time. Reactions were halted by adding 1 ml ice-cold BSS, rapidly sedimenting the cells at 4° C, removing the supernatant by aspiration for histamine assay and cell pellets for protein kinase C assay. Before the assay, the cell pellets were immediately suspended in a cold solution (50 mM Tris/HCl pH 7.3, 50 mM NaF, 50 mM sodium pyrophosphate, 10 mM EGTA and 2 mM PMSF) and were frozen by dryice and acetone treatment. To the supernatant 4 % $HClO_4$ were added in a final concentration. Experiments were performed in triplicate.

Protein kinase assay: Protein kinase C activity was assayed by measuring the incorporation of ^{32}P from (gamma^{32}P) ATP into lysine-rich histone. The reaction mixture contained 2 mM $CaCl_2$, 20 mM Tris/HCl pH 7.5, 6 ug/ml 1,2-diacylglycerol (as diolein), 24 ug/ml phosphatidylserine, 200 ug/ml lysine-rich histone, 10 M (gamma^{32}P) ATP (diluted to 5 x 10^7 cpm/umol with unlabeled ATP) and the cell pellets after thawing in 37°C water bath just before the assay. Data on ^{32}P incorporation into lysine-rich histone represent the mean of triplicate values. Differences between triplicates were less than 8 %.

Histamine assay: Histamine was assayed by the fluorometric technique described by Shore (14). Data on histamine release represent the mean of triplicate values. Differences between triplicates were less than 9 %.

Measurement of PI kinase activity in the granules: PI kinase activity was measured by the methods previously described by us (11). Standard incubation mixtures contained 20 mM Tris/HCl pH 7.4, 20 mM $MgCl_2$, 10 uM (gamma ^{32}P) ATP (diluted to 5 x 10^9 cpm/umol with unlabeled ATP) mixed with suspended mast cell granules in BSS. Each tube contained intact membrane granules from 1.5-2.0 x 10^6 mast cells. Incubations were conducted at 30°C for 15 min and the reaction was stopped by the addition of organic solvents to the entire granule suspension. Lipids in the mast cell granules were extracted with acidic medium and phospholipids were separated by thin layer chromatography on 1 % (w/v) oxalic acid impregnated silica gel *plates. Radioactivity in DPI was quantitated by liquid scintillation counting. Experiments were performed in duplicate and data on ^{32}P incorporation into DPI represent the mean of duplicate values. Differences between duplicates were less than 10 %.*

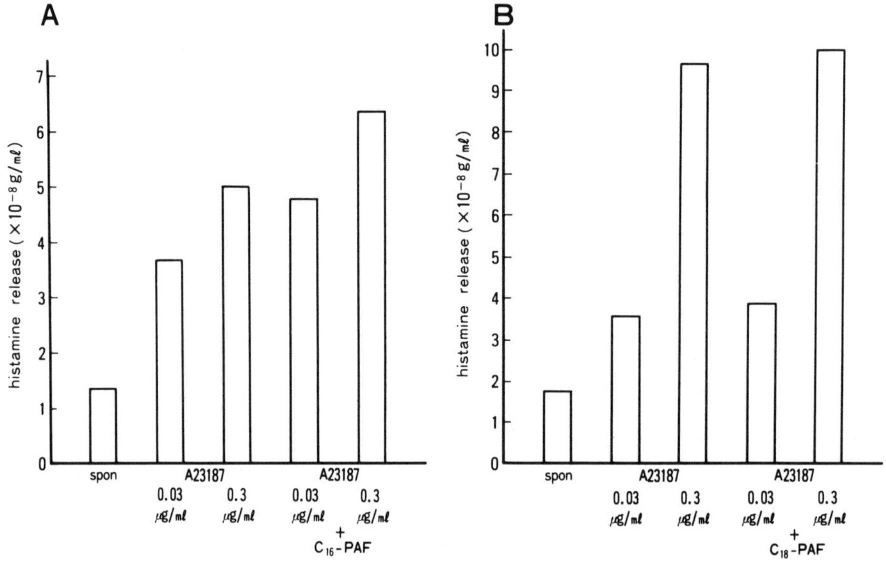

Fig.2.: Effect of PAF on calcium ionophore A23187-induced histamine release from rat mast cells. Calcium ionophore A23187 concentration was 0.03 and 0.3 ug/ml. A, C_{16}-PAF; B, C_{18}-PAF.

Results and discussion

When mast cells were incubated with anti-IgE for 15 min, the amount of histamine release was enhanced when PAF, especially C_{16}-PAF, was added to the incubation medium (Fig. 1). Also PAF, especially C_{16}-PAF, enhanced the histamine release from A23187 stimulated mast cells (Fig. 2). On the other hand the amount of histamine release from compound 48/80 stimulated mast cells was not enhanced by C_{16}-PAF (Fig. 3). Among the secretagogues which activate mast cells, anti-IgE requires extracellular calcium for its *action and calcium ionophore A23187 directly elevates intracellular calcium levels by carrying calcium across the cell membrane. Since compound 48/80 activates mast cells without extracellular calcium (5), PAF could enhance the histamine release from mast cells by increasing intracellular calcium levels. In fact, there is experimental evidence which suggests that PAF could exert its biological effects by increasing the permeability of membranes to calcium in platelets (10). The differences between* C_{16}*- and* C_{18}*-PAF effects on histamine release could be due to their biological activities.*

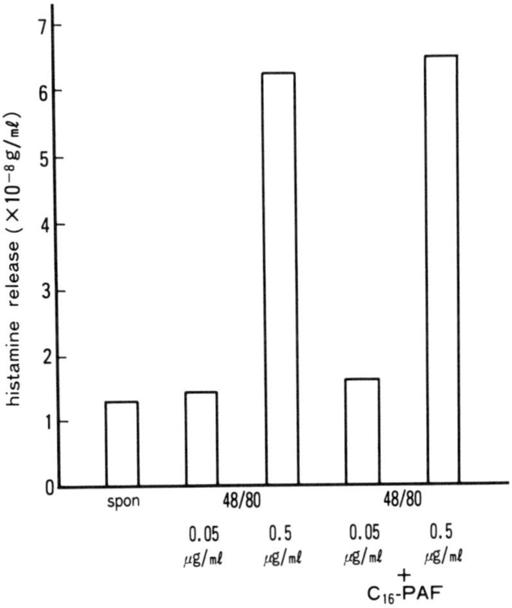

Fig.3.: Effect of C_{16}*-PAF on compound 48/80-induced histamine release from rat mast cells. Compound 48/80 concentrations was 0.05 and 0.5 ug/ml.*

When mast cells were stimulated by 0.3 ug/ml A23187, the amount of histamine release showed maximum at 1 min after the challenge with the elevation of protein kinase C activity (Fig. 4). To investigate the possible mechanism of PAF on mast cell activation, mast cells were incubated with 100 ng/ml PAF for 1 min and then incubated with 0.3 ug/ml A23187 for the additional 1 min and the amount of histamine release and protein kinase C activity were measured. As shown in figure 5, even the amount of histamine release was enhanced by C_{16}*-PAF. There were no significant changes of protein kinase C activities, indicating no possible involvement* *of protein kinase C activation as the mechanism of biological effects of PAF.*

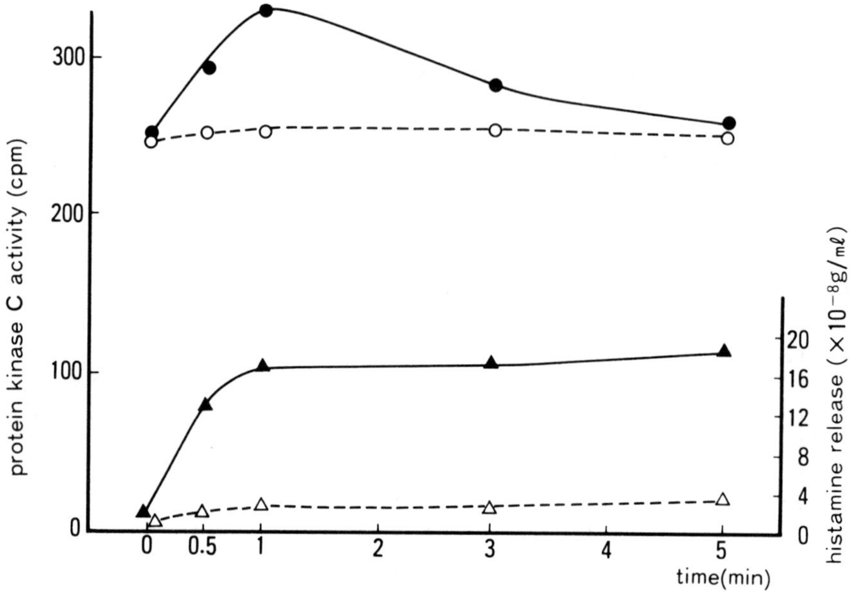

Fig.4.: Time courses of protein kinase C activity in and histamine release from rat mast cells after challenge with calcium ionophore A23187.
○ ,● :protein kinase C activity; △, ▲ :histamine release; —— : with challenge; - - - - : without challenge.

Rat mast cell granules were shown to contain a highly active PI kinase which catalyzes the formation of DPI from endogenous PI in the granule membrane (11). The enzyme was inhibited by adenosine, AMP, ADP and cyclic AMP (16), suggesting possible roles of DPI in granule secretion process from rat mast cells as energy charge regulation. When effects of phospholipids on the PI kinase were investigated, the enzyme activity was enhanced by exogenous PI and the rate of DPI synthesis was dependent on its concentration (100 pg/ml - 100 ng/ml). Phosphatidylcholine (PC) was less effective and phosphatidylethanolamine and PS were inactive on the enzyme stimulation.

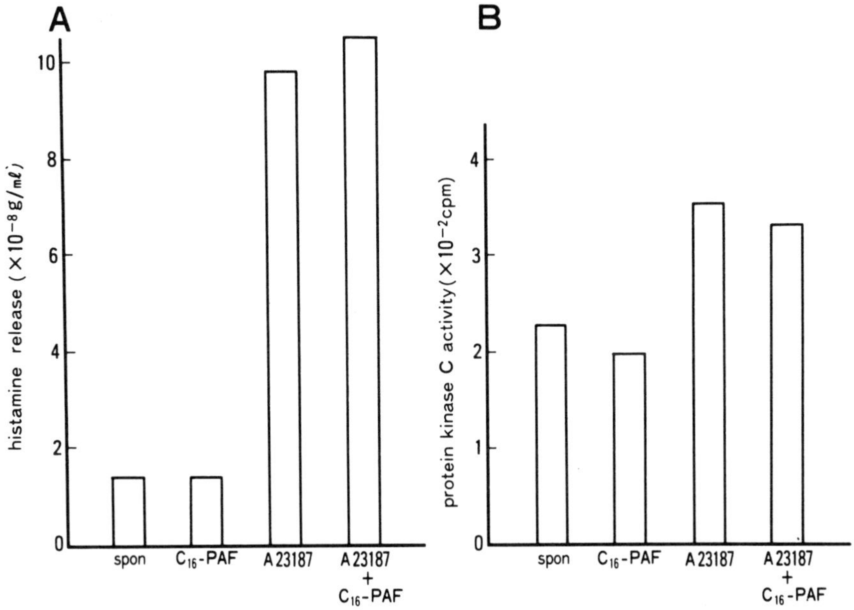

Fig.5.: Effect of C_{16}-PAF on calcium ionophore A32187-induced changes of protein kinase C activity in and histamine release from rat mast cells. A, histamine release; B, protein kinase C activity.

Interestingly PAF, especially C_{16}-PAF (100 pg/ml - 100 ng/ml) showed the tendency of enhancing the enzyme activity. In contrast to several other studies, the PI kinase in mast cell granules has been studied in situ within the granule membrane with membrane PI as the substrate. Because of the rapid ^{32}P incorporation into DPI, rat mast cell granules may contain abundant endogenous PI (11). This will explain why exogenous PI did not enhance the enzyme activity so dramatically as is usually seen in other tissues (17). The reason why PC enhanced the granule enzyme activity was unknown. The most likely explanation for this effect on the enzyme is activation of phospholipase A_2 producing PC breakdown, followed by PI resynthesis. In support of this possibility, absolute levels of diacylglycerol, one of the cleavage products of this enzyme, increase rapidly, followed by less rapid PI resynthesis after mast cells are stimulated (8,18). The significance of the effect of C_{16}-PAF on the enzyme *activity remains uncertain and the mechanisms of the effects of PAF on the granule enzyme is still obscure even the possible activation of phospholipase A_2 by PAF has been suggested (9).*

We have already reported that changes in polyphosphoinositide metabolism may be an intrinsic part of the biochemical mechanism that control mediator release from mast cells (19) and ^{32}P incorporation into DPI in mast cell supernatants as well as pellets was increased by stimulation (20). So, the PI kinase activity in mast cell granules can be modified by PAF even after the secretion.

Even though mast cells may be not the main cells which release PAF, these results mentioned above suggested the possible mast cell and PAF interaction in allergic reactions.

Reference

1. Chap, H., Mauco, G., Simon, M.F., Benveniste J. and Douste-Blazy, L. (1981) Biosynthetic labelling of platelet activating factor from radioactive acetate by stimulated platelets. Nature 289: 312-314.

2. Roubin, R., Mencia-Huerta, J.M., Landes, A. and Benveniste, J. (1982) Biosynthesis of platelet-activating factor (PAF-acether) IV. Impairment of acetyltransferase activity in thioglycolate-elicited mouse macrophages. J. Immunol. 129: 809-813.

3. Lee, T.C., Lenihan, D.J., Malone, B., Roddy, L.L. and Wassermann, S.I. (1984) Increased biosynthesis of platelet-activating factor in activated human eosinophils. J. Biol. Chem. 259: 5526-5530.

4. Mueller, H.W., O'Flaherty, J.T. and Wykle, R.L. (1983) Biosynthesis of platelet activating factor in rabbit polymorphonuclear neutrophils. J. Biol. Chem. 258: 6213-6218.

5. Henson, P.M. and Pinckard, R.N. (1977) Basophil-derived platelet-activating factor (PAF) as an in vivo mediator of acute allergic reactions: Demonstration of specific desensitization of platelets to PAF during IgE induced anaphylaxis in the rabbit. J. Immunol. 119: 2179-2184.

6. Camussi, G., Mencia-Huerta J.M. and Beneviste, J. (1977) Release of platelet-activating factor and histamine I. Effect of immune complexes, complement and neutrophils on human and rabbit mastocytes and basophils. Immunology 33: 523-534.

7. Mencia-Huerta, J.M. and Benveniste, J. (1979) Platelet-activating factor and macrophages I. Evidence for the release from rat and mouse peritoneal macrophages and not from mastocytes. Eur. J. Immunol. 9: 409-415.

8. *Kennerly, D.A., Sullivan, T.J., and Parker, C.W. (1979) Activation of phospholipid metabolism during mediator release from stimulated rat mast cells. J. Immunol. 122: 152 - 158.*

9. *Benveniste, J., Chignard, M., Le Couedic, J.P., and Vargaftig, B. (1982) Biosynthesis of platelet-activating factor (PAF-acether) II. Involvement of phospholipase A_2 in the formation of PAF-acether and lyso-PAF-acether from rabbit platelets. Thromb. Res. 25: 375 - 385.*

10. *Lee, T.C., Malone, B., Blank, M.L., and Snyder F. (1981) 1-alkyl-2-acetyl- sn - glycero-3-phosphocholine (platelet-activating factor) stimulates calcium influx in rabbit platelets. Biochem. Biophys. Res. Commun. 102: 1262 - 1268.*

11. *Kurosawa, M. and Parker, C.W. (1986) A phosphotidylinositol kinase in rat mast cell granules. J. Immunol 136: 616 - 622.*

12. *Enerback, L., and Svenson, I. (1980) Isolation of rat peritoneal mast cells by centrifugation on density of Percoll. J. Immunol. Methods 39: 135 - 145.*

13. *Kruger, P.G., Lagunoff, D., and Wan, H. (1980) Isolation of rat mastcell granules with intact membranes. Exp. Cell Res. 129: 83 - 93.*

14. *Shore, P., Burkhalter A., and Cohn Jr., V. (1959) A method for the fluorometric assay of histamine in tissues. J Pharmacol. Exp. Ther. 127: 182 - 186.*

15. *Baxter, J.H., and Adamik, R. (1978) Biochem. Pharmacol. 27: 497 - 508.*

16. *Tanaka, T., Aoki, S., Igarashi, Y., Ishizuka, T., and Kurosawa, M. (1986) Effect of adenine nucleotides and anti-allergic drugs on phosphatidylinositol (PI) kinase in rat mast cell granules. Japan. J. Pharmacol. (Suppl.) 40: 68P.*

17. *Collins, C.A., and Wells W.W. (1983) Identification of phosphatidylinositol kinase in rat liver lysosomal membranes. J. Biol. Chem. 258: 2130 - 2134.*

18. *Kennerly, D.A., Sullivan, T.J., Silwester, P. and Parker C.W. (1979) Diacylglycerol metabolism in mast cells; a potential role in membrane fusion and arachidonic acid release. J. Exptl. Med. 150: 1039 - 1044.*

19. *Kurosawa, M., Nemoto, T., Fueki, R., and Kobayashi, S. (1985) Studies of phosphorylation in rat mast cells (seventh report) - histamine release and metabolism of polyphosphoinositides. Japan. J. Allergy 34: 198 - 203.*

20. *Kurosawa, M. (1985) Studies of phosphorylation in rat mast cells (eighth report) - polyphosphoinositide (PPI) release from stimulated mast cells and localization of PPI response. Japan. J. Inflammation 5: 211 - 214.*

AAS 21:
PAF, Platelets, and Asthma

PAF AND AIRWAY HYPERREACTIVITY; PROSPECTS FOR NOVEL PROPHYLACTIC ANTI-ASTHMA DRUGS.

John Morley, Preclinical Research, Sandoz Ltd., 4002 Basel

AIRWAY HYPERREACTIVITY IN ASTHMA

It is generally accepted that airway hyperreactivity is characteristic of asthma, notwithstanding the occurrence of occasional patients with asthma who do not exhibit this phenomenon. However, airway hyperreactivity is not restricted to asthma and this phenomenon may be evident in other respiratory diseases such as bronchitis. In asthma patients, persisting airway hyperreactivity coexists with periods during which airway hyperreactivity is enhanced, as after an upper respiratory tract infection or following exposure to allergen in atopic patients. Such clinical evidence implies that the phenomenon of hyperreactivity is heterogeneous and that clinical hyperreactivity most probably represents an interaction between a number of distinct mechanisms. Nonetheless, it has been widely presumed that hyperreactivity in asthma is a single entity and much confusion stems from this false premise.

Study of the role of PAF in asthma has led to an emphasis of the importance of direct investigation of hyperreactivity and has led to the recognition of distinct and unrelated agencies of hyperreactivity (1). Furthermore, PAF formation has emerged as a plausible mechanism whereby acute changes of airway reactivity, as seen in association with infection or exposure to allergen, can be linked to persisting hyperreactivity of the type that characterises clinical asthma.

PAF AS AN INFLAMMATORY MEDIATOR

PAF was recognised as an allergic mediator with a prominent capacity to activate platelets (2). A possible role in asthma was intimated when it was shown that PAF was a potent stimulus to acute bronchospasm in guinea-pigs (3). However, evidence of spasmogenic activity cannot be considered of great significance, since diverse spasmogens are released in quantities sufficient to contract airway smooth muscle during an acute allergic reaction. This assessment can be supported by direct experimental evidence, for acute allergic bronchospasm of the guinea-pig is only diminished to a minor extent by selective PAF antagonists (4) which accords with the evidence that histamine and SRS-A have quantitatively greater significance as mediators of acute allergic bronchospasm in this species. It may be presumed that similar considerations apply to acute allergic responses in asthma, since these responses are diminished substantially by histamine (H1) antagonists (5) or by inhibitors of mast cell activation (6).

The first indication that PAF might be involved in hyperreactivity came as a result of studying the effects of intracutaneous injection of PAF. In the guinea pig, PAF produces intense, but transient, increased vascular permeability (7). This process is accompanied by an accumulation of platelets and neutrophils at the injection site (8), a phenomenon that is consistent with the potency of PAF as stimulus of platelet (9) and neutrophil (10) activation in vitro. Whilst these acute effects might reasonably have been anticipated, the protracted accumulation of inflammatory cells at the injection site was exceptional and distinguishes PAF from other autocoids (purines, amines, peptides, eicosanoids) released during allergic and other inflammatory reactions. In the guinea-pig, injection of PAF causes acute intravascular margination of platelets and neutrophils is succeeded by an emigration of both platelets and neutrophils into extravascular sites, so that by 4-8 hours there is a neutrophil-rich inflammatory reaction (8). At 24 hours, the inflammatory cell infiltrate is undiminished, although neutrophils become less prominent having been superceded by mononuclear cells, including substantial numbers of activated macrophages (8). The ability of PAF to effect sequential accumulation of neutrophils and mononuclear cells is impressive when compared with that of lymphokines (11) and must bring into question the presumption that lymphokines have an important role as chemattractants in vivo.

It seems likely that platelets have a crucial role in determining persisting cellular accumulation, since intracutaneous injection of PAF does not induce a persisting inflammatory reaction in the rat, a species whose platelets lack PAF receptors. In man, there is no direct evidence of platelet involvement during the inflammatory reaction to PAF; however, the clinical appearance of the skin reaction has a time course that is comparable with that which has been reported to follow intracutaneous injection of products of platelet activation in man (12). Biopsy at sites of intracutaneous injection of PAF reveals a neutrophil-rich inflammatory cell infiltrate at 4 hours and, at 32 hrs, a mixed cell infiltrate in which mononuclear cells are prominent (13). Consequently, it might be presumed that, in man as in the guinea-pig, PAF and platelets play a central role in determining persisting inflammation. This conclusion is strengthened by the recent report that intracutaneous injection of PAF causes a preferential accumulation of eosinophils in atopic but not normal subjects (14). Thus, intracutaneous injection of PAF induces a reaction that corresponds to an allergic response, both by clinical and histological criteria.

The capacity of PAF to elicit a late-onset reaction in human skin constituted an observation of major significance, since this was the first defined allergic mediator to reveal such a property. Furthermore, an analogous effect was evident in lung of the rabbit, for intratracheal instillation of PAF could be shown to cause airway obstruction of delayed onset, that was susceptible to inhibition by DSCG (15). This circumstantial evidence was considered decisive and led to proposal of PAF as the primary agency of increased airway reactivity in allergic and other forms of asthma exacerbation (16).

PAF AND AIRWAY HYPERREACTIVITY

Clinical investigations have established an association between inflammation of the airways such as the late onset reaction to allergen or upper respiratory tract infection and the occurrence of increased airway reactivity. The ability of cromoglycate to abrogate sustained inflammation as well as the acute bronchospasm of an allergic reaction had led to the propsal that mast cell activation was central to asthma and by implication the primary determinant of increased airway reactivity. However, neither mast cell activation nor application of products of mast cell activation suffice to induce late-onset reactions or to induce airway hyperreactivity. Two possibilities emerge: either the changes of airway hyperreactivity that follow allergen inhalation are not due to the release of one or more autocoids, but rather reflect a reduction of airway dimensions following oedema and occlusion of the lumen by mucus; alternatively, an allergic mediator, originating in cell types other than mast cells, must determine increased airway reactivity.

The recent recognition that cells such as eosinophils or macrophages (17) could be activated by IgE-dependent processes and release appreciable quantities of PAF (18) favors the latter possibility, provided that it can be established that PAF has the capacity to induce airway hyperreactivity. In the guinea-pig, acute exposure to a single dose of PAF induces pronounced bronchoconstriction without effecting appreciable hyperreactivity. However, study of acute responses to PAF gave the first indication that hyperreactivity does develop in response to PAF, since repeated intravenous injection of PAF evidences consistent bronchoconstrictor responses. Reproducibility of the response of airway to PAF (which is platelet dependent) is in marked contrast with the tachyphylaxis that is evident when platelets aggregate in response to repeated intravenous injection of PAF. The paradox can be accommodated by considering that the consistent bronchoconstrictor response to bolus infection of PAF represents a diminished constrictor reaction to PAF whose tachyphylaxis has been offset by increased airway reactivity. In that event, it follows that repeated injection or infusion of PAF must induce non-selective airway hyperreactivity. This phenomenon can be demonstrated in the guinea-pig by repeated injection of PAF, by intravenous infusion of PAF, or by inhalation of PAF as an aerosol (19). A noticeable feature of the hyperreactivity that follows exposure to PAF is the protracted nature of such changed lung function. This is most clearly evidenced in man, for inhalation of PAF on a single occasion induces hyperreactivity that can remain evident 4 weeks after exposure (20).

The mechanism that underlies altered hyperreactivity is not known. In the guinea-pig, the phenomenon is dependent upon platelets since expression of acute increased hyperreactivity is wholly prevented by destruction of circulating platelets by lytic antiserum, whereas destruction of neutrophils appears inconsequential. It is possible that platelets rapidly modify the function of airway smooth muscle by release of an intermediary substance during PAF-induced bronchospasm but that more protracted changes of airway reactivity may depend upon platelet migration into airway tissue to influence smooth muscle growth by release of mitogens. The relationship of these events to eosinophil accumulation remains unresolved.

PROPHYLACTIC DRUGS IN ASTHMA THERAPY

Generation of PAF in lung tissue offers the first credible mechanism whereby an allergic mediator might effect long-lasting inflammatory reactions together with associated airway hyperreactivity in pulmonary tissue. Release of PAF could effect cumulative pathology of the type depicted by Cockcroft (21), and provide a rationale for allergen avoidance as a therapeutic approach in asthma. Avoidance of allergen, and hence avoidance of successive periods of PAF formation, is a logical approach but may be impracticable when allergens are ubiquitous, as in certain occupational or domestic environments. Moreover, the benefit of protracted periods of allergen avoidance can be nullified by intermittent accidental exposure, which remains a constant hazard. Consequently, there is a need to supplement allergen avoidance by the use of drugs which prevent the adverse effects of allergen exposure.

PHARMACOLOGY OF PROPHYLAXIS

The testing of drugs that might exhibit properties appropriate to asthma prophylaxis has been limited by the absence of a convenient animal model which exhibits hyperreactivity following allergen exposure. Consequently, the identification of PAF as an allergic mediator capable of inducing hyperreactivity comparable with that evoked in asthma patients by allergen, offers an opportunity to evaluate novel prophylactic drugs by a test that closely corresponds to clinical provocation by allergen. If this test is to be predictive, those drugs which are known to be effective in asthma prophylaxis might be expected to inhibit development of PAF-induced hyperreactivity, whereas drugs which have proved ineffectual in asthma should not influence development of altered lung function formation.

In the guinea-pig, infusion of PAF causes hyperreactivity, with an intensity that is related to the dose of PAF employed. 600 ng/kg over 1 hour represents a near maximal dose of PAF that consistently produces an enhanced response of the airway and hence is suitable for detecting inhibitory effects (22). This preparation has been used to test a wide range of compounds, whose effects can be grouped into three distinct categories.

a) <u>Inhibitory</u> Established prophylactic anti-asthma drugs (cromoglycate, theophylline, glucocorticosteroids and ketotifen) will markedly suppress the induction of hyperreactivity, when given by intravenous infusion coincidentaly with an infusion of PAF. Pronounced inhibition may also be achieved by compounds that have been designated as selective PAF antagonists (e.g. CV 9288, L-652-731 Kadsurenone, ginkgolide B, SRI 63-441)

b) <u>Ineffective</u> The known prophylactic anti-asthma drugs exhibit other pronounced pharmacological actions, including amine antagonism, SRS-A antagonism, mast cell stabilisation, inhibition of arachidonate metabolism and relaxation of airway smooth muscle. However, when compounds were selected by reference to such properties, it became evident that none of these activities could account for inhibition of the response to PAF by anti-asthma drugs. Thus, PAF-induced hyperreactivity was not inhibited by histamine (H1) antagonists (mepyramine, clemastine, azelastine, astemizole or oxatomide); nor by serotonin antagonists (methysergide, ketanserin and ICS 205-930); nor SRS-A antagonists (FPL 55712, azelastine, amaxanox); nor mast cell stabilising agents (tranilast, zaprinast, AA 861, azelastine, oxatomide); nor by lipoxygenase inhibitors (QA 208-199, AA 861). Some inhibition was observed when using the mast cell stabilising agent lodoxamide tromethamine, but this may be discounted because pronounced cardiovascular affects follow intravenous administration. It has recently been reported that OKY-046 and FCE-22178 have an inhibitory effect on PAF-induced hyperreactivity which has been attributed to thromboxane synthetase inhibition (23,24). The presumption that these drugs lack PAF antagonism should be investigated rather than disregarded.

c) <u>Additive</u> Of the compounds so far tested, three categories have augmented the hyperreactivity response to PAF. Indomethacin causes an enhancement of the response, but this property of indomethacin is evident to a similar extent with other spasmogens. Consequently, the augmented response should be regarded not as a modification of the response to PAF, *but rather as an interaction with an unrelated form of airway sensitisation. This interpretation is with earlier studies of indomethacin and airway hyperreactivity (25). More unexpected has been the observation that (±) isoprenaline consistently enhanced the hyperreactivity that follows exposure to PAF (26), despite inhibiting the acute bronchoconstrictor action of PAF. This has led us to examine the effect of (±) isoprenaline in the absence of PAF. It is now apparent that (±) isoprenaline per se will induce hyperreactivity and that the enhanced response to PAF represents an additive effect between these two independent mechanisms (1). This prompted us to examine (±) propranolol, which as could be anticipated also enhanced the response to PAF, since it is well known that beta-adrenoceptor antagonists enhance constrictor responses of the guinea-pig airway (27). It is possible that the effect of bet-adrenoceptor on the airway is due to a mechanism that is identical with, or closely related to, that responsible for the induction of hyperreactivitiy by (±) isoprenaline.*

CONCLUSION

The evidence that implicates PAF and hence platelet activation in asthma pathology is now substantial. PAF has a number of properties appropriate to asthma and amongst the putative mediators of asthma PAF is unique in causing substantial eosinophil and platelet accumulation within airways together with persisting airway hyperreactivity. Existing prophylactic anti-asthma drugs inhibit such consequences of PAF exposure, hence it would seem prudent to establish this type of property as an obligatory component when selecting novel prophylactic anti-asthma drugs.

REFERENCES

1. Morley, J., Sanjar, S. and Mazzoni, L. Evidence of distinct mechanism of airway hyperreactivity by isoprenaline and platelet activating factor (PAF) in the guinea-pig. (Submitted).

2. Benveniste, J., Henson, P.M. and Cochrane, C.G. (1972) Leucocyte dependent histamine release from rabbit platelets: The role of IgE, basophil and a platelet activating factor. J. Exptl. Med. 136:1356-1377.

3. Vargaftig, B.B., Lefort, J., Chingard, M. and Benveniste, J. (1980) Platelet-activating factor induces a platelet dependent

bronchoconstriction unrelated to the formation of prostaglandin derivatives. Europ J Pharmacol 65:185-192

4. *Morley, J., Sanjar, S. and Doran, J. The role of arachidonate metabolites in the response of giunea-pig airways to platelet activating factor (PAF). Agents and Actions (Supplement). (In press).*

5. *Holgate, S.T., Emanuel, M.B. and Howarth, P.H.(1985) Astemizole and other (H1) antihistaminic drug treatment of asthma. J Allergy Clin Immunol 76:375.*

6. *Stokes, T.C., and Morley, J. (1981) Prospects for an oral Intal. Brit J Dis Chest 75:1-14.*

7. *Morley, J., Page, C.P. and Paul, W.(1983) Inflammatory actions of platelet activating factor (PAF-acether) in guinea-pig skin. Brit J Pharmacol 80:503-509.*

8. *Dewar, A., Archer, C.B., Paul, W., Page, C.P., MacDonald, D.M. and Morley, J. (1984) Cutaneous and pulmonary histopathological responses to platelet activating factor (PAF-acether) in the guinea-pig. J Path 144: 24-24.*

9. *Schneider, M.W. and Drazen, J.M. (1980) Comparitive in vitro effects of arachidonate acid metabolites on tracheal strips and parenchymal strips. Am Rev Respir Dis 121:835.*

10. *O'Flaherty, J.T., Wykle, R.L., Miller, C.H., Lewis, J.C., Waite, M., Bass, D.A., McCall, C.E. and De Chatelet, L.R. (1981) 1-O-alkyl-2 -acetyl- sn -glyceryl-3-phosphorylcholines: A novel class of neutrophil stimulants. Am J Path 103:70-79.*

11. *Franco, M.F., Kelly, R.H. and Morley, J. (1978) A comparison of the hematogenous cell infiltrate evoked by lymphokine injection with that of delayed hypersensitivity reactions. Am J Path 93:117-130*

12. *Dolovich, J., Hargreave, F.E., Chalmers, R., Shier, K.J., Gauldie, J. and Bienenstock, J. (1973) Late cutaneous allergic response in isolated IgE-dependent reactions. J Allergy Clin Immunol 52:38-46*

13. *Archer, C.B., Page, C.P., Morley, J. and MacDonald, D.M. (1985) Accumulation of inflammatory cells in response to intracutaneous platelet activating factor (PAF-acether) in man. Brit J Dermatol 112:285-290*

14. *Henocq, E. and Vargaftig, B.B. (1986) Accumulation of eosinophils in response to intracutaneous PAF-aceth er and allergens in man. Lancet i:1378-1379.*

15. *Page, C.P., Tomiak, R.H.H., Sanjar, S. and Morley, J. (1985) Suppression of PAF-acether responses: an anti-inflammatory effect of anti-asthma drugs. Agents and Actions 16:33-345.*

16. *Morley, J., Page, C.P. and Sanjar, S. (1985) Platelets in asthma.*

Lancet ii:726-727.

17. *Capron, A., Dessaint, J.P., Capron, M., Joseph, M., Ameisen, J.C. and Tonnel, A.B. (1986) From parasites to allergy: a second receptor for IgE. Immunology Today 7:15-18.*

18. *Snyder, F. (1985) Chemical and biochemical aspects of platelet activating factor: A novel class of acetylated ether-linked choline phospholipids. Med Res Rev 5:107-140.*

19. *Mazzoni, L., Morley, J., Page, C.P. and Sanjar, S. (1985) Induction of hyperreactivity by platelet activating factor in the guinea-pig. J Physiology 365:107P.*

20. *Cuss, F.M., Dixon, C.M.S. and Barnes, P.J. (1986) Effects of inhaled platelet activating factor on pulmonary function and bronchial responsiveness in man. Lancet ii:189-192.*

21. *Cockcroft, D.W. (1983) Mechanism of perennial allergic asthma. Lancet ii:253-255.*

22. *Morley, J., Page, C.P., Mazzoni, L. and Sanjar, S. (1985) Anti-allergic drugs in asthma. Triangle 24:59-70.*

23. *Giorgetti, C., Cadelli, G.C., Baroldi, P. and Fabbri, L.M. A thromoboxane-synthetase inhibitor reduces airway hyperresponsiveness induced by platelet activating factor (PAF-acether) in guinea-pigs. Agents and Actions (Supplement). (In press).*

24. *Chung, K.F., Aizawa, H., Becker, A.B., Frick, O., Gold, W.M. and Nadel, J.A. (1986) Inhibition of antigen-induced airway hyperresponsiveness by a thromboxane synthetase inhibitor (OKY-046) in allergic dogs. Am Rev Respir Dis 134:258-261.*

25. *Garland, L.G.(1984) The pharmacology of airway hyperreactivity. Trends in Pharmacological Science 338-340.*

26. *Mazzoni, L., Morley, J., Page, C.P. and Sanjar, S. (1985) Prophylactic anti-asthma drugs impair the airway hyperreactivity that follows exposure to platelet activating factor (PAF). Brit J Pharmacol 86:571P.*

27. *Omini, C., Folco, G.C., Vigano, T., Rossoni, G., Brunelli, G. and Berti, F. (1981) Leukotriene C4 induces generation of PGI2 and TXA2 in guinea-pig in vivo. Pharmacol Res Comm 13:633-640.*

THE ROLE OF PAF-ACETHER IN ANAPHYLAXIS DEMONSTRATED WITH THE USE OF THE ANTAGONIST BN 52021

Pierre Braquet, Philippe Guinot and Caroline Touvay
I.H.B. Research Labs, 17 avenue Descartes, F-92350 Le Plessis Robinson (France)

INTRODUCTION

Released by various immune and chemical stimuli from inflammatory cells (basophils, neutrophils, eosinophils, macrophages, platelets) as well as from vascular endothelium, Platelet Activating Factor (PAF-acether) is a potential mediator of anaphylaxis and inflammatory reactions *(Benveniste et al., 1972)*. PAF-acether increases vascular permeability and causes sustained hypotension and thrombosis *(reviewed in Braquet et al., 1986a ; Vargaftig and Braquet, 1986)*. It may also participate in various hypersensitivity reactions including bronchial asthma which cannot be fully accounted for by the known inflammatory mediators, including peptido-leukotrienes *(reviewed in Vargaftig et al., 1985)*.

PAF-acether involvement in airway hypersensitivity is suggested by different lines of evidence :

(i) cyclooxygenase and anti-histamine-independent bronchoconstriction follows human or animal exposure to PAF-acether or to antigen ;

(ii) aerosolized PAF-acether causes platelet-independent bronchoconstriction in the guinea-pig *(Lefort et al., 1984)*. Guinea-pigs which are desensitized to bronchoconstriction following the intra-pulmonary aerosolization of PAF-acether retain their responsiveness to intravenous injections *(Lefort et al., 1984)*, indicating that different cells are involved when the two routes are used, platelets on the one hand and a component of the alveolar lining, on the other. This component may be the alveolar macrophages which can be activated by PAF-acether *(Maridonneau-Parini et al., 1985)* and can release lyso-PAF-acether itself when exposed to specific antigen *(Arnoux et al., 1980)*. Parente and Flower (1985) demonstrated that hydrocortisone and its mediator protein, lipocortin, inhibit the formation of lyso-PAF by zymosan-stimulated macrophages and by antigen-stimulated guinea-pig lungs, and it is possible that anti-allergic glucocorticosteroids may act by inhibiting direct or indirect macrophage activation in which PAF-acether is involved.

(iii) the late reaction of asthma, characterized by bronchial hyper-responsiveness and by the migration of inflammatory cells into the lungs can be duplicated by PAF-acether administration (see below).

(iv) guinea-pigs desensitized to aerosolized antigen maintain their responsiveness to aerosol, whereas guinea-pigs desensitized to PAF-acether do not respond to aerosolized antigen, even though the systemic response persists *(Lefort et al,. 1984)*.

(v) PAF-acether is released during systemic anaphylaxis in the rabbit *(Kravis and Henson, 1975)* and antigen-challenged perfused guinea-pig lungs release its lyso precursor and/or catabolite *(Rotilio et al., 1983 ; Fitzgerald et al., 1986)*.

Intensive research for specific PAF-acether receptor antagonists was therefore undertaken in the mid 80's in order to assess the exact role of this mediator in hypersensitivity reactions and with the aim to develop new drugs of potential therapeutical implications *(reviewed in Braquet and Godfroid, 1986)*.

In this regard a new compound, BN 52021 (Gingkolide B ; Fig 1), isolated and purified from a crude *Gingko biloba* extract has been shown to display a potent and specific inhibition of the binding of [^{3}H] PAF-acether to its receptor in rabbit platelets (Ki $\simeq$ 1.2 X 10^{-7} M ; *Braquet 1984 ; reviewed in Braquet et al., 1986b)*.

This phenomenon also characterized by Page et al. (1982), using radio-labelled platelets, is specific to PAF-acether and antigen ; thus, bronchoconstriction induced by another cell-stimulating agent, the tripeptide f-met-leu-phe, is not inhibited by BN 52021 and is also accompagnied by pulmonary leukocyte accumulation, whereas platelets are only marginally accumulated, in contrast to radio-labelled leukocytes *(Boukili et al., 1985)*. In contrast, BN 52021 antagonizes both platelet accumulation and contraction of pulmonary microvessels induced by PAF-acether. This may account for the anti-anaphylactic effect of BN 52021 (see below) since pulmonary recruitment of platelets, particularly to the extravascular compartment where they are lodged in apposition to bronchial smooth muscle, was described for PAF-acether *(Lellouch-Tubiana et al., 1985)* and antigen *(Lellouch-Tubiana et al., 1986)*. This may also suggest the prophylactic value of the treatment by BN 52021 since platelet may be implicated in smooth muscle hyperplasia by releasing smooth muscle mitogens, such as platelet-derived growth factor *(PDGF, Ross and Vogel, 1978)* : accordingly, the observation of PAF-acether-induced platelet accumulation in close proximity to the bronchial muscle may have important implications for the pathogenesis of bronchial smooth muscle hyperplasia observed in asthma.

Eosinophil infiltration is a major feature of asthma and allergic reactions *(De Monchy et al., 1985)*. Eosinophils are not frequent during the acute phase response, but increase in number, to account for 10→80% of the total cell infiltrate during the late phase. Furthermore, released granules are found in lung from asthmatic patients, and may participate in bronchial hyperreactivity *(Gleich et al., 1976)*. These granules contain Major Basic Protein (MBP) which, together with other toxic materials, is found in the sputum of asthmatics. MBP is said to induce destructive changes similar to those found in chronic asthma *(Filley et al., 1982)*.

Since PAF-acether appears to be a potent activator of eosinophil functions (Fig 6), BN 52021 as an antagonist may interfere with the late phase response. Indeed :

(a) Systemic PAF-acether injections induce hemoconcentration and increased total leukocyte counts ; the underlying eosinophil and monocyte subsets are decreased by up to a third, which is suppressed by BN 52021 (table 3 ; *Etienne and Braquet, unpublished)*.

(b) PAF-acether is one of the most potent chemotactic agents for human eosinophils *(Wardlaw and Kay, 1986)*. This effect is receptor-mediated and BN 52021 dose-dependently inhibits eosinophil locomotion *(Wardlaw and Kay, 1986 ; Braquet and Vargaftig, 1987)*.

(c) Eosinophils from patients with eosinophilia, including asthmatics, have an increased capacity to release PAF-acether, as compared to those from normal individuals *(Lee et al., 1984)*. Intracutaneous injections of PAF-acether cause a marked eosinophilic infiltration exclusively in allergic patients, a large number of these cells being degranulated *(Henocq and Vargaftig, 1986)*. In addition, PAF-acether induces LTC_4 formation by human eosinophils ; this phenomenon is increased in patients with parasite infestations *(Borgeat et al., 1984)*. BN 52021 antagonizes both LTC_4 and 5-HETE production in PAF-acether and zymosan-stimulated eosinophils (table 4 ; *Bruynzell et al., 1986 ; Braquet and Vargaftig, 1986*).

(d) PAF-acether induces $O_2^{\bullet -}$ production and chemoluminescence in various cell systems. BN 52021 selectively inhibits this effect in human eosinophils (table 5 ; *Bruynzeel et al., 1986 ; Koenderman and Bruynzeel, 1986*), human and rabbit neutrophils (table 5 ; *Braquet, 1984 ; Hoshikawa-Fujimura et al., 1986 ; Baggiolini and Dewald, 1986*) and guinea-pig macrophages *(Desquand et al., 1986)*. BN 52021 also significantly inhibits aggregation and degranulation of isolated human neutrophils stimulated by PAF-acether *(Braquet et al., 1984)*. BN 52021 also inhibits the PAF-acether induced adherence of human leukocytes in various systems *(Fink et al., 1986 ; Jacob et al., 1986)*.

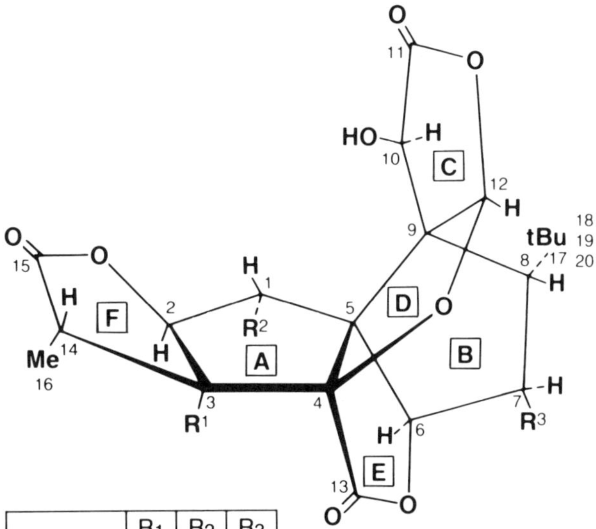

	R_1	R_2	R_3
BN 52021	OH	OH	H

Fig 1 : Chemical structure of BN 52021 (Ginkgolide B)

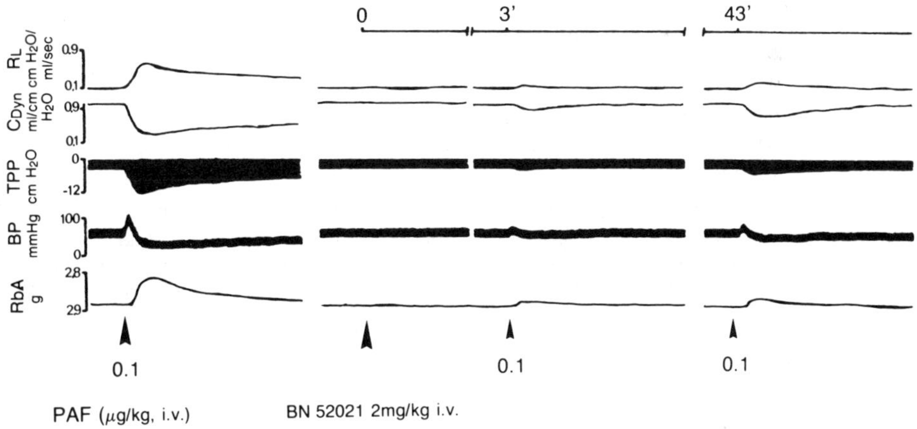

Blood (extracorporal circulation) superfuses a strip of rabbit aorta (Rba) to monitor TXA_2-like activity

Fig 2 : Effect of PAF-acether on lung resistance (R_L), dynamic compliance (C_{DYN}), transpulmonary pressure (TPP) and arterial blood pressure (BP) in anaesthetized guinea-pigs. Effect of BN 52021 *(from Berti et al., 1986).*

BN 52021 specifically inhibits human *(Braquet, 1984 ; Nunez et al., 1986 ; Küster et al., 1986)* and rabbit *(Braquet et al., 1985a)* platelet aggregation and the related events *(Lachachi et al., 1985 ; Baroggi et al., 1986 ; Simon et al., 1986)*. It antagonizes the renal *(Hebert et al., 1986 ; Plante et al., 1986)*, cerebral *(Plotkine et al., 1986)* and the cardiovascular *(Baranes et al., 1986 ; Thievant et al., 1986)* impairments due to PAF-acether in various models. BN 52021 also inhibits PAF-acether-induced tissue-type plasminogen activator release *(Fernandez Gallardo et al., in preparation ; Emeis, 1987)* and ion transport impairments in macrophages *(Garay and Braquet, 1986)* or in guinea-pig ventricle muscle fibers *(Delgado and Tamargo, 1986)*. Finally BN 52021 blocks specifically rat paw oedema induced by PAF-acether *(Cordeiro et al., 1986a ; 1986b)*.

BN 52021 is also effective in complex immune disorders : (i) it inhibits the lethality *(Etienne et al., 1986)*, the hemodynamic changes *(Adnot et al., 1986)* and the gastric ulcerations *(Wallace et al., 1986 ; Clostre et al., in preparation)* induced by endotoxin ; (ii) it prolongs graft survival in rats *(Foegh et al., 1985 ; 1986)* ; (iii) it antagonizes lethality induced by mycotoxins *(Feuerstein et al., 1986)* ; (iv) it inhibits IgG aggregate-induced shock in rats *(Sanchez Crespo et al., 1985)* and the related appearance, in plasma of lysosomial enzymes *(Fernandez Gallardo et al., in preparation)* ; (v) it significantly reduces in rats proteinuria induced by both immune challenge (anti-GBM nephritis) and adriamycin (anthracyclin-induced nephropathy *(Ortiz et al., 1986)*. In the latter model, ginkgolide B also abolishes lethality induced by adriamycin ; (vi) it blocks the hemodynamic changes of experimental cirrhosis in rats *(Villamediana et al., 1986)* ; (vii) it protects the rat intestinal mucosa against ischaemic damage *(Tagesson, pers. com.)*.

BN 52021 is also a potent inhibitor of PAF-acether effects in man : it dose-dependently antagonizes both wheal and flare (Guinot et al., 1986 ; Barnes et al., 1986) and *ex vivo* platelet aggregation (Barnes et al., 1986) induced by the autacoid.

In this paper the effects of BN 52021 on lung anaphylaxis and airway hyperresponsiveness are reviewed.

1. INHIBITION OF PAF-ACETHER-INDUCED PULMONARY IMPAIRMENTS BY BN 52021

The i.v. administration of PAF-acether to guinea-pigs induces a dose-dependent fall in systemic blood pressure and heart rate associated with an increase in lung resistance (R_L) and marked decrease in dynamic compliance (C_{DYN}) which indicates bronchoconstriction of the more peripheral airways (Fig 2). This is also accompanied by an increase in non specific bronchial responsiveness both in animals and in humans, a property not exhibited by other pro-inflammatory mediators *(Patterson et al., 1983 ; Cuss et al., 1986)*. The severity of bronchoconstriction also correlates with the modification of the values of blood lactate, pH, p CO_2 and p O_2 (Fig 3).

BN 52021 given i.v. (0.5 $\rightarrow$ 2 mg/kg) or orally (5 $\rightarrow$ 15 mg/kg) dose-dependently antagonizes both (i) the cardiovascular and pulmonary changes (table 1) and (ii) the increase in bronchial responsiveness induced by PAF-acether *(Braquet, 1984 ; Braquet et al., 1985b ; Touvay et al., 1985 ; 1986a ; Desquand et al., 1986 : Berti et al., 1986 ; Vilain et al., 1986)* : e.g. BN 52021 administered at the dose of 2 mg/kg i.v. prevents almost completely the lowering of blood pressure and heart rate, and the bronchoconstrictive effect of PAF-acether (Figs 2 & 3). It also dose-dependently prevents thrombopenia, leucopenia and the increase in circulating thromboxane (at a dose of 2 mg/kg i.v., it keeps this parameter in normal range). The antagonistic activity of BN 52021 seems to be long lasting since bronchoconstriction is still markedly inhibited after 40 min *(Berti et al., 1986)*.

In an interesting study Arnoux and Gillis (1986) studied the effects of BN 52021 against PAF-acether-induced vasoconstriction and bronchoconstriction in isolated rabbit lung. Given 60 sec before challenge, ginkgolide B like SRI 63-072 [another PAF-acether antagonist derived from

table 1 : Effects of BN 52021 on PAF-acether-induced bronchoconstriction in guinea-pigs

PAF-acether (dose, route)			BN 52021			Reference
			route	dose	inhibition	
33	ng / kg	i.v.	i.v.	3 mg / kg	– 100 %	*Desquand et al., 1986*
60	ng / kg	i.v.	i.v.	1 mg / kg	– 89 %	*Braquet et al., 1985b*
100	ng / kg	i.v.	i.v.	1 mg / kg	– 67 %	*Touvay et al., 1986a*
45 - 100	ng / kg	i.v.	oral	2 mg / kg	– 59 %	*Touvay et al., 1986c*
100	ng / kg	i.v.	i.v.	1 mg / kg	– 62 %	*Berti et al., 1986*
100	ng / kg	i.v.	i.v.	2 mg / kg	– 94 %	
300 μg/ml for 2 min., aerosol			i.v.	3 mg / kg	– 91 %	*Desquand et al., 1986*

table 2 : Antagonistic activity of BN 52021 against PAF-acether-induced contraction in lung parenchymal strip (PS), spirally cut large bronchus (BS) and main pulmonary artery (PAS) *(from Berti et al., 1986).*

TISSUES	TREATMENT	CONTRACTION (mm)	
		M ± SEM	% inhib.
PS	PAF (100 ng)	27.3 ± 6.3	—
	BN 52021 (1.2 μg/ml) + PAF-acether	6.4 ± 2.3	77**
BS	PAF (100 ng)	14.1 ± 2.3	—
	BN 52021 (1.2 μg/ml) + PAF-acether	4.0 ± 1.4	69**
PAS	PAF (100 ng)	38.0 ± 8.9	
	BN 52021 (1.2 μg/ml) + PAF-acether	8.3 ± 4.4	79*

The figures represent the mean values (M) ± standard error of the mean (SEM) of at least 5 experiments. ** $p<0.01$; * $p<0.05$ as compared to the agonist effect.

table 3 : Effect of BN 52021 on PAF-acether (1μg / kg, i.v. ; single dose) -induced changes of white cell subsets in the rat*

Cells	BN 52021 (mg / kg,po)	% change
Neutrophils	—	– 10.0
	5	– 2.2
Eosinophils	—	– 33.3
	5	– 6.7
Monocytes	—	– 44.0
	5	– 8.1
Lymphocytes	—	+ 15.0
	5	+ 1.3

* 15 min after the challenge ; BN 52021 is given 30 min before PAF-acether

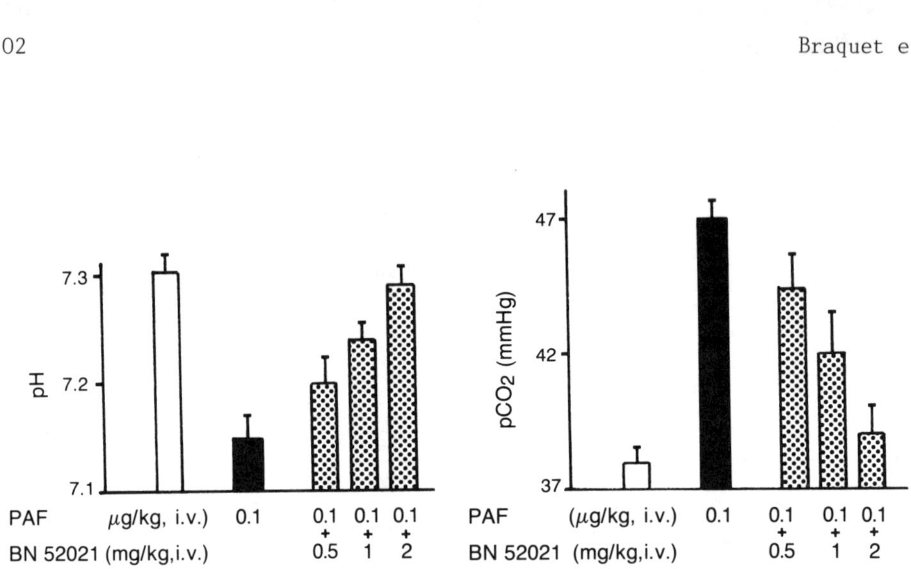

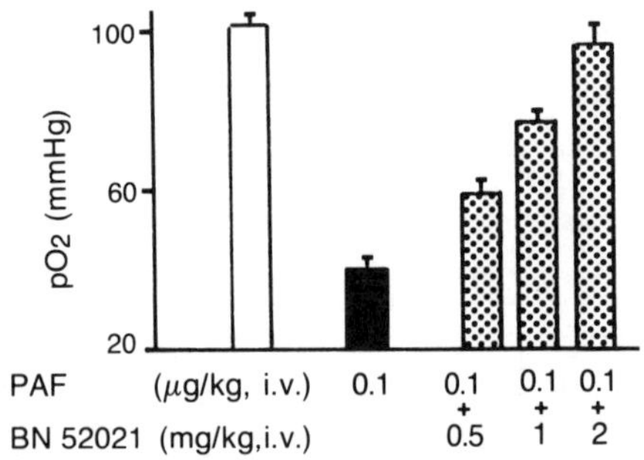

Vertical bars = standard error of the mean of the least 5 experiments

Open columns = control

Fig 3 :

Modification of blood pH, pO_2 and pCO_2 during bronchoconstriction (peak effect) induced by PAF-acether (0.1µg/kg, i.v.) in anaesthetized guinea-pigs and their prevention by graded doses of BN 52021 *(from Berti et al., 1986).*

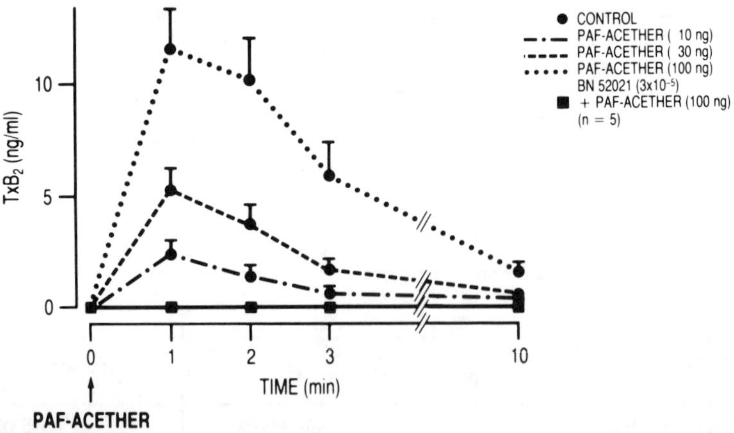

Fig 4 : Inhibition by BN 52021 of the PAF-acether-induced release of thromboxane from the guinea-pig perfused lung *(from Desquand et al., 1986).*

the mediator framework, *(Winslow et al., 1985)*], totally blocks the deleterious effects of PAF-acether. In contrast, when given simultaneously with PAF-acether, only BN 52021 prevents the vasoconstriction and the bronchoconstriction of the isolated lung suggesting that the affinity of ginkgolide B for lung PAF-acether receptors is higher than that of SRI 63-072. Given curatively 40 sec after the challenge, BN 52021 significantly reverses the effects of PAF-acether. Conversely only a slight improvement is observed when the antagonist is given 90 sec after PAF-acether.

These data suggest that BN 52021 can reverse the effects of PAF-acether if the subsequent events underlying the cellular effects of the mediator have not yet developped.

Aerosolized PAF-acether also induces bronchoconstriction *(Lefort et al., 1984)*. Here again BN 52021 blocks this phenomenon provided doses of above 3 mg/kg were used (table 1; *Desquand et al., 1986)*.

BN 52021 also blocks bronchoconstriction and thrombopenia induced by various PAF-acether analogs where the polar head is replaced by isosteric groups e.g. morpholinium, piperidinium etc ... *(Coeffier et al., 1986)*. This inhibition is correlated with the blockade by BN 52021, of aggregation and hypotension induced by the various agonists.

The antagonist activity observed with BN 52021 seems to be rather specific against PAF-acether since ginkgolide B does not affect in a significant way the bronchoconstriction and the lowering of the systemic blood pressure caused by acetylcholine, the tripeptide f-met-leu-phe, serotonin, histamine, collagen, arachidonic acid and LTC_4 *(Berti et al., 1986 ; Desquand et al., 1986)*.

In isolated perfused lungs, PAF-acether activates the arachidonic cascade with a dose-dependent and pronounced generation of thromboxane (Fig 4), suggesting that the lungs stimulated by PAF-acether participate in generating lipidic substance which are detrimental for the cardiovascular and respiratory functions. BN 52021 suppresses the PAF-acether-induced generation of thromboxane (Fig 4) without affecting the conversion of arachidonic acid *(Berti et al., 1986 ; Desquand et al., 1986)*. Therefore BN 52021 does not seem to interfere with cyclooxygenase but may act at an early step involving PAF-acether receptors and phospholipase activation.

Since a variety of effects of PAF-acether in guinea-pigs are platelet-dependent, it is reasonable to presume that the protecting activity of BN 52021 may be primarily ascribed to a prevention of platelet activation and suppression of thromboxane and other eicosanoid generation. However a direct activation of bronchial and vascular smooth muscles cannot be ruled out : PAF-acether induces contraction of guinea-pig lung parenchymal strips ; BN 52021 inhibits the response to the autacoid in a dose-dependent manner *(Touvay et al., 1986a, 1986b ; Desquand et al., 1986)*. This effect is specific since the contractions of the lung tissue by histamine, LTB_4 and LTD_4 are not significantly affected by BN 52021 *(Touvay et al., 1986c)*.

BN 52021 also inhibits PAF-acether-induced contractions of spirally cut large bronchi and of main pulmonary arteries (table 2 ; *Berti et al., 1986*) ; this phenomenon should not be underestimated since these PAF-acether-induced impairments contribute to the alteration of the local circulation which may be further aggravated by accumulation of thrombi in pulmonary arterial and capillary vessels and infiltration by inflammatory cells *(Page et al., 1985 ; Bourgain et al., 1985)*. Indeed, morphological studies in rabbits *(Mac Manus and Pinckard, 1985)*, guinea-pigs *(Lellouch-Tubiana et al., 1985)* or baboons *(Arnoux et al., 1986)* had shown that PAF-acether induces platelet and neutrophil aggregation within the pulmonary microvessels accompanied by eosinophil infiltration and contraction of small muscular arteries and bronchioles. Most importantly, activated platelets can be seen near the respiratory smooth muscle, as in systemic passive anaphylaxis (Fig 5) *(Lellouch-Tubiana et al., 1985)*.

(e) BN 52021 blocks in a dose-dependent manner the increase in eosinophil cytotoxicity induced by PAF-acether in the presence of *Schistosoma mansoni* previously coated with C_{3b} and specific antibodies *(Mac Donald et al., 1986)*. More interestingly, BN 52021 inhibits IgE-induced cytotoxicity of rat and human eosinophils *(M. Capron, pers. com.)*.

(f) Finally, preliminary studies using electronic microscopy demonstrate that BN 52021 antagonizes eosinophil lung recruitment induced by PAF-acether in guinea-pigs (Fig 7). This may partially explains the BN 52021-induced inhibition of bronchial hyperresponsiveness following PAF-acether administration.

These lines of evidence demonstrate the PAF-acether may participate in eosinophil (and macrophages) recruitment and granule release may account for bronchial hyperreactivity (Fig 6), particularly since the removal of epithelial layer from respiratory smooth muscle *in vitro* leads to hyperresponsiveness of the smooth muscle to a range of spasmogens in animals *(Barnes et al., 1985)* and in humans *(Rubin et al., 1986)*.

BN 52021, as PAF-acether antagonist counteracts these processes and could therefore antagonize airway hyperresponsiveness.

II - INHIBITION OF ANTIGEN-INDUCED PULMONARY IMPAIRMENTS BY BN 52021.

BN 52021 given i.v. (0.1 → 2 mg/kg) or orally (10 → 15 mg/kg) significantly antagonizes both homologous *(Vilain et al., 1986 ; Lagente et al., 1985 ; 1986)* and heterologous *(Braquet, 1984 ; Braquet et al., 1985b ; Touvay et al., 1985 ; 1986a)* passive anaphylaxis in guinea-pigs (table 6). The PAF-acether antagonist (2 → 4 mg/kg, i.v.) also totally protects the animals from death and counteracts the sustained bronchoconstriction observed in actively sensitized guinea-pigs (Fig 8) *(Berti et al., 1986)*. Nevertheless its efficiency is more variable in active shock since (table 6) :

(i) More important doses are required in active bronchoconstriction

(ii) In certain procedure of active sensitization using low doses of antigen, BN 52021 is sligthly or not effective whereas anti-H1 (e.g. mepyramine) are very effective *(Lagente et al., 1985 ; Touvay et al., unpublished)* suggesting a more pronounced involvement of histamine in such anaphylactic shock.

The protective effect of BN 52021 on immune bronchoconstriction is associated with the recovery of blood pH, p O_2 and TxB_2 level impaired by antigen challenge *(Berti et al., 1986)*. Interestingly in passive anaphylaxis, BN 52021 antagonizes the antigen-induced thrombopenia but the accompanying leukopenia is unaffected *(Lagente et al., 1986 ; Touvay et al., 1985)*. These results are in agreement with those of Adnot et al. (1986) and Beijer et al. (1986) who respectively showed that BN 52021, in guinea-pigs, (i) antagonizes the hypotensive response to i.v. *Salmonella typhimurium* endotoxin without interfering with leukopenia and (ii) counteracts lung platelet accumulation induced by endotoxin aerosol.

BN 52021 also antagonizes immune bronchoconstriction when antigen is given by aerosol in passively sensitized guinea-pigs (Fig 9) ; interestingly in the same experiment, another PAF-acether antagonist Ro 19-3704 *(Barner et al., 1985)* is also effective (althought uneffective when antigen is given i.v. ; *Cirino et al., 1986)*.

Suppression by BN 52021 of TxB_2 , 6-keto $PGF_{1\alpha}$, PGE_2 formation by isolated lungs from both passively *(Lagente et al., 1986)* or actively *(Harczy et al., 1986 ; Sirois et al., 1986)* sensitized guinea-pigs is not accounted for by thromboxane synthetase or cyclooxygenase inhibition since BN 52021 is completely inactive against arachidonic acid under similar conditions *(Desquand et al., 1986)*. In active anaphylaxis of guinea-pig isolated lung, LTB_4 and LTD_4 formation is also antagonized by BN 52021 (Fig 10; *Sirois et al., 1986*). Furthermore it is quite surprising to note that

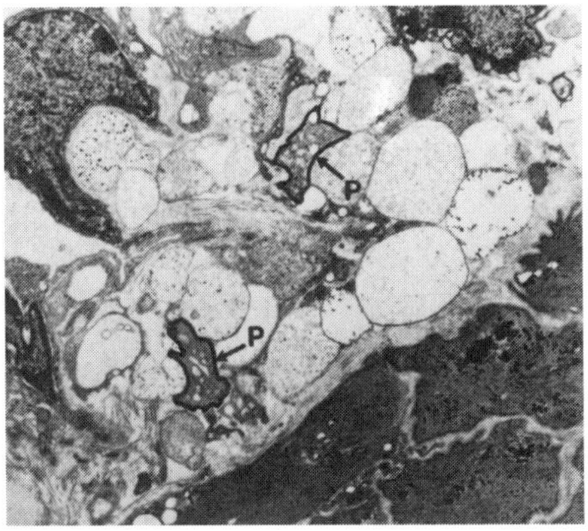

Fig 5 :

Infiltration of degranulated platelets near the respiratory smooth muscle cells following PAF-acether - or antigen -induced anaphylaxis in guinea-pigs *(from Lellouch-Tubiana et al., 1985 ; 1986).*

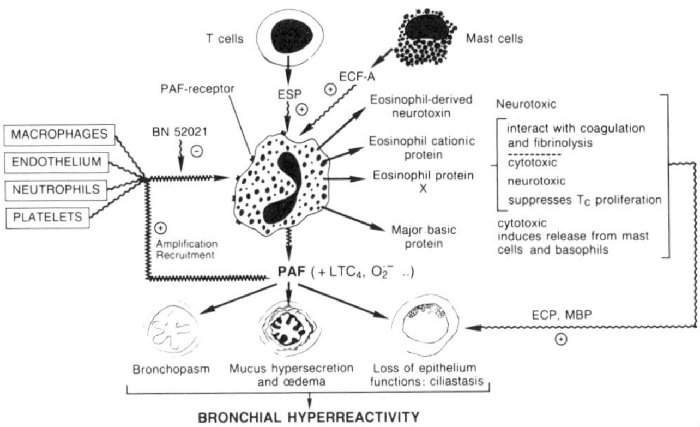

Fig 6 : Putative role of eosinophils and PAF-acether in the amplification process of bronchial hyperreactivity *(from Braquet and Vargaftig, 1987).*

Fig 7 :

Presence of eosinophil granules in lung tissue in PAF-acether- or antigen-induced anaphylaxis in guinea-pigs *(from Lellouch-Tubiana et al., 1985 ; 1986).*

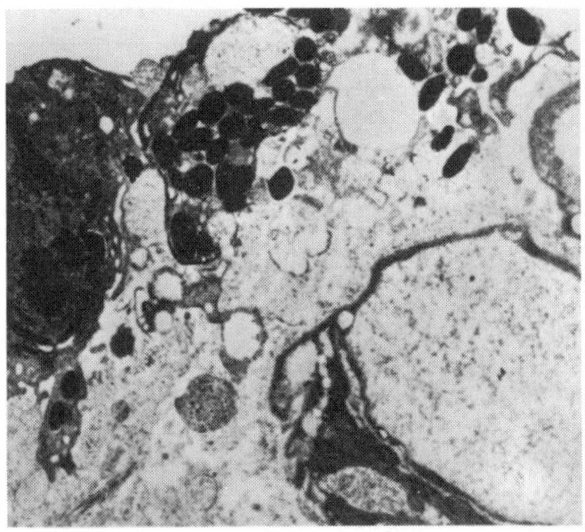

table 4 : 5-HETE* and LTC_4* formation induced by PAF-acether (3 μM) in eosinophils from patient with eosinophilia - inhibition by BN 52021.

PAF-ANTAGONIST (M)	5 - LO metabolites (picomoles / 10^6 cells)	
	5 - HETE	LTC_4
—	277 ± 48	147 ± 36
BN 52021, 5 x 10^{-5} M	134 ± 41	76 ± 30
BN 52021, 5 x 10^{-6} M	170 ± 38	84 ± 37
BN 52021, 5 x 10^{-7} M	237 ± 47	120 ± 41

* RP - HPLC system (ternary gradient) (n = 8)

table 5 : Stimulation of $O_2^{\bullet -}$ release by PAF-acether in human neutrophils : inhibition by BN 52021

PAF-acether (x 10^{-6} M)	BN 52021 (x 10^{-6} M)	Superoxide release (nmol / 10^7 cells / 5 min)
—	—	1.5 ± 1.2
0.01	—	2.3 ± 1.0
	0.5	2.1 ± 1.3
	1.0	1.4 ± 1.3
0.10	—	2.7 ± 1.1
	5	2.1 ± 1.3
	10	1.5 ± 1.1
1.00	—	3.3 ± 1.6
	50	2.5 ± 1.7
	100	1.9 ± 1.5

(from Braquet et al., 1984).

table 6 : Effects of BN 52021 on anaphylactic bronchoconstrictions in guinea-pigs

Sensitization procedure	Challenge (OA)		BN 52021		Reference
	Route	Dose	Route	Dose and effect	
passive, homologous	i.v.	1 mg/kg	i.v.	1 mg/kg, 93 % inh. (inh. suppressed by propranolol)	*Lagente et al., 1986*
	aerosol	1-10 mg/kg	i.v.	3 mg/kg, 85 % inh. (inh. suppressed by propranolol)	*Cirino et al., 1986*
passive, heterologous	i.v.	1 mg/kg	i.v.	1 mg/kg, 85% inh. 2 mg/kg, 78% inh.	*Braquet et al., 1985b* *Touvay et al., 1986a*
	i.v.	1 mg/kg	oral	20 mg/kg, 55% inh.	*Touvay et al., 1986c*
active, OA 100 mg/kg i.v. + 100 mg/kg SC	i.v.	5 mg/kg	i.v.	ED_{50} = 1,71 mg/kg	*Berti et al., 1986*
active, OA – 10μg/animal i.v. + Al $(OH)_3$	i.v.	1 mg/kg	i.v. and oral	inactive	*Lagente et al., 1985* *Touvay et al., 1986a*

histamine secretion is also blocked by the PAF-acether antagonist (Fig 11 ; *Lagente et al., 1986*), even though PAF-acether is known not to activate lung mast cells and accordingly, fails to release histamine from normal isolated guinea-pig lungs *(Vargaftig, pers. com.)*. The protection exerted by BN 52021 result either (i) from a specific, PAF-acether independent effect since it blocks IgE-induced histamine release in rat mast cells *(Stanworth et al., 1986)* or (ii) from a PAF-acether dependent phenomenon since *Pretolani et al. (in preparation)* showed that PAF-acether and LTD_4 are turned into histamine-releasing agents when injected to lungs dissected from sensitized animals ; formation of PAF-acether by a lung component may thus account for histamine release in anaphylaxis and accordingly, BN 52021 may interfere as a PAF-acether antagonist.

Of interest, BN 52021 is also effective in active shock in mice *(Etienne, unpublished)*, in cardiac anaphylaxis in both passively *(Koltai et al., 1986)* and actively *(Piper et al., 1986)* sensitized isolated guinea-pig hearts and in IgG aggregate-induced hypotension *(Sanchez Crespo et al., 1985)*, three immune challenges where PAF-acether may also be involved.

Is BN 52021 effective against immune bronchoconstriction strictly because of its anti-PAF-acether properties, or does it display additionnal anti-allergic effects ? It is too early to provide a final statement, but some dissociation may occur since :

(a) other PAF-acether antagonists like SRI 63-119 *(Stenzel et al., 1986a)*, 48 740 RP *(Stenzel et al., 1986b)*, Ro 19-3704 *(Vargaftig et al., in preparation)* do not block antigen-induced anaphylaxis although the latter compound is more effective in blocking PAF-acether-induced platelet activation than BN 52021.

(b) Propanolol removes the *in vivo* anti-anaphylactic activity of BN 52021 in passive shock *(Lagente et al., 1986)* even though the anti-PAF-acether activity was poorly affected by beta adrenergic blockade. As BN 52021 does not interfere with the binding of beta adrenergic ligands to their receptor *(Braquet et al., 1985a)* this suggest an undirect effect which remains to be elucidated. Nevertheless it may be argued that propanolol may produce a distortion of the relative importance of mediators of anaphylactic bronchoconstriction, turning the shock less PAF-acether-dependent and accordingly less inhibitable by BN 52021 *(Lagente et al., 1986)*.

(c) One further complication is the failure of BN 52021 to reduce the in vivo contractions of the parenchyma lung strip and the accompanying release of histamine and thromboxane triggered by antigen *(Lagente et al., 1986)* even though BN 52021 blocks the contraction of lung strips induced by PAF-acether *(Touvay et al., 1986c ; Desquand et al., 1986)*. This is also in apparent contradiction with the fact that the release of thromboxane and histamine are significantly reduced when antigen is given intraarterially to the lungs (see above). In fact, it is difficult to compare results obtained in perfused lungs and isolated strips, since much more PAF-acether is required to induce contraction of the strips than to active the perfused lungs : in the former case the contractions are long lasting and tachyphylaxis is readily obtained *(Detsouli et al., 1985)*, whereas concentration-dependent activation of perfused lungs is obtained with nanograms of PAF-acether injected intraarterially at short intervals *(Lefort et al., 1984)*.

Finally, BN 52021 reaches the isolated strip by diffusion and the perfused lung by the vascular route to interact with endothelium in a first instance : it is thus likely that the mechanisms accounting for smooth muscle contraction and mediator release may differ, at least partly, in these two preparations of the same tissue. Whatever the explanation for the differences between both preparations, failure of BN 52021 at effective anti-PAF-acether concentrations, to block passive anaphylaxis triggered on lung parenchymal strips and its effectiveness on isolated perfused lungs, suggests again some degree of dissociation between PAF-acether antagonism and anti-anaphylactic activity.

(d) PAF-acether induces a rapid and transient increase in plasma tryptic-like activity which returns

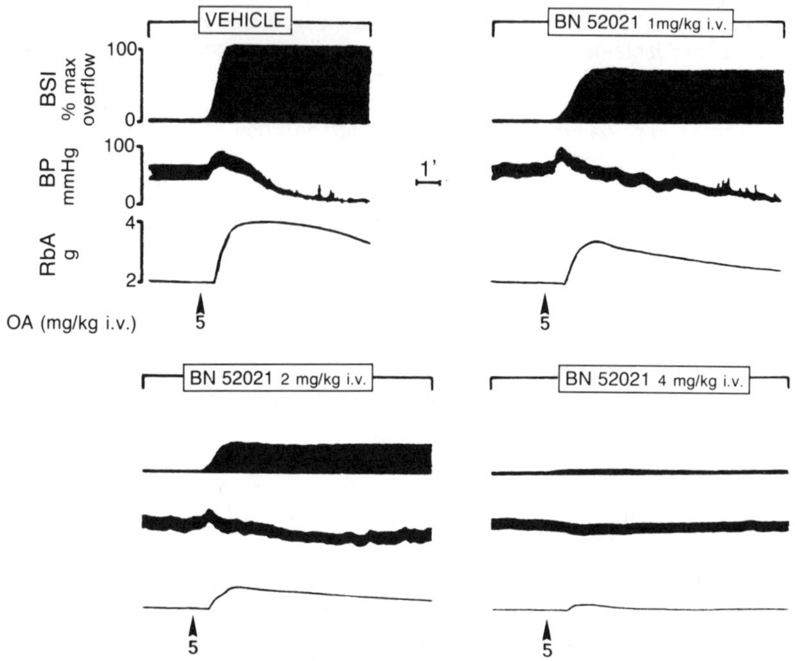

OA = ovalbumin. BN 52021 has been injected intravenously 5 min before OA
BSI = immunological bronchospasm.
BP = arterial blood pressure.
RbA = strip of rabbit aorta superfused with blood, monitoring TxA_2-like activity

Fig 8 : Dose-dependent inhibition of immune bronchoconstriction by BN 52021 in actively sensitized guinea-pigs *(from Berti et al., 1986).*

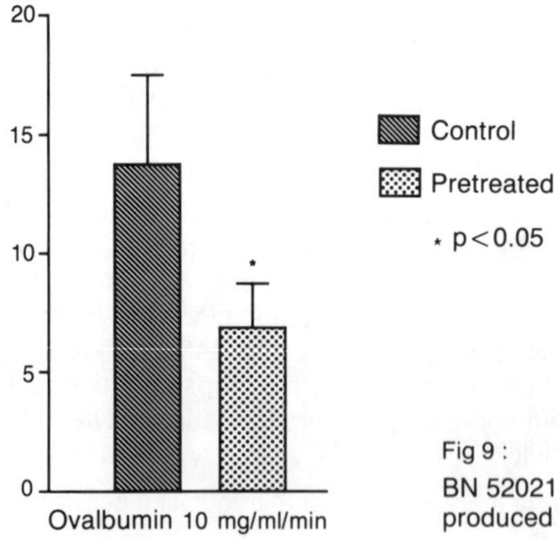

Fig 9 :
BN 52021 reduces the bronchoconstriction produced by aerosolized antigen.

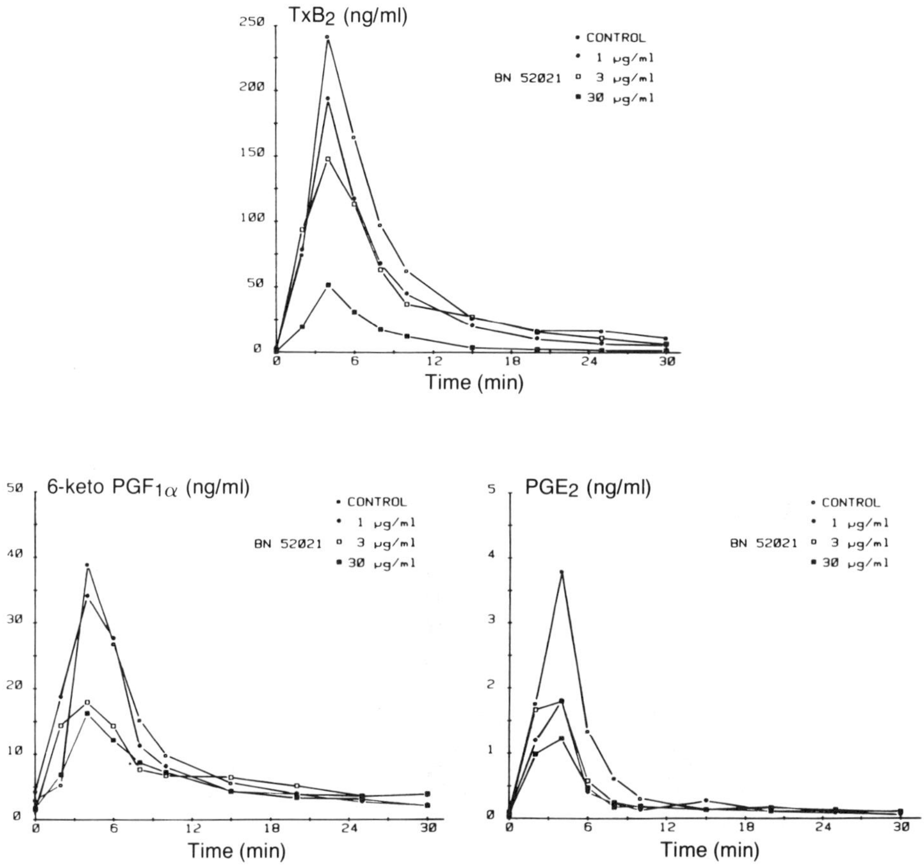

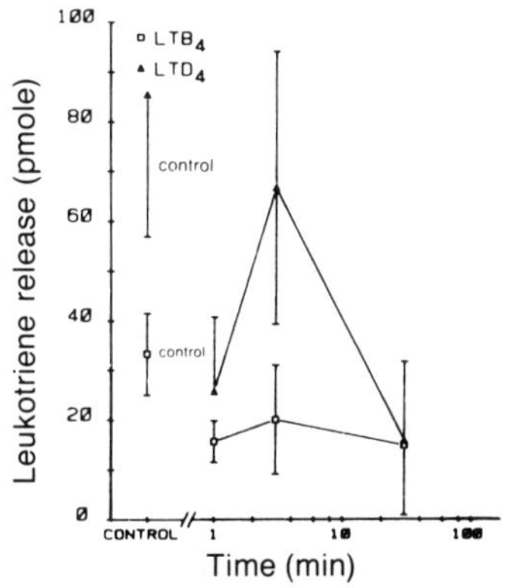

Fig 10 :

Effect of BN 52021 on the release of various eicosanoids from isolated guinea-pig lung challenged with antigen (actively-sensitized animals) *(from Harczy et al., 1986 ; Sirois et al., 1986).*

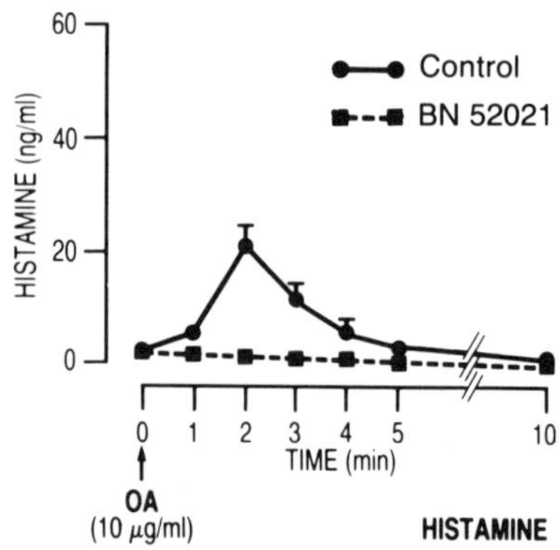

Fig 11 :

Effect of BN 52021 on histamine release from isolated guinea-pig lung challenged with antigen (passively - sensitized animals - homologous serum; *from Lagente et al., 1986*)

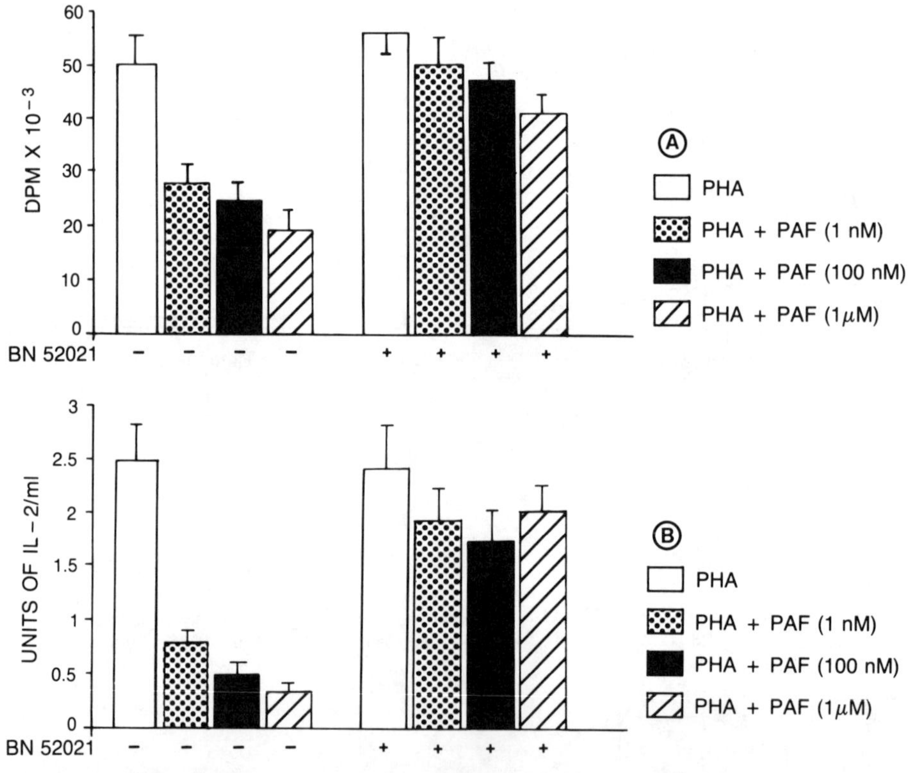

Fig 12 : Effect of PAF-acether on PHA-induced human lymphocyte proliferation (A) and Interleukin-2 production (B) and their prevention by BN 52021 *(from Rola-Pleszczynski et al., 1986).*

to normal level at about 30 min *(Etienne et al., 1986)*. In comparison, *Salmonella anteridis* endotoxin induces a slower but higher and more durable increase in plasama proteasic activity. BN 52021 does not exhibit any *in vitro* significant anti proteasic effect. In contrast, when given i.v. or orally, BN 52021 induces a dose-dependent and very significant decrease in plasma tryptic-like activity triggered in rats by either PAF-acether or endotoxin *(Etienne et al., 1986)*. Since proteasic activity is increased in blood *(for inst. Neuman et al., 1984)* or bronchial lavage fluid *(Püsa and Tchörzewski, 1985)* of asthmatic patients, the antiproteasic activity displayed *in vivo* by BN 52021 may account for its anti-anaphylactoid property, this activity being totally or partially related to its PAF-acether antagonist property.

It is therefore difficult to provide a final statement on the mechanisms underlying the anti-anaphylactoid effect of BN 52021. Nevertheless a recent paper of Cazals Stenzel (1986) demonstrate than another PAF-acether antagonist WEB 2086, a triazolobenzodiazepine, has an anti-anaphylactic profile very similar to that of BN 52021 : WEB 2086 inhibits significantly passive anaphylaxis (heterologous serum) in guinea-pigs. Lethality is abolished only in animals treated concomitantly with the anti-H_1 mepyramine. In active anaphylaxis [OA : 40 μg/kg, Al $(OH)_3$] WEB 2086 does not prevent lethaly whereas mepyramine is effective suggesting here again a major role for histamine in this shock. Furthermore using kadsurenone *(Shen et al., 1985)* and Alprazolam *(Kornecki et al., 1984),* Darius et al., (1986) confirmed our findings that PAF-acether antagonists can counteract immune bronchoconstriction. If these data reinforce the possible involvement of PAF-acether in immune bronchoconstriction and mainly in passive anaphylaxis, the mechanisms underlying anaphylaxis inhibition totally remain to be elucidated.

III - EFFECTS OF PAF-ACETHER AND BN 52021 ON THE T CELL SYSTEM. POSSIBLE RELATIONSHIPS WITH BRONCHIAL HYPERRESPONSIVENESS.

T lymphocytes are known to modulate IgE production *(Kyle et al., 1982)* and therefore play an important role in the pathogenesis of atopic diseases . The circulating T cell system appears to be impaired in atopic states : Several studies suggest a decreased suppressor cell functions with a reduction of OKT 3 + cell and a raised OKT 4 + / OKT 8 + ratio due to a drop in suppressor cells *(Engel et al., 1984 ; Kus et al., 1985 ; Hwang KC et al., 1985)*. In contrast Gerblich et al. (1984) observed a decrease in T helper cells and an increase in activated T lymphocytes in the peripheral blood of patients with bronchial asthma challenged with the relevant antigen but not with methacholine or non specific antigen.

Both in humans and animals, the inflammatory response following antigen challenge involves a rise in helper T cells in bronchoalveolar lavage *(BAL ; Metzger et al., 1986)*. Similar impairment is classically recorded in sarcoidosis *(Rossi et al., 1984 ;1986 ; Costabel et al., 1986 ; Van der Bosh et al., 1986)* or in hypersensitivity pneumonitis *(Mornex et al., 1984)*. An increase of both OKT 4 + and OKT 8 + subsets has also been recorded in BAL of patients suffering from extrinsic allergic alveolitis (Van der Bosh et al., 1986).

PAF-acether [and therefore PAF-acether antagonists] may regulate the lymphocyte functions :

(i) either undirectly since PAF-acether produces leukotrienes formation in lungs *(Voelkel et al., 1984)* which in turn are potent modulators of lymphocyte functions *(Rola-Pleszczynski et al., 1984)* ;

(ii) either directly since when human lymphocytes are cultured in presence of the mitogen phytohemagglutinin, their proliferation is markedly impaired by nanomolar concentrations of (R) PAF-acether *(Rola-Pleszczynski et al., 1986)*. A similar suppression is observed with ethoxy-PAF at higher concentrations but lyso-PAF and (S) PAF-acether, the inactive enantiomer of the mediator, are inactive *(Braquet et al., 1986c)*. Several cyclooxygenase metabolites of arachidonic acid, and in particular prostaglandins of the E series, can exert a powerful suppressive effect on lymphocyte proliferation. Indeed, while indomethacin has no significant effect per se, its concomitant use in the proliferation assay completely prevented the PAF-acether-induced suppression, indicating that PAF-acether may exert its effect through some cyclooxygenase metabolites e.g. PGE_2.

BN 52021 and the related compound BN 52020 (Ginkgolide A) at micromolar concentrations completely reversed the inhibition caused by (R) PAF-acether or ethoxy-PAF (Fig 12 ; *Braquet et al., 1986c*). Furthermore, by themselves, these compounds are slightly stimulatory. A similar effect of (R) PAF-acether and ethoxy-PAF was observed when production of IL-2 by human lymphocytes was measured following mitogen stimulation, using the IL-2-dependent CTLL cells line *(Rola-Pleszczynski et al., 1986)*. The inhibition by PAF-acether was also reversed by the concomitant use of BN 52021 (Fig 12). All those effects were more evident when neutrophils were added to the lymphocyte cultures at a 1 : 1 ratio *(Rola Pleszczynski et al., 1986)*.

When exogenous IL-2 is added on human T lymphoblast preparations, BN 52021 does not inhibit [^{3}H]-Thymidine incorporation. In contrast, L-652,731 and CV 3988, two PAF-acether antagonists deriving respectively from lignan series *(Hwang et al., 1985)* and PAF-acether framework *(Terashita et al., 1983)* produced dose-related inhibition of sub-optimal IL-2-induced [^{3}]-thymidine incorporation *(Barret et al., 1986)*. A similar result was obtained with the PAF-acether synthesis inhibitor L-648,611 *(Robbins et al., 1985)* but not with BN 52021 *(Barret et al., 1986)*.

Conversely PAF-acether and related agonist structures (e.g. PR 1501 and PR 1502) produced a dose-related and marked potentiation of IL-2-induced T cell proliferation *(Barret et al., 1986)*.

The above results clearly shown that PAF-acether may be involved in T cell system regulation *in vitro*. Nevertheless it is too early to conclude about the existence of relationship between bronchial asthma, impairment of lymphocyte function and PAF-acether.

REFERENCES

Adnot, S., Lefort, J., Lagente, V., Braquet, P. and Vargaftig, B.B (1986). Interference of BN 52021, a PAF-acether antagonist, with endotoxin-induced hypotension in the guinea-pig. Pharmacol. Res. Commun. **18 (Supp.)**, 197-200.

Arnoux, B., Duval, D. and Benveniste, J. (1980). Release of platelet-activating factor (PAF-acether) from alveolar macrophages by the calcium ionophore A23187 and phagocytosis. Eur. J. Clin. Invest. **10**, 437-441.

Arnoux, B., Page, C.P., Denjean, A., Nolibe, D., Morley, J. and Benveniste, J. (1986) submitted.

Arnoux, B. and Gillis, C.N. (1986). Role of fatty acids and BN 52021 on vascular and airway actions of platelet-activating factor (PAF) in isolated rabbit lung in situ. Int. Joint Meeting of European Societies of Pneumology Paris Sept. 3-6 1986, Abst. 556, p 85s.

Baggiolini, M. and Dewald, B. (1986). Stimulus amplification by PAF and LTB_4 in human neutrophils. Pharmacol. Res. Commun. **18 (Supp.)**, 51-60.

Baranes, J., Hellegouarch, A., Le Hegarat, M., Viossat, I., Auguet, M., Chabrier, P.E., Clostre, F. and Braquet, P. (1986). The effects of PAF-acether on the cardiovascular system and their inhibition by a new highly specific PAF-acether receptor antagonist BN 52021. Pharmacol. Res. Commun., **18**, 737-758.

Barnes, P.J., Cuss, F.M. and Palmer, J.B. (1985). The effect of airway epithelium on smooth muscle contractility in bovine trachea. Br. J. Pharmacol. **86**, 685-691.

Barnes, P.J., Dent, G., Guinot, Ph., Mac Cusker, M. and Page, C.P. (1986). Effectiveness of a specific antagonist of platelet-activating factor, BN 52063, in man. Brit. J. Pharmacol. (Abst.), In press.

Barner, R., Hadvary, P., Burri, K., Hirth, G., Cassal, J.M. and Muller, K. (1984). Glycerin derivatives Eur. Pat Appl. EP 147,768, 12.18.84 [see CA **104**, 889390, (1986)].

Baroggi, N., Etienne, A. and Braquet, P. (1986). Changes in cytosolic free calcium induced by platelet activating factor in rabbit platelets : specific inhibition by BN 52021 and structurally related compounds. Agents Actions, In press.

Barrett, M.L., Lewis, G.P., Ward, S. and Westwick, J. (1986). Platelet activating factor modulates interleukin-2-induced proliferation of human T-lymphoblasts. Brit. J. Pharmacol. Abst. In press.

Beijer, L., Botting, J., Oyekan, A.O., Page, C. and Rylander, R. (1986). The involvement of PAF in endotoxin-induced pulmonary recruitment. Brit. J. Pharmacol. (Abst.), In press.

Benveniste, J., Henson, P.M. and Cochrane, C.G. (1972). Leukocyte-dependent histamine release from rabbit platelets. The role of IgE, basophils, and a platelet-activating factor. J. Exp. Med. **136**, 1356-1377.

Berti, F., Omini, C., Rossoni, G. and Braquet, P. (1986). Protection by two ginkgolides, BN 52020 and BN 52021, against guinea-pig lung anaphylaxis. Pharmacol. Res. Commun. **18**, 775-793.

Borgeat, P. Fruteau de Laclos, B., Rabinovitch, H., Picard, S., Braquet, P., Hebert, J. and Laviolette, M. (1984). Eosinophil-rich human polymorphonuclear leukocyte preparations characteristically release leukotriene C_4 on ionophore A 23187 challenge. J. Allergy Clin. Immunol. **74**, 310-315.

Boukili, M.A., Lagente, V., Lefort, J. and Vargaftig, B.B. (1985). Bronchoconstriction by F-MET-LEU-PHE may involve cyclooxygenase and leukotriene-independent mechanisms, Int. J. Immun. **7**, 382-389.

Bourgain, R.H., Maes, L., Braquet, P., Andries, R., Touqui, L. and Braquet, M. (1985). The effect of 1-O-alkyl-2-acetyl-sn-glycero-3-phosphocholine (PAF-acether) on the arterial wall. Prostaglandins **30**, 185-197.

Braquet, P. (1984). Treatment or prevention of PAF-acether disorders provoked by a new series of highly specific inhibitors, GB Patent, 84/18, 424 (July 19, 1984) Belg. BE 901, 915 [see CA **103** : 189808d, (1985)].

Braquet, P., Spinnewyn, B., Braquet, M., Bourgain, R.H., Taylor, J.E., Etienne, A. and Drieu, K. (1985a). BN 52021 and related compounds : a new series of highly specific PAF-acether receptor antagonists isolated from *Ginkgo biloba*, Blood and Vessels, **16**, 559-572.

Braquet, P., Etienne, A., Touvay, C., Bourgain, R.H., Lefort, J. and Vargaftig, B.B. (1985b). Involvement of platelet activating factor in respiratory anaphylaxis, demonstrated by PAF-acether inhibitor BN 52021, Lancet **i**, 1501.

Braquet, P. and Godfroid, J.J. (1986). PAF-acether specific binding sites : 2. Design of Specific antagonist. TIPS **7** **(10)**, 397-403.

Braquet, P., Touqui, L., Vargaftig, B.B. and Shen, T.Y. (1986a). Perspectives in platelet-activating factor research. Pharmacol. Rev. In press.

Braquet, P., Drieu K. and Etienne, A. (1986b). Le ginkgolide B (BN 52021) : un puissant inhibiteur du PAF-acether isolé du *Ginkgo biloba*. L. Actualités de Chimie Thérapeutique (Paris) **13**, 237-254.

Braquet, P., Pignol, B. and Rola-Pleszczynski, M. (1986c). Modulation of interleukin 2 synthesis by platelet activating factor. Brit. J. Pharmacol. Abst. In press.

Braquet, P. and Vargaftig, B.B. (1987). Platelet-activating factor today. ISI Atlas of Sciences, In press.

Bruynzeel, P.L.B., Koenderman, L., Kok, P.T.M., Hameling, M.L. and Verhagen, J. (1986). Platelet-activating factor (PAF-acether)-induced leukotriene C4 formation and luminol dependent chemiluminescence by human eosinophils. Pharmacol. Res. Commun., **18**, 61-69.

Casalz-Stenzel, J. (1986). Effects of WEB 2086, a novel antagonist of platelet activating factor, in active and passive anaphylaxis. Immunopharmacology. In press.

Cirino, M., Lagente, V., Lefort, J. and Vargaftig, B.B. (1986). A study with BN 52021 demonstrates the involvement of PAF-acether in IgE-dependent anaphylactic bronchoconstriction. Prostaglandins. July issue.

Clostre, F., Etienne, A. and Braquet, P. (1986). The role of platelet-activating factor in gastro-intestinal ulcerations. In preparation.

Coeffier, E., Borrel, M.C., Lefort, J., Chignard, M., Broquet, C., Heymans, F., Godfroid, J.J. and Vargaftig, B.B. (1986). Effects of PAF-acether and structural analogues on platelet activation and bronchoconstriction in guinea-pigs. Eur. J. Pharmacol. In press.

Cordeiro, R.S.B., Silva, P.M.R., Martins, M.A. and Vargaftig, B.B. (1986a). Effects of potential antagonists on the rat paw oedema induced by PAF-acether. Prostaglandins. In press.

Cordeiro, R.S.B., Martins, M.A., Silva, P.M.R., Castro Faria Neto, H.C., Castanheira, J.R.C. and Vargaftig, B.B. (1986b). Desensitization to PAF-induced rat paw oedema by repeated intraplantar injections. Life Sciences. In press.

Costabel, U., Bross, K.J., Guzman, J., Nilles, A., Ruhle, K.H. and Matthys, H. (1986). Predictive value of bronchoalveolar T cell subsets for the course of pulmonary sarcoidosis. Ann. NY Acad. Sci. **465**, 418-426.

Cuss, F.M., Dixon, C.M. and Barnes, P.J. (1986). Effects of inhaled platelet activating factor on pulmonary function and bronchial responsiveness in man. Lancet **ii**, 189-192.

Darius, H., Lefer, D.J., Smith, J.B. and Lefer, A.M. (1986). Role of platelet-activating factor-acether in mediating guinea-pig anaphylaxis. Science, **232**, 58-60.

Delgado, D. and Tamargo, D.Y. (1986). Efectos electrofisiologicos del L 652,731 y BN 52021 en fibras musculares de cobaya. IIIrd meeting of eicosanoid club. Madrid (Spain) Sept. 19-20, Abst.

De Monchy, J.G., Kauffman, H.F., Vense, P., Koeter, G.H., Jansen, H.M., Sluiter, H.J., De Vries, K. (1985). Bronchoalveolar eosinophilia during allergen-induced late asthmatic reactions. Am. Rev. Respir. Dis. **135**, 373-376.

Desquand, S., Touvay, C., Randon, J., Lagente, V., Vilain, B., Maridonneau-Parini, I., Etienne, A., Lefort, J., Braquet, P. and Vargaftig, B.B. (1986). Interference of BN 52021 (ginkgolide B) with the bronchopulmonary effects of PAF-acether in the guinea-pig. Eur. J. Pharmacol., **127**, 83-95.

Detsouli, A., Lefort, J. and Vargaftig, B.B. (1985). Histamine and leukotriene-independent guinea-pig anaphylactic shock unaccounted for by PAF-acether. Br. J. Pharmacol. **84**, 801.

Emeis, J.J. (1987). The role of lipid mediators in blood fibrinolysis. In : Lipid mediators in immunology of burn and sepsis M. Paubert-Braquet et al. eds, Plenum Press (New York) NATO ASI Series, In press.

Engel, P., Huguet, J., Sanosa, J., Sierra, P., Cols, N., Garcia-Calderon, P.A. (1984). T cell subsets in allergic respiratory disease using monoclonal antibodies. Ann. Allergy **53**, 337-340

Etienne, A., Hecquet, F., Soulard, C., Spinnewyn, B., Clostre, F. and Braquet, P. (1985). In vivo inhibition of plasma protein and *salmonella enteritidis*-induced mortality in the rat by a specific PAF-acether antagonist : BN 52021. Agents Actions, **17** , 368-370.

Etienne, A., Hecquet, F., Guilmard, C., Soulard, C. and Braquet, P. (1986). Inhibition of rat endotoxin-induced lethality by BN 52021 and BN 52063 compounds with PAF-acether antagonistic effect and protease inhibitory activity. Int. J. Tissue Reactions In press.

Feuerstein, G., Leader, P., Siren, A.L. and Braquet, P. (1986). Protective effect of a PAF-acether antagonist, BN 52021, in trichothecene toxicosis. J. Appl. Pharmac. Toxicol. In press.

Filley, W.V., Kephart, G.M., Holley, K.E. and Gleich, G.J. (1982). Identification by immunofluorescence of eosinophil granule major basic protein in lung tissues of patients with bronchial asthma Lancet **ii**, 11-15.

Fink, A., Afek, A., Shalev, Y., Eliraz, A. and Bentwich, Z. (1986). The sensitivity of peripheral blood leukocytes of ischemic heart patients to PAF-acether and cysteinyl containing leukotrienes : determination by the tube leukocyte adherence inhibition assay. 6th Int. Conference on prostaglandins and related compounds, Abst. p. 301.

Fitzgerald, M.F., Moncada, S. and Parente, L. (1986). The anaphylactic release of platelet-activating factor from perfused guinea-pig lungs. Br. J. Pharmac. **88**, 149-153.

Foegh, M., Alijani, M.R., Helfrich, G.B., Khirabadi, B.S. and Ramwell, P. (1985). Prolongation of cardiac allograft survival with the PAF antagonist BN 52021 and with the thromboxane receptor antagonists L640035 and L636499. Advances in Prostaglandin, Thromboxane and Leukotriene Research, Raven press, New York, **15**, 381-399.

Foegh, M.L. Khirabadi, B.S., Rowles, J.R., Braquet, P. and Ramwell, P.W. (1986). Prolongation of cardiac allograft survival with BN 52021 a specific antagonist of platelet activating factor. Transpl. **42**, 86-88.

Garay, R. and Braquet, P. (1986). Involvement of K^+ movements in the membrane signal induced by PAF-acether. Biochem. Pharmacol., **35**, 2811-2815.

Gerblich, A.A., Campbell, A.E. and Schuyler, M.R. (1984). Changes in T-lymphocyte subpopulations after antigenic bronchial provocation in asthmatics. New Engl. J. Med. **310**, 1349-1356.

Gleich, G.J., Loegering, D.A., Mann, K.G. and Maldonado, J.E. (1976). Comparative properties of the Charcot-Leyden crystal protein and the major basic protein from human eosinophils. J. Clin. Invest. **57**, 633-640.

Guinot, Ph, Braquet, P., Duchier, J. and Cournot, A. (1986). Inhibition of PAF-acether induced weal and flare reaction in man by a specific PAF antagonist. Prostaglandins. July issue.

Harczy, M., Maclouf, J., Pradelles, P., Braquet, P., Borgeat, P. and Sirois, P. (1986). Inhibitory effects of a novel platelet activating factor (PAF) antagonist (BN 52021) on antigen-induced prostaglandin and thromboxane formation by the guinea-pig lung. Pharmacol. res. Com. **18 (Supp)**, 111-119.

Hebert, R.L., Sirois, P., Braquet, P. and Plante, G.E. (1986). Hemodynamic effects of PAF-acether on the dog kidney. Prostagl. Leukot. Med. In press.

Henocq, E. and Vargaftig, B.B. (1986). Accumulation of eosinophils in response to intracutaneous PAF-acether and allergens in man, Lancet **i**, 1378-1379.

Hoshikawa-Fujimura, A.Y., Chamone, D.A.F. and Jancar, S. (1986). Effect of BN 52021 on human PMN superoxide anion production. 6 th Int. Conference on Prostaglandins and related compounds Florence (Italy) June 3-6, Abst. p. 388.

Hwang, K.C., Fikrig, S.M., Fridman, H.M. and Gupta, S. (1985). Deficient concanavalin-A-induced suppressor-cell activity in patients with bronchial asthma, allergic rhinitis and atopic dermatitis. Clin. Allergy 15, 67-72.

Jacob, H.S., Vercelotti, G. and Stroncek, D. (1986). The role of PAF in vascular damage syndromes. Evidence from inhibitor studies with BN 52021 . 6 th Int. Conference on Prostaglandins and Related Compounds Florence (Italy) June 3-6, Abst.

Koenderman, L. and Bruijnzeel, P.L.B. (1986). The luminol dependent chemiluminescent response pattern of eosinophils and neutrophils from normal individuals after challenge with opsonized zymosan, the calcium ionophore A23187, N-formyl-methionyl-leucyl-phenylalanine, leukotriene B_4 and platelet activating factor. Infect. Immun. In press.

Koltai, M., Lepran, I., Szekeres, L., Viossat, I., Chabrier, E. and Braquet, P. (1986). Effect of BN 52021 , a specific PAF-acether antagonist, on cardiac anaphylaxis in Langendorff hearts isolated from passively sensitized guinea-pigs. Eur. J. Pharmacol. In press.

Kornecki, E., Ehrlich, Y.H. and Lenox, R.H. (1984). Platelet-activating factor-induced aggregation of human platelets specifically inhibited by triazolobenzodiazepines, Science 226, 1454-1456.

Kravis, T.C. and Henson, P.M. (1975). IgE-induced release of platelet activating factor from rabbit lung. J. Immunol. 115, 1677-1684.

Kus, J., Tse, K.S., Vedal, S. and Chan-Yeung, M. (1985). Lymphocyte sub-populations in patients with allergic and non-allergic asthma. Clin. Allergy 15, 523-529.

Küster, L.J., Filep, J. and Frölich, J.C. (1986). Mechanisms of PAF-induced platelet aggregation in man. Thromb. Res., 43, 425-433.

Kyle, R.A., Pajak, T.F. and Henderson, E.S. (1982). Multiple myeloma resistant to melphalan : treatment with doxorubicin, cyclophosphamide, carmustine (BCNU) and prednisone. Cancer Treat. Rep. 66, 451-456.

Lachachi, H., Plantavid, M., Simon, M.F., Chap, H., Braquet, P. and Douste Blazy, L. (1985). Inhibition of transmembrane movement and metabolism of platelet-activating factor (PAF-acether) by a specific antagonist, BN 52021, Biochem. Biophys. res. Commun. 132, 460-466.

Lagente, V., Desquand, S., Randon, J., Lefort, J. and Vargaftig, B.B. (1985). Interference of PAF-acether antagonists with the effects of PAF itself and of anaphylactic shock *in vitro* and *in vivo* guinea-pig bronchopulmonary preparations. Prostaglandins 30, 703.

Lagente, V., Touvay, C., Randon, J., Desquand, S., Cirino, M., Vilain, B., Lefort, J., Braquet, P. and Vargaftig, B.B. (1986). Interference of the PAF-acether antagonist BN 52021 with passive anaphylaxis in the guinea-pig. Prostaglandins. In press.

Lee, T.C., Lenihan, D.J., Malone, B., Roddy, L.L. and Wasserman, S.I. (1984). Increased biosynthesis of Platelet-activating Factor in activated human eosinophils. J. Biol. Chem. 259, 5526-5530.

Lefort, J., Rotilio, D. and Vargaftig, B.B. (1984). The platelet-independent release of thromboxane A_2 by PAF-acether from guinea-pig lungs involves mechanisms distinct from those for leukotriene C_4 and bradykinin. Br. J. Pharmacol. 82, 525-531.

Lellouch-Tubiana, A., Lefort, J., Pirotzky, E., Vargaftig, B.B. and Pfister, A. (1985). Ultrastructural evidence for extravascular platelet recruitment in the lung upon intravenous injection of platelet-activating factor (PAF-acether) to guinea-pigs. Br. J. Exp. Path. 66, 345-352.

Lellouch-Tubiana, A., Lefort, J., Pfister, A. and Vargaftig, B.B. (1986). Interactions between granulocytes and platelets in the lung in passive anaphylaxis shock. Correlations with PAF-acether-induced lesions. Int. Arch. All. Appl. Immunol. In press.

McDonald, A.J., Moqbel, R., Wardlaw, A.J. and Kay, A.B. (1986). Platelet-activating factor (PAF-acether) enhances eosinophil cytotoxicity in vitro. J. Allergy Clin. Immunol., 77, 227.

McManus, L.M. and Pinckard, R.N. (1985). Kinetics of acetyl glyceryl ether phosphorylcholine (AGEPC)-induced acute lung alterations in the rabbit. Am. J. Pathol. 121, 55-68

Maridonneau-Parini, I., Lagente, V., Lefort, J., Randon, J., Russo-Marie, F. and Vargaftig, B.B. (1985). Desensitization to PAF-induced bronchoconstriction and to activation of alveolar macrophages by repeated inhalations of PAF in the guinea-pig. Biochem. Biophys. Res. Commun. 131, 42-50.

Metzger, W.J., Moseley, P., Richerson, H.B., Spoerdsma, K., Monick, M. and Hunninghake, G.W. (1986). Platelets in bronchoalveolar lavage from asthmatics with allergen-induced late phase responses. Platelets, analgesics and asthma, IIIrd Int. Symposium Davos (Switzerland) Sept. 7-9. p. 24.

Mornex, J.F., Cordier, G., Pages, J., Vergnon, J.M., Lefevre, R., Brune, J. and Revillard, J.P. (1984). Activated lung lymphocytes in hypersensitivity pneumonitis. J. Allergy Clin. Immunol. **74**, 719-727.

Neuman, I., Inbar, O., Creter, D. (1984). The kinin system in exercice-induced asthma. Ann. Alleregy, **53**, 351-354.

Nunez, D., Chignard, M., Korth, R., Le Couedic, J.P., Norel, X., Spinnewyn, B., Braquet, P. and Benveniste, J. (1986). Specific inhibition of PAF-acether-induced platelet activation by BN 52021 and comparison with the PAF-acether inhibitors Kadsurenone and CV-3988. Eur. J. Pharmacol., **123**, 197-205.

Ortiz, R., Robles, R., De Nicolas, R. and Egido, J. (1986). Papel de los antagonistos farmacologicos del PAF-acether en las nefropatias experimentales. IIIrd meeting of eicosanoid club. Madrid (Spain) Sept. 19-20, Abst.

Page, C.P., Paul, W. and Morley, J. (1982). An in vivo model for studying platelet aggregation and disaggregation. Thrombos Haemostas **47**, 210-213.

Page, C.P., Paul, W., Basran, G.S. and Morley. J. (1985). In : Weiss E.B., Segal M.S., Stein M. eds. Bronchial asthma, Mechanisms & Therapeutics Little, Brown & Co., pp. 266-270.

Parente, N. and Flower, R.J. (1985). Hydrocortisone and macrocortin inhibit the zymosan-induced release of lyso-PAF from rat peritoneal leucocytes. Life Sci. **36**, 1225-1231.

Patterson, R. and Harris., K.E. (1983). The activity of aerosolized and intracutaneous synthetic platelet activating factor (AGEPC) in rhesus monkeys with IgE-mediated airway responses and normal monkeys. J. Lab. Clin. Med. **102**, 933-938.

Piper, P.J. and Stewart, A.G. (1986). Evidence of a role for platelet-activating factor in antigen-induced coronary vaso-constriction in guinea-pig perfused hearts. Brit. J. Pharmacol., **88**, 238.

Plante, G.E., Hebert, R.L., Lamoureux, C., Braquet, P. and Sirois, P. (1986). Hemodynamic effects of PAF-acether. Pharmacol. Res. Commun., **18 (Supp.)**, 173-180.

Plotkine, M., Massad, L., Allix, M., Capdeville, C. and Boulu, R.G. (1986). Cerebral effects of PAF-acether in rats. 6 th Int. Conference on prostaglandins and related compounds Florence (Italy) June 3-6, Abst. p. 300.

Püsa, T. and Tchörzewski, H. (1985). Analysis of proteolytic enzymes and their natural inhibitors in serum and bronchial lavage fluid in atopic bronchial asthma. Allerg. Immunol. **31**, 169-178.

Robbins, J.C., MaChoy, B.H., Lam, M.J., Ponpipom, M., Rupprecht, K.M. and Shen, T.Y. A synthetic phospholipid inhibitor of platelet-activating factor (PAF) biosynthesis. Fed. Proc., **44**, 1269.

Rola-Pleszczynski, M., Gasnon, L., Rudzinskia, M., Borgeat, P. and Sirois, P. (1984). Human natural cytotoxic cell activity : enhancement by leukotrienes (LT) A_4, B_4 and D_4, but not by stereoisomers of LTB_4 or HETEs. Prostaglandins Leukotrienes Med., **13**, 113-117.

Rola-Pleszczynski, M., Pignol, B., Pouliot, C. and Braquet, P. (1986). Inhibition of human lymphocyte proliferation and interleukin 2 production by platelet activiting factor (PAF-acether) : reversal by a specific antagonist BN 52021. Biochem. Biophys. Res. Commun. In press.

Ross, R. and Vogel, A. (1978). The platelet derived growth factor cell, **14**, 203-210.

Rossi, G.A., Sacco, O., Cosulich, E., Damiani, G., Corte, G., Bargellesi, A and Ravazzoni, C. (1984). Pulmonary sarcoidosis : excess of helper T lymphocytes and T cell subset imbalance at sites of disease activity. Thorax **39**, 143-149.

Rossi, G.A., Sacco, O., Cosulich, E., Risso, A., Balbi, B. and Ravazzoni, C. (1986). Helper T-lymphocytes in pulmonary sarcoidosis. Functional analysis of a lung T-cell subpopulation in patients with active disease. Am. Rev. Respir. Dis. **133**, 1086-1090.

Rotilio, D., Lefort, J., Detsouli, A. and Vargaftig, B.B. (1983). Absence de contribution du PAF-acether à la reponse anaphylactique pulmonaire in vitro chez le cobaye. J. Pharmac. (Paris) **14 (Suppl. 1)**, 97-109.

Rubin, A.E., Smith, L.J. and Patterson, R. (1986). Am. Rev. Resp. Dis. **133**, A91.

Sanchez-Crespo, M., Fernandez-Gallardo, S., Nieto, M.L., Baranes, J. and Braquet, P. (1985). Inhibition of the vascular actions of IgE aggregates by BN 52021, a highly specific antagonist of PAF-acether. Immunopharmacology **10**, 69-75.

Shen, T.Y., Hwang, S.B., Chang, M.N., Doebber, T.W., Lam, M.H., Wu, M.S., Wang, X., Han, G.Q., Li, R.Z. (1985). Characterization of a platelet-activating factor receptor antagonist isolated from haifenteng (Piper futokadsura) : specific inhibition of in vitro and in vivo platelet-activating factor-induced effects, Proc. Natl. Acad. Sci. USA **82** : 672-676 (see also Patent JP 60 97,972 [85 97, 972] 31 May 1985, US Appl. 541,806 13 Oct. 1983).

Simon, A.F., Chap, H., Braquet, P. and Douste-Blazy, L. (1986). Effect of BN 52021, a specific antagonist of platelet-activating factor (PAF-acether) in Ca^{2+} mobilization and phosphatidic acid production induced by PAF-acether in human platelets, Thromb. Res. In press.

Sirois, P., Harczy, M., Robidoux, C., Borgeat, P. and Braquet, P. (1986). Lipid mediators in lung anaphylaxis. In : Lipid Mediadors in immunology of burn and sepsis, a NATO ASI, Helsingor (Denmark) July 20-25, Abst. p. **40**.

Stanworth, D.R., Griffiths, H.R. and Braquet, P. (1986). Effect of PAF-acether antagonists on pre-formed mediator secretion from mast cells. In : 2nd world conference on inflammation, Monte Carlo, March 19-22, Abst. A 193.

Stenzel, H. Hümmer, B. and Halm, H.L. (1986a). Effect of the PAF-antagonist SRI 63-441 on the allergic reaction in awake dogs with natural asthma. Platelets, analgesics and asthma, IIIrd Int. Symposium Davos (Switzerland) Sept. 7-9. Abst. p. 50.

Stenzel, H., Sannwal, U. and Haln, H.L. (1986b). Effect of the PAF-antagonist RP 48740 on allergic reactions in awake dogs. 6 th international Conference on Prostaglandins, Florence (Italy) June 3-6, Abst., p. 306.

Terashita, Z., Tsushima, S., Yoshioka, Y., Nomura, H., Inada, Y. and Nishikawa, K. (1983). CV 3988 - a specific antagonist of platelet activating factor (PAF), Life Sci. **32**, 1975-1982.

Touvay, C., Etienne, A. and Braquet, P. (1985). Inhibition of antigen-induced lung anaphylaxis in the guinea-pig by BN 52021 a new specific PAF-acether receptor antagonist isolated from *Ginkgo biloba*. Agents Actions **17**, 371-372.

Touvay, C., Vilain, B., Taylor, J.E., Etienne, A. and Braquet, P. (1986a). Proof of the involvement of platelet-activating factor (PAF-acether) in pulmonary complex immune systems using a specific PAF-acether receptor antagonist : BN 52021. Prog. Lip. Res. In press.

Touvay, C., Vilain, B., Etienne, A., Sirois, P., Borgeat, P. and Braquet, P. (1986b). Characterization of platelet-activating factor (PAF-acether)-induced contractions of guinea-pig lung strips by selected inhibitors of arachidonic acid metabolism and by PAF antagonists. Immunopharmacology. In press.

Touvay, C., Vilain, B., Carré, C., Etienne, A. and Braquet, P. (1986c). Comparative effects of three orally active PAF-receptor antagonists extracted from *Ginkgo biloba* on *in vivo* bronchoconstrictions and *in vitro* lung strips contractions induced by PAF-acether. 6 th Conference on prostaglandins and related compounds. Abst. Florence, June 3-6, p. 316.

Van der Bosh, J.M., Heye, C., Wagenaar, S.S. and van Velzen-Blad, H.C. (1986). Bronchoalveolar lavage in extrinsic allergic alveolitis. Respiration **49**, 45-51.

Vargaftig, B.B., Borgeat, P., Braquet, P., Braquet, M., Brocklehurst, W.E., Dahlen, S.E., Drazen, J.M., Etienne, A., Fitzpatruck, F.A., Henson, P.M., Holgate, S.T., Israel, E., Mencia-Huerta, J.M., Murphy, R.C., Robinson, C., Shore, S. (1985). Ann. Inst. Pasteur/Immunol. 136D, 175-228.

Vargaftig, B.B. and Braquet, P. (1986). PAF-acether to day : relevance for acute experimental anaphylaxis. Brit. J. Med. In. press.

Vilain, B., Lagente, V., Touvay, C., Desquand, S., Randon, J., Lefort, J., Braquet, P. and Vargaftig, B.B. (1986). Pharmacological control of the in vivo passive anaphylactic shock by the PAF-acether antagonist compound BN 52021. Pharmacol. res. Commun., **18 (Supp.)**, 119-126.

Villamediana, L.M., Sanz, E., Fernandez-Gallardo, S., Caramelo, C., Sanchez-Crespo, M., Braquet, P. and Lopes-Novoa, J.M. (1986). Effects of the platelet-activating factor antagonist BN 52021 on the hemodynamics of rats with experimental cirrhosis of the livers. Life Sciences, **39**, 201-205.

Voelkel, N.F., Worche, S., Reeves, J.T., Henson, P.M. and Murphy, R.C. (1982). Nonimmunological production of leukotrienes induced by platelet activating factor. Science. **218**, 286-288.

Wallace, J.L., Stell, G., Whittle, B.J.R., Lagente, V. and Vargaftig, B.B. (1986). Evidence for platelet activating factor (PAF) as a mediator of endotoxin-induced gastro intestinal damage in the rat : effects of three PAF antagonists. Gastroenterology. In press.

Wardlaw, A.J. and Kay, A.B. (1986) PAF-acether is a potent chemotactic factor for human eosinophils, J. Allergy Clin. Immunol., **77**, 236.

Winslow, C.M., Anderson, R.C., D'Aries, F.J., Frish, G.E., Dellilo, A.K., Lee, M.L. and Saunders, R.N. (1985). Toward understanding the mechanism of action of PAF receptor antagonists, in : New Horizons in Platelet Activating Factor Research (M.L. Lee and C.M. Winslow, eds.) John Wiley (in press).

EVIDENCE FOR PLATELET ACTIVATION IN ALLERGIC ASTHMA

P. Gresele, E. Ribaldi, S. Grasselli, T. Todisco, G. G. Nenci

Istituto di Semeiotica Medica, University of Perugia, Italy

Introduction

Several experimental studies in animals have shown that platelets are involved in allergic responses. The exposure to an antigen induces, in sensitized rabbits or guinea pigs, bronchoconstriction associated with intravascular aggregation of platelets, release of platelet factor 4 (PF4), a platelet-specific protein, and pulmonary sequestration of platelet aggregates (1-3). Platelet depletion of the experimental animals abrogates allergic bronchoconstriction (1,4). A series of responses similar to those evoked by allergen challenge can be reproduced by the intravenous injection or intratracheal instillation of the ether-linked phospholipid PAF-acether into experimental animals (3-6). Platelets play a central role in these effects of PAF-acether: in the rat, whose platelets do not respond to PAF-acether, the intravenous injection of the ether-linked phospholipid does not induce bronchoconstriction; platelet depletion of guinea-pigs or rabbits abolishes the effects of PAF-acether on lung function; intravenous injection of prostacyclin, at doses which prevent platelet activation but do not influence by themselves bronchus tone, contrasts the bronchoconstrictor activity of PAF-acether (7). Exposure to PAF-acether provokes the release of platelet granules (7), and substances able to inhibit the platelet release reaction suppress the bronchoconstriction induced by antigen or PAF-acether in experimental animals (3,7). Exposure of platelets to PAF-acether induces a temporary refractoriness to this inducer (7): in sensitized rabbits, platelets exhibit a hypoaggregability to PAF-acether in the period following exposure to the allergen (8).

Although most of the evidence available on participation of platelets to allergic bronchoconstriction derives from animal studies, a number of reports exist which may indicate that similar phenomena are also operative in man.

Platelets and Clinical Asthma: Literature Studies

The studies concerning platelet involvement in asthma in man can be divided in three main groups: those reporting on abnormalities of the aggregation of platelets of asthmatic subjects when studied in vitro with the photometric method of Born; those trying to detect a condition of platelet activation in vivo concomitant to asthmatic attacks; and studies reporting on other aspects possibly relevant to platelet participation in asthma.

Numerous studies have attempted to establish whether the platelets from patients with asthma present a special pattern of aggregation in vitro (table I). Various platelet agonists have been tested and both normal and abnormal aggregation responses have been reported (9-16). In one of the most complete of these studies, Maccia and coworkers found that abnormal platelet responses to ADP and epinephrine were significantly more frequent in the patient population, and especially in those cases with a well identified immunologic basis for their disease (14). The main abnormality was the absence of the second wave of platelet aggregation; a similar abnormality is observed in a number of conditions in which the platelets overstimulated in vivo become partially refractory to a subsequent stimulation in vitro (17). Interestingly, Maccia and coworkers reported that in some of their atopic patients the platelet abnormality disappeared when the studies were repeated several months after the end of the allergy season (14).

Table I. Platelets and asthma - human studies. Platelet aggregation studies.

Patients (no.)	Aggregating agent	Results	Reference
N.S.	ADP	Abnormal (2nd phase)	Fishel et al., 1970
26	Epinephrine	Abnormal (2nd phase)	Solinger et al., 1973
10	Epinephrine ADP Streptoc.M Prot.	Normal	Harwell et al., 1973
15	Collagen	↑ sensitivity to aspirin	Schwartz et al., 1973
41	Epinephrine	Normal	McDonald et al., 1974
33	Epinephrine ADP Thrombin Collagen	Abnormal Abnormal Abnormal(±) Abnormal(±)	Maccia et al., 1977
12	PAF Collagen	Abnormal Normal	Thompson et al., 1984
6	ADP	Normal	Greer et al., 1984

Other authors did not find any significant abnormality of platelet aggregation in patients with asthma (11,13,16). These conflicting results may be explained by one of the following: different characteristics of the patient population (indeed, it must be considered that under the general definition of asthma several separate clinical entities may be collected); the use of supramaximal concentrations of aggregation inducers, able to overcome the platelet functional defect; improper selection of the control group; improper selection of the period of the study.

Another particularly interesting observation is the report by Thompson et al. of a transient, selective hypoaggregability to PAF-acether, following spontaneous or antigen-challenge-induced asthma but not following aspecific (cold air-induced) bronchospasm (15). This finding suggests an exposure of platelets to PAF-acether in vivo during the specific allergic bronchoconstriction determining the observed in vitro refractoriness.

More recently, a series of studies has addressed the problem of platelet participation in human asthma by trying to detect platelet activation in vivo using different methods (18-26)(table II). In four different studies involving a total of 57 patients, a significant elevation of PF4 and/or β-thromboglobulin (β-TG) in plasma, two platelet specific proteins released upon platelet activation (27), was detected concomitantly to antigen-or exercise-challenge-induced asthma (18,19,23,25,26). In three other studies involving a total of 27 patients, however, the changes in β-TG and PF4 during antigen-bronchoprovocation did not attain the level of significance (21,22,24). It must be noted that even in those studies where a significant elevation of these markers of platelet-activation was found, a wide variability from patient to patient was observed, with some subjects even presenting a pattern of PF4/β-TG release not differing from that seen in normal volunteers studied under the same conditions (18,25). The small numbers of patients studied, different clinical characteristics of the patient population, differences in the conditions of the study (such as antigen-challenge technique) and in the methodologies applied may explain these contrasting results.

The activation of platelets in vivo during provoked or spontaneous asthmatic attacks has also been shown by using different techniques, such as the detection of circulating platelet aggregates (19) or the morphological characterization of activated platelets in the circulation (20).

Finally, a series of disparate reports may be taken as a support to the hypothesis of platelet involvement in human allergic asthma (14,23,28-31) (table III). Among these, of particular interest are the finding of platelets, some of which degranulated, present in the bronchoalveolar lavage fluid of asthmatic patients challenged with antigen (23) or the detection of platelet activation, indicated by the liberation of a burst of oxygen and cytotoxic activity, of platelets from asthmatic patients challenged in vitro with the specific antigen (31).

Table II. Platelets and asthma - human studies. Detection of platelet activation.

Patients (no.)	Clinical condition	Parameter studied	Results	Reference
13	Antigen challenge	PF4	↑	Knauer et al., 1981
5	Antigen challenge	βTG CPA	↑	Gresele et al., 1982
8	Spontaneous attack	Circulating activated platelets	↑	Traietti et al.,1984
6	Antigen challenge	βTG TxB_2	= =	Greer et al., 1985
13	Antigen challenge	βTG PF4	= =	Durham et al., 1985
20	Antigen challenge	FPA βTG PF4	↑ ↑ =(±)	Metzger et al.,1985
8	Antigen challenge	βTG TxB_2	= ↑	Shephard et al.,1985
15	Antigen challenge	βTG CPA	↑ ↑	Gresele et al.,1985
9	Exercise challenge	βTG PF4	↑ ↑	Johnson et al.,1986

Platelets and Clinical Asthma: Personal Studies

In a first series of experiments we have studied a total of 15 patients with allergic asthma (dyspnea and wheezing during the pollination season, positive immediate skin-reaction to the specific allergen). Plasma βTG and circulating platelet aggregates (CPA) (32) were measured before and at various intervals, up to 30 min., after antigen inhalation (19,25). We found that following specific bronchoprovocation a drop of the forced expiratory volume during 1 sec. (FEV_1) was associated with a significant rise of plasma βTG and of circulating platelet aggregates. Although both these parameters were significantly modified by antigen challenge in the group as a whole, the size of the alterations was very variable from patient to patient, with some subjects even showing no modifications. The changes in FEV_1 and plasma βTG

Table III. Platelets and asthma - human studies. Other evidence of platelet involvement.

Patients (no.)	Parameter studied	Results	Reference
29	platelet count (allergen challenge)	↓	Storck et al., 1955
2	intraplatelet nucleotides	↓	D'Souza & Glueck, 1977
33	release of 5HT, PF4 (by collagen, epinephrine, ADP)	↓	Maccia et al., 1977
3	pulmonary megakaryocytes (status asthmaticus)	↑	Slater et al., 1985
12	platelets in broncho-alveolar lavage fluid (antigen challenge)	↑ (degranulated)	Metzger et al., 1985
N.S.	oxygen generation by platelets challenged with antigen	↑	Capron et al., 1985

followed a similar temporal pattern, reaching peak alterations at 10 min and then tending to return toward basal values (19,25). Control experiments, carried out in 6 healthy volunteers to evaluate whether the blood sampling procedures could affect plasma β-TG levels, excluded an artifactual increase of β-TG in asthmatics (25); aspecific bronchoconstriction, obtained with methacholine inhalation in asthmatic subjects, was not accompanied by a significant platelet activation. The administration of aspirin (500 mg x 2) or sulphinpyrazone (400 x 2) to four asthmatics did not inhibit either the β-TG rise or the drop of FEV_1 induced by allergen-challenge (25).

In a second series of experiments we studied a total of 7 patients with allergic asthma during a period of symptomatic spontaneous bronchoconstriction (pollination season). Six of these patients were studied again on a later occasion, when they were asymptomatic. Care was taken to select patients with no history of allergy to aspirin; no drugs were allowed during the study period except for β2-stimulants by inhalation when strictly necessary. After a determination of the FEV_1 was carried out, blood was taken for the determination of platelet production of malondialdehyde (MDA), a byproduct of the arachidonic acid metabolism through the cyclooxygenase pathway in platelets, according to a previously described method (33). After the basal evaluation, each patient ingested 500 mg of aspirin and the platelet regeneration time (PRT) was indirectly evaluated by daily determinations of MDA recovery (34). Six age and sex matched controls were simultaneously studied in the same way. PRT was significantly shortened in asthmatic patients during periods of bronchoconstriction (mean FEV_1 reduction of around 40%) as compared to healthy controls. When studied again in an asymptomatic period (mean FEV_1 reduction of around 15%) the patients no longer showed a shortened PRT (Fig. 1).

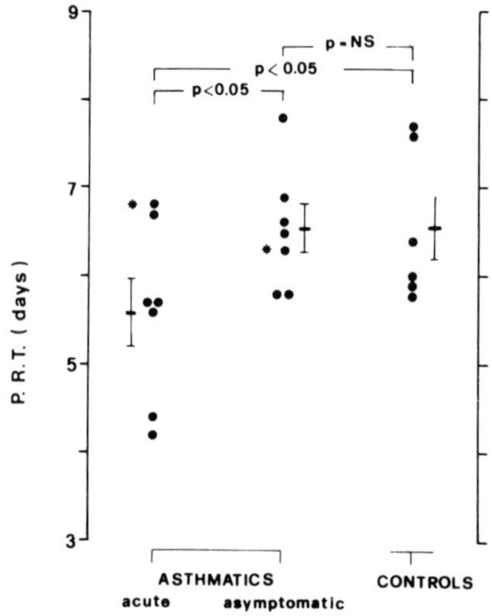

Fig. 1. Platelet regeneration time (PRT) in 7 asthmatic patients during a spontaneous attack and during an asymptomatic period and in 6 normal controls. One patient was studied only during the period of spontaneous bronchoconstriction, and another only during the asymptomatic phase (asterisks).

A shortening of the PRT is considered as an index of in vivo platelet activation leading to an accelerated platelet consumption (35).

Platelets and Clinical Asthma: Possible Connections

Some recent experimental findings seem to corroborate the hypothesis that platelets are not simply involved as innocent bystanders in the phenomenon of asthma but actively participate in it. Human bronchial surgical specimens are strongly contracted by PAF-acether in the presence of platelets, but neither platelets nor PAF-acether alone exert a spasmogenic activity (36). The intratracheal administration of PAF-acether in humans presenting a cerebral death induces bronchoconstriction and thrombocytopenia (37). A factor released by activated platelets, possibly PF4, induces the release of histamine from human basophils in a concentration-dependent way (38,39).

Conclusions

Although some controversy still exists, the evidence involving platelet activation in allergic asthma in man is rapidly growing. A possible sequence of events is the following: the interaction between an allergen and sensitized lung cells (basophils? macrophages?) induces the formation of PAF-acether, and the latter activates platelets to release a still-unidentified component contributing to bronchoconstriction.

The extension of the studies on platelet involvement in human asthma and the possible characterization of patient subgroups or clinical settings where this involvement is particularly relevant may help to understand the pathophysiology of asthma and, possibly, to develop more active drugs for the management of this disease.

Acknowledgements

This work was supported in part by grant. no. 840082744 from the Consiglio Nazionale delle Ricerche (Progetto finalizzato Oncologia, sottoprogetto 9.2) and by grant no. 85/0227144.

Dr. P. Gresele, Istituto di Semeiotica Medica, Università di Perugia, Via Enrico dal Pozzo, I-06100 Perugia, Italy.

References

1. Pinckard, R.N., Halonen, M., Palmer, J.D., Butler, C., Shaw, J.O., Henson, P.M. (1977) Intravascular aggregation and pulmonary sequestration of platelets during IgG-induced systemic anaphylaxis in the rabbit:abrogation of lethal anaphylactic shock by platelet depletion. J. Immunol. 119, 2185-2193.

2. McManus, L.M., Morley, C.A., Levine, S.P., Pinckard, R.N. (1979) Platelet activating factor (PAF) induced release of platelet factor 4 (PF4) *in vitro* and during IgE anaphylaxis in the rabbit. J. Immunol. 123, 2835-2841.

3. Page, C.P., Paul, W., Morley, J. (1984) Platelets and bronchospasm. Int. Arch. Allergy Appl. Immunol. 74, 347-350.

4. Vargaftig, B.B., Lefort, J., Chignard, M., Benveniste, J. (1980) Platelet-activating factor induces a platelet-dependent bronchoconstriction unrelated to the formation of prostaglandin derivatives. Eur. J. Pharmacol. 55, 185-192.

5. Halonen, M., Palmer, J.D., Lohman, C., McManus, L.M., Pinckard, R.N. (1981) Differential effects of platelet depletion on the physiologic alterations of IgE anaphylaxis and acetyl ether phosphorylcholine infusion in the rabbit. Am. Rev. Respir. Dis. 124, 416-419.

6. Denjean, A., Arnoux, B., Masse, R., Lockhart, A., Benveniste, J. (1983) Acute effects of intratracheal administration of platelet-activating factor in baboons. J. Appl. Physiol. 55, 799-804.

7. Vargaftig, B.B., Benveniste, J. (1983) Platelet-activating factor today. Trends Pharmacol. Sci. 4, 341-343.

8. Henson, P.M., Pinckard, R.N. (1977) Basophil-derived platelet-activating factor (PAF) as an in vivo mediator of acute allergic reactions:demonstration of specific desensitization of platelets to PAF during IgE-induced anaphylaxis in the rabbit. J. Immunol. 119, 2179-2184.

9. Fishel, C.W., Zwemer, R.J. (1970) Aggregation of platelets from B.pertussis-infected mice and atopically sensitive human individuals. Fed. Proc. 29, 640.

10. Solinger, A., Bernstein, I.L., Glueck, H.I. (1973) The effect of epinephrine on platelet aggregation in normal and atopic subjects. J. Allergy Clin. Immunol. 51, 29-34.

11. Harwell, W.B., Patterson, J.T., Lieberman, P., Beachey, E. (1973) Platelet aggregation in atopic and normal patients. J. Allergy Clin. Immunol. 51, 274-284.

12. Schwartz, H.J., Bennett, B. (1973) The differential effect of acetylsalicytic acid on in vitro aggregation of platelets from normal, asthmatic and aspirin-sensitive subjects. Int. Arch. Allergy 45, 899-904.

13. McDonald, J.R., Tan, E.M., Stevenson, D.D., Vaughan, J.H. (1974) Platelet aggregation in asthmatic and normal subjects. J. Allergy Clin. IMmunol. 54, 200-208.

14. Maccia, C.A., Gallagher, J.S., Ataman, G., Glueck, H.I., Brooks, S.M., Bernstein, I.L. (1977) Platelet thrombopathy in asthmatic patients with elevated immunoglobulin E. J. Allergy Clin. Immunol. 59, 101-108.

15. Thompson, P.J., Hanson, J.M., Bilani, H., Turner-Warwick, M., Morley, J. (1984) Platelets, platelet activator factor and asthma. Am. Rev. Resp. Dis. 129, A3.

16. Greer, I.A., Winter, J.H., Gaffney, D., McLoughlin, K., Belch, J.J.F., Boyd, G., Forbes, C.D. (1984) Platelets in asthma. Lancet 2, 1479.

17. Rao, A.K., Walsh, P.N. (1983) Acquired qualitative platelet disorders. Clin. Haematol. 12, 201-238.

18. Knauer, K.A., Lichtenstein, L.M., Adkinson, N.F., Fish, J.E. (1981) Platelet activation during antigen-induced airway reactions in asthmatic subjects. N. Engl. J. Med. 304, 1404-1407.

19. Gresele, P., Todisco, T., Merante, F., Nenci, G.G. (1982) Platelet activation and allergic asthma. N. Engl. J. Med. 306, 549.

20. Traietti, P., Marmaggi, S., Dardes, N., Moscatelli, B., Bologna, E., Vulterini, S. (1984) Circulating platelet activation in respiratory diseases: differences between arterial and venous blood in COLD and asthmatic patients. Respiration 46 (Suppl. 1), 62-63.

21. Greer, I.A., Winter, J.H., Gaffney, D., McLoughlin, K., Belch, J.J.F., Boyd, G., Forbes, C.D. (1985) Platelet activation in allergic asthma. Thromb. Haemost. 53, 438.

22. Durham, S.R., Dawes, J., Kay, A.B. (1985) Platelets in asthma. Lancet 2, 36.

23. Metzger, W.J., Hunninghake, G.W., Richerson, H.B. (1985) Late asthmatic responses:inquiry into mechanisms and significance. Clin. Rev. Allergy 3, 145-165.

24. Shephard, E.G., Malan, L., Macfarlane, C.M., Mouton, W., Joubert, J.R. (1985) Lung function and plasma levels of thromboxane B_2, 6-ketoprostaglandin $F_{1\alpha}$ and β-thromboglobulin in antigen-induced asthma before and after indomethacin pretreatment. Brit. J. Clin. Pharmacol. 19, 459-470.

25. Gresele, P., Grasselli, S., Todisco, T., Nenci, G.G. (1985) Platelets and asthma. Lancet 1, 347.

26. Johnson, C.E., Belfield, P.W., Davis, S., Cooke, N.J., Spencer, A., Davies, J.A.(1986) Platelet activation during exercise induced asthma:effect of prophylaxis with cromoglycate and salbutamol. Thorax 41, 290-294.

27. Messmore, H.L., Walenga, J.M., Fareed, J. (1984) Molecular markers of platelet activation. Semin. Thromb. Hemost. 10, 264-269.

28. Storck, H., Hoigné, R., Koller, F. (1955) Thrombocytes in allergic reactions. Int. Arch. Allergy 6, 372-384.

29. D'Souza, L., Glueck, H.I. (1977) Measurement of nucleotide pools in platelets using high pressure liquid chromatography. Thromb. Haemost. 38, 990-1001.

30. Slater, D., Martin, J., Trowbridge, A. (1985) The platelet in asthma. Lancet 1, 110.

31. Capron, A., Ameisen, J.C., Joseph, M., Auriault, C., Tonner, A.B., Caen, J. (1985) New functions for platelets and their pathological implications. Int. Arch. Allergy Appl. Immunol. 77, 107-114.

32. Wu, K.K., Hoak, J.C. (1974) A new method for the quantitative detection of platelet aggregates in patients with arterial insufficiency. Lancet 2, 924-926.

33. Nenci, G.G., Parise, P., Capodicasa, E., Berrettini, M. (1983) Platelet malondialdehyde production kinetics after cyclooxygenase block. A study performed with a modified high sensitivity assay. Haemostasis 13, 53-60.

34. Stuart, M.J., Murphy, S., Oski, F.A. (1975) A simple nonradioisotope technique for the determination of platelet life span. N. Engl. J. Med. 292, 1310-1313.

35. Harker, L.A. (1978) Platelet survival time:its measurement and use. Progr. Hemost. Thromb. 4, 321-347.

36. Schellenberg, R.R., Walker, B., Snyder, F. (1983) Platelet-dependent contraction of human bronchus by platelet-activating factor. J. Allergy Clin. Immunol. 71, 145.

37. Gateau, O., Arnoux, B., Deriaz, H., Viars, P., Benveniste, J. (1984) Acute effects of intratracheal administration of PAF-acether (platelet-activating factor) in humans. Am. Rev. Resp. Dis. 129, A3.

38. Brindley, L.L., Sweet, J.M., Goetzl, E.J. (1983) Stimulation of histamine release from human basophils by human platelet factor 4. J. Clin. Invest. 72, 1218-1223.

39. Kagey-Sobotka, A., Lichtenstein, L.M., Orchard, M.A., Proud, D. (1985) Supernatants from stimulated platelets induce histamine release from human basophils. Brit. J. Pharmacol. 85, 345P.

PLATELET ABNORMALITIES IN ASTHMA - DO THEY EXIST IN HUMANS?

R.S. Farr, R.E. Chang, M.L. Wardlow, J.L. Schul, and K.E. Grandel
National Jewish Center for Immunology and Respiratory Medicine, Department of Medicine, Denver, CO, USA.

Background

MORLEY et al. (1) proposed that "platelet-dependent events determine exacerbation of asthma" and that "exacerbations of asthma symptoms arise as a consequence of PAF-acether (PAF) formation within the lung." Quite naturally and reasonably, much of the data to support this concept have been drawn from experiments performed on guinea pigs, rabbits, and rats. There are, however, some significant differences between results concerning PAF among species. For example, human saliva contains significant amounts of a PAF-like lipid (PAF-LL) (2) whereas rat saliva does not (3). Another example is the platelet accumulation in the lungs of guinea pigs following the i.v. infusion of PAF (4,5) whereas there was no evidence of platelet trapping in the lungs of humans during asthma provoked by inhalation challenge with an allergen (6). Further, we are aware of differences between sexes within species, e.g. serum levels of PAF-acylhydrolase (7) are approximately 30% higher in men than in women (8). Because of these intra- and interspecies differences, this report concerns itself with data regarding the relationship between platelets, PAF and asthma in human subjects.

There have been at least three studies that indicate platelets are activated during allergen-induced asthma after bronchial provocation tests. KNAUER et al. (9) showed 7/13 patients had a greater than 100% increase in plasma platelet factor 4 (PF4) 10 minutes following positive inhalation challenges with ragweed extract. None of five non-allergic control subjects had such an elevation in PF4 after antigen or methacholine challenge. GRESELE et al. (10) reported an increase in beta-thromboglobulin (BTG) of "around 450%" during falls (of "around 55% of baseline values") in forced expiratory volume during one second (FEV_1) in 22 patients during bronchospasm after specific antigen bronchial challenge. These changes occurred 10 minutes after the end of the challenges. Control experiments were done on 6 healthy volunteers and they observed lesser elevations of BTG which occurred 30 minutes after the end of the challenge.

METZGER et al. (11) challenged 20 mildly seasonal allergic asthmatic subjects and seven normal subjects with Alternaria. They found a highly significant group difference for BTG between asthmatics and controls. The analysis for PF4 did not reach statistical significance, due to the large variability among the normal population. These elevations occurred during the late asthmatic response (12). The authors (11) also examined bronchoalveolar lavage fluid 24 hours following positive bronchial challenges with Alternaria. Electron microscopy revealed activated alveolar macrophages, platelet granules and free platelets.

In addition to the studies that indicate platelets are activated during bronchial antigen challenge, there are at least two reports that platelets are altered during naturally occurring or antigen-induced asthma. MALMGREN et al. (13) demonstrated the severe impairment of serotonin (5-HT) uptake by platelets tested during symptomatic endogenous asthma. Further, serum and whole blood from asthmatic patients contained higher amounts of 5-HT than that of normal subjects. THOMPSON et al. (14) measured the amount of PAF and collagen required to aggregate platelets from four normal subjects, four asthmatics during antigen challenge, four during cold air challenge, and four during spontaneous acute asthma. Reduced sensitivity to PAF but not to collagen was associated with acute asthma (2 to 8 fold) and allergen-induced bronchoconstriction (2 to greater than 20 fold). These changes were not observed after cold air challenges.

In contrast to the studies cited above indicating that platelets are activated during early or late asthmatic responses, there are at least three studies that failed to detect evidence of activation. GREER et al. (15) challenged six house-dust-mite allergic subjects with antigen and histamine. The FEV_1's were reduced greater than 20% of pre-inhalation values within 30 minutes in all subjects. They did not demonstrate any significant differences in BTG or in platelet aggregation to adenosine diphosphate in blood drawn 5-15 minutes after challenge. SHEPHARD et al. (16) challenged eight patients to an antigen to which they had positive skin tests and previously demonstrated positive bronchial challenge tests as measured by a greater than 20% decrease from baseline in the area below the maximum expiratory flow-volume curve ($A\dot{V}/V$). Two challenges resulted in an early asthma response only, four patients had a biphasic asthma response, and two had a delayed response only. Each patient was challenged after both placebo or indomethacin treatment. Blood samples for BTG, platelet counts and other mediators were taken prior to antigen challenge and then every 15 minutes for 1.5 hr after challenge. Other samples were obtained 2.5, 6.5 and 7.5 hr after challenge. They found no increase in plasma BTG levels or any significant changes in platelet counts after antigen challenge while on either placebo or indomethacin. They did report changes in levels of thromboxane B_2 and other metabolites of the cyclooxygenase pathway, and they concluded that their data indicated that platelets played a minimal role in the process. DURHAM et al. (17) studied 19 patients for BTG and PF4 release after inhalation challenge. Thirteen patients underwent specific allergen inhalation challenge and nine received methacholine (four received both forms of challenge). They found no significant differences in pre-challenge and post-challenge BTG or PF4 concentration after antigen or methacholine challenges. These authors emphasized the need for extreme care with venosection techniques and that an indwelling cannula must be avoided. Further, they suggested that "allergen-induced asthma may reduce the threshold of platelet activation, increasing the tendency of platelets to release *in vitro*; this could explain the discrepancies between reports by different investigators."

Current Experiments

Most of the positive data cited above constitute indirect evidence that platelets and presumably PAF are involved in human asthma. As part of a study of primary acquired cold urticaria (PACU), GRANDEL et al. (18) developed methodology to extract PAF (1-0-alkyl-2-acetyl-sn-glycero-3-phosphocholine) from human blood. This methodology was successful in demonstrating the release of PAF-LL into plasma during the inflammatory reaction that results when the hands of patients with PACU are immersed in ice water. It was therefore decided to look for PAF-LL in the plasma of patients during both the early and late asthma phases induced following specific antigen bronchial provocation tests of allergic subjects. Although the entire study is not complete at the time of this Symposium, this report briefly describes the lack of correlation we found between pulmonary function data, peripheral blood platelet counts and PAF-LL release after antigen bronchial provocation tests in humans.

Materials and Methods

Patient Selection:

One man and seven women ages 24 to 39 with clear histories of asthma when exposed to environmental antigens were selected for study. None of the patients were receiving "around the clock medications" for their asthma and none were taking glucocorticosteroids. Each had a positive intradermal skin test to the antigen in question at a dilution of 1:100,000 w/v. Five were allergic to cat dander, and one each to dog dander, Bermuda grass and Alternaria. Each of the patients had an FEV_1 at least 70% of predicted value at the time of study and had received no medications in the previous 12 hours. The patients were then tested for methacholine reactivity according to the protocol proposed by the American Academy of Allergy (19). Each had a fall in FEV_1 of greater than 20% (PC20) after five breaths of equal to or less than 1.71 mg methacholine/ml saline.

Experimental Procedures

A week after the methacholine challenge test, the patients returned for antigen bronchial provocation tests. An arterial line was placed in the radial artery and kept patent by frequent flushings with normal saline containing 3 units heparin/ml. Baseline timed vital capacities (TVC's) were performed and the FEV_1's were $\pm$ 10% of the FEV_1 prior to the methacholine challenge test the week before. In each instance, the antigen challenge began with 5 breaths of 1:100,000 w/v dilution of the specific antigen. TVC's were repeated each 5 minutes thereafter for 15 minutes and if the FEV_1 was greater than 80% of baseline, the challenges were repeated with 1:10,000 w/v, TVC's were repeated, and the process continued until the FEV_1 was less than 80% of baseline. The maximum dose given was 5 breaths of 1:100 w/v. The patients were not treated with inhaled bronchodilators after the early fall in FEV_1 and were moved to a Special Care Unit for further observation. TVC's were taken every hour for a total of 12 hours or until a late drop in FEV_1 to less than 80% of baseline occurred. When a late fall in FEV_1 occurred, the patient was treated with inhaled beta-2 agonists and a 3-4 day course of oral theophylline and prednisone. The treatment was given because past experience has shown that this type of patient tends to have recurrent asthma for up to a week after a positive late antigen challenge without further treatment. Separate blood samples were drawn for PAF determinations and platelet counts each time a TVC was done. The blood was processed and assayed for PAF as previously described (18). Separate serum and plasma samples were also collected for future determinations of PF4, histamine and neutrophil chemotactic activity levels (NCA) and these results are not yet available.

Results

Seven of the eight subjects had an early fall in FEV_1 at antigen concentrations of 1:1,000-1:100 w/v. One subject did not have a significant fall in FEV_1 after 5 breaths of a 1:100 w/v dilution of cat dander during a 12 hr period of observation. Instead, she developed rhinitis. This negative result occurred despite a good history of asthma when exposed to cats, a positive intradermal skin test to 1:100,000 w/v of the same bottle of cat dander extract to which she had been challenged, and a positive methacholine test with a PC20 of 1.71 mg. The intradermal skin test to 1:100,000 w/v extract remained positive the morning following the negative bronchial challenge. Of the seven subjects with an early fall in FEV_1 of greater than 20%, six tended to return to pre-challenge levels and then had a late response with a second fall in FEV_1 of greater than 20%. One subject did not have a late response when challenged with 1:1,000 w/v of cat dander. This subject was rechallenged 5 weeks later with 1:100 w/v and this resulted in an early response in FEV_1 of 34% of baseline and a late response of 68% of baseline 9.5 hr after the initial challenge.

PAF analysis revealed three patients had one sporadic peak of PAF activity of between 5 and 9 pg equivalents of authentic PAF/ml plasma. These patients had both an early and late FEV_1 reduction and the positive PAF samples were completely unrelated to the FEV_1 or platelet count data. One subject had three peaks, two of which occurred during the antigen challenge period and one occurred 5 hr post-challenge, with the late fall in FEV_1 occurring 1 hr later. Two subjects had seven separate peaks, again unrelated to either the FEV_1's or the platelet counts. For unknown reasons, the blood from a seventh subject had mild hemolysis in some samples taken during the first hour of the experiment using our extraction technique. During this first hour, there were nine peaks of PAF activity, including an 80 pg equivalent peak in a pre-challenge sample. The eighth patient with the negative provocation test to cat dander, described above, had 3 positive PAF peaks during the first 26 minutes after inhaling the 1:100,000 w/v and 1:10,000 w/v dilution of antigen. There were no subsequent peaks of PAF activity until 1 to 4 hrs post-challenge when 3 peaks occurred. Subjectsseven and eight demonstrated how difficult it is to remove blood from patients without releasing PAF from either platelets or leukocytes *in vitro* at a time when PAF was almost certainly not present *in vivo*.

There were no significant or consistent changes in the platelet counts or PAF activity associated with the FEV_1 changes or the sporadic peaks of PAF activity. Of particular interest, thrombocytopenia was not observed in the seventh patient with nine peaks of PAF activity.

Discussion

Our data failed to indicate a correlation between fall in FEV_1, a thrombocytopenia or the detection of PAF. We did detect PAF and saw falls in platelet counts from time to time during the course of our 6-12 hr experiments. In accordance with DURHAM et al. (7), we feel these sporadic changes were probably due to technical problems that resulted in pertubation of either polymorphonuclear leukocytes or platelets that resulted in occasional *in vitro* release of PAF or platelet count changes. When the data from our PF4, histamine and NCF studies become available, they will be correlated with pulmonary function, PAF and platelet results.

We do not interpret our failure to detect PAF during either the early or delayed asthma induced by specific allergen as evidence that PAF is not involved in human asthma. We performed these experiments in this manner because, using the same blood extraction technique, we did find PAF was released during cold challenge of the hands of patients with PACU (18). However, there are major differences between the PACU experiments and the present experiments: 1) the basic mechanisms involved in PACU may not be the same as the mediators involved in asthma; 2) in the PACU experiments, the entire hand is immersed in cold water whereas during bronchial challenge the lung is exposed to only five breath increments of increasing antigen concentrations. It is possible, even probable, that only a small portion of the total lung area was stimulated by antigen and the rest of the lung participated in bronchoconstriction on the basis of neurologic reflex; 3) a greater proportion of the total blood perfusate of the hand is probably delivered to the antecubital vein during the PACU experiment than the proportion of the total perfusate of the lung delivered to the peripheral radial artery. Thus, if PAF were released during antigen induced asthma, it would have been greatly diluted in the radial artery. Further, we know our extraction technique may be only 50% efficient when known amounts of authentic ^{3}H-labeled PAF are added to whole blood *in vitro*.

There are at least two other possible reasons why we failed to detect PAF in the present study. First, the mediator release and the subsequent events leading to bronchospasm may be a local event without systemic PAF release. The systemic release of even histamine after antigen bronchoprovocation tests has been questioned

(20). Secondly, a PAF other than AGEPC with more specific reactivity with human lung PAF receptors than with rabbit PAF receptors could have been involved. PINCKARD et al. (21) have demonstrated that just one cell type, the human neutrophilic polymorphonuclear leukocyte, is capable of producing at least five different species of PAF molecules with the capacity to stimulate rabbit platelets. This entire area of the heterogeneity among the PAFs will require a great deal of study before it is completely understood.

Conclusion

We do not interpret our results as evidence that PAF is not involved in human asthma, nor do we feel the evidence is overwhelming that PAF is involved. As indicated in the literature cited in Background (see above), evidence for platelet activation in human asthma is conflicting and this question needs to be resolved to everyone's satisfaction. Also, some of the key experiments for (13,14) or against (6) platelet alteration and presumably PAF involvement need to be confirmed.

Despite the attractiveness of the hypothesis of MORLEY et al. (1), we believe many more experiments must be done on human subjects before it can be established that PAF is the major mediator and platelets are the predominant formed blood element involved in human asthma.

Acknowledgements

We thank Ms. Gloria Edwards for her skillful technical assistance and Ms. Margaret Hammond for the careful preparation of the manuscript.

References

1. Morley, J., Sanjar, S. and Page, C.P. (1984) The platelet in asthma. Lancet 2, 1142-1144.

2. Cox, C.P., Wardlow, M.L., Jorgensen, R. and Farr, R.S. (1981) The presence of platelet-activating factor (PAF) in normal human mixed saliva. J. Immunol. 127, 46-50.

3. Cox, C.P. and Quissell, D.D. (1985) A novel platelet activating protein derived from rat submandibular glands. Thrombin Res. 39, 343-353.

4. Lellouch-Tubiana, A., Lefort, J., Pirotsku, E., Vargaftig, B.B. and Pfister, A. (1985) Ultrastructural evidence for extravascular platelet recruitment in the lung upon intravenous injection of platelet activating factor (PAF-acether) in guinea pigs. Br. J. Exp. Pathol. 66, 345-352.

5. Morley, J., Page, C.P. and Sanjar, S. (1985) Platelets in asthma. Lancet 2, 726-727.

6. Ind, P.W., Peters, A.M., Malik, F., Lavender, J.P. and Dollery, C.T. (1985) Pulmonary platelet kinetics in asthma. Thorax 40 412-417.

7. Wardlow, M.L., Cox, C.P., Meng, K.E., Greene, D.E. and Farr, R.S. (1986) Substrate specificity and partial characterization of the PAF-acylhydrolase in human serum that rapidly inactivates platelet-activating factor. J. Immunol. 136, 3441-3446.

8. Farr, R.S., Howell, S.E. and Wardlow, M.L. (1986) Platelet activating factor-acylhydrolase (PAF-ase) activity is higher in serum of men than women and is related to levels of low density lipoprotein (LDL). Fed. Proc. 45, 856 (abstract).

9. Knauer, K.A., Lichtenstein, L.M., Adkinson, N.F., Jr., and Fish, J.E. (1981) Platelet activation during antigen-induced airway reactions in asthmatic subjects. New Eng. J. Med. 304, 1404-1407.

10. Gresele, P., Todisco, T., Merante, F. and Nenci, G.G. (1982) Platelet activation in allergic asthma. New Eng. J. Med. 306, 549.

11. Metzger, W.J., Hunninghake, G.W. and Richerson, H.B. (1985) Late asthmatic responses: Inquiry into mechanisms and significance. Clin. Rev. Allergy 3, 145-165.

12. Metzger, W.J., Henricksen, R.A., Zaleski, T. and Donnelly, A. (1983) Evidence for platelet release and thrombin generation in late asthmatic responses. Clin. Res. 31, 164A (abstract).

13. Malmgren, R., Grubbstrom, J., Olsson, P., Theorell, H., Tornling, G. and Unge, G. (1982) Defective serotonin (5-HT) transport mechanisms in platelets from patients with endogenous and allergic asthma. Allergy 37, 29-39.

14. Thompson, J.M., Hanson, H., Bilani, H., Turner-Warwick, M. and Morley, J. (1984) Platelets, platelet activating factor and asthma. Am. Rev. Respir. Dis. 129 A3 (abstract).

15. Greer, I.A., Winter, J.H., Gaffney, D., McLoughlin, K., Belch, J.J.F., Boyd, G. and Forbes, C.D. (1984) Platelets in asthma. Lancet 2, 1479.

16. Shepard, E.G., Malam, C.M., Macfarlane, C.M., Mouton, W. and Joubert, J.R. (1985) Lung function and plasma levels of thromboxane B2, 6-ketoprostaglandin F1 alpha and beta-thromboglobulin in antigen-induced asthma before and after indomethacin pretreatment. Br. J. Clin. Pharm. 19, 459-470.

17. Durham, S.R., Dawes, J. and Kay, A.B. (1985) Platelets in asthma. Lancet 2 36.

18. Grandel, K.E., Farr, R.S., Wanderer, A.A., Eisenstadt, T.C. and Wasserman, S.I. (1985) Association of platelet-activating factor with primary acquired cold urticaria. New Eng. J. Med. 313, 405-409.

19. Chai, H., Farr, R.S., Froehlich, L.A., Mathison, D.A., McClean, J.A., Rosenthal, R.R., Sheffer, A.L., Spector, S.L., and Townley, R.G. (1975) Standardization of bronchial inhalation challenge procedures. (Report of the panel selected by program directors of allergy disease centers; sponsored by NIAID). J. Allergy Clin. Immunol. 56, 323-327.

20. Marone, G. (1985) The role of basophils and mast cells in the pathogenesis of pulmonary diseases. Int. Archs Allergy Appl. Immunol. suppl. 1, 76, 70-82.

21. Pinckard, R.N., Jackson, E.M., Hoppens, C., Weintraub, S.T., Ludwig, J.C., McManus, L.M. and Mott, G.E. (1984) Molecular heterogeneity of platelet-activating factor produced by stimulated human polymorphonuclear leukocytes. Biochem. Biophys. Res. Comm. 122, 325-332.

Prof. Richard S. Farr, Department of Medicine, National Jewish Center for Immunology and Respiratory Medicine, 1400 Jackson Street, Denver, Colorado 80206, USA.

After 15 November 1986, Dr. Farr's address will be: Department of Molecular Biology, Research Institute of Scripps Clinic, 10666 North Torrey Pines Road, La Jolla, California 92037, USA.

LACK OF PAF RELEASE IN EXTRINSIC ASTHMA

G. Menz, M. Schmitz-Schumann, J. Böttiger, and Chr. Virchow

Hochgebirgsklinik Davos-Wolfgang, CH-7265 Davos-Wolfgang

Introduction

Platelet activating factor (PAF, PAF-acether) has been shown to be a potent agent at inducing bronchial constriction and bronchial hyperreactivity (2,11). As such PAF has been proposed as being an important mediator in the pathogenesis of bronchial asthma and that exacerbations of asthma symptoms arise as a consequence of PAF formation within the lung (2,8). In IgE-sensitized rabbits it has been demonstrated that following antigen challenge there is intravascular release of PAF associated with a drop in the number of circulating basophils, platelets and leukocytes (9). More recently preliminary clinical studies have indicated that platelet activation and PAF release accompany exacerbations of asthma (1,7, reviewed by Gresele et al. in this suppl.).

Methods

The present study has attempted to find evidence of PAF release in allergic asthma by utilising the bioassay technique described by Henson and Pinckard (5) where by prior exposure of platelets to PAF renders them selectively desensitized to further stimulation by PAF. This bioassay technique has been adapted for use by increasing the sensitivity as a result of looking at so called threshold synergism between PAF and collagen. Von Felten and Beer (1) have used this technique to demonstrate the release of PAF in a limited group of allergic asthmatics. This technique has been utilised in the present study. In brief, aggregation was induced by increasing concentrations of PAF (1, 1.5, 2, 3, 4 and 5 x 10^{-8} M) in the *presence of 0.15 ug/ml of collagen . Synergistic doses that induced an increase of light transmission of 70% of the maximum aggregation amplitude where defined as the threshold dose of the synergism of PAF and collagen (10).*

Measurements of the threshold synergism between PAF and collagen were carried out in the platelet rich plasma (200.000 platelets/ul) of 10 patients with allergic bronchial asthma against house dust mite, Dermatophagoides pteronyssinus. The patients underwent inhalative bronchoprovocation with a standardized inhalation device (Pari Provotest) applying biologically defined allergen extracts (Pharmalgen, Pharmacia). The inhalation challenges were performed in house dust mite free high mountain area (1600 m) after two weeks of continuous allergen avoidance. The results of the provocations are expressed as PC_{20} for forced expiratory volume in 1st second (FEV_1) versus the individual allergen threshold (log BU, biological unit).

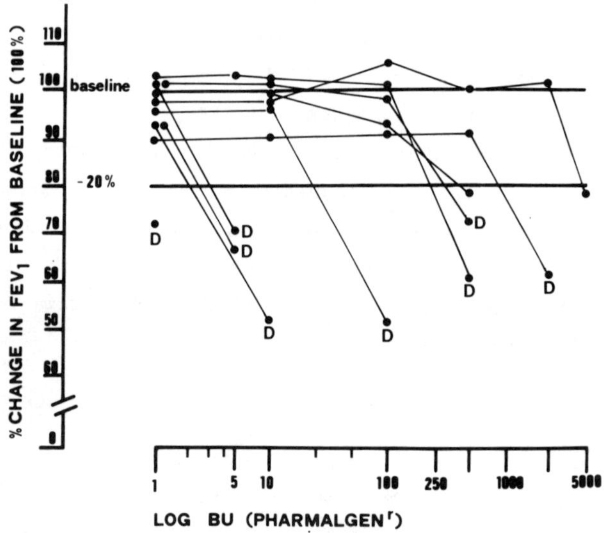

Fig. 1.: PC_{20} (biological units) and outcome of inhalative bronchial allergen challenge in 10 atopic patients. D = dual reaction.

Results

All patients underwent positive inhalative house dust allergen challenge (Fig.1). Eight of them developped a dual (late) response (D). The lung function values at the time of blood collection are given in

Fig.2. The antigen dose necessary to induce a significant bronchoconstriction varied between 1 and 5000 BU (Fig.3).
There was no significant spontaneous platelet aggregation or unspecific response to saline at the beginning of the test as well as 60 minutes and 240 minutes after bronchoprovocation. Neither at 60 minutes nor at 240 minutes any significant changes in the dose response behaviour of the threshold synergism between PAF and collagen could be observed.
These results fail to demonstrate a detectable desactivation of the threshold synergism between PAF and collagen as an indicator of endogenous PAF release after allergen-induced bronchoconstriction in man.

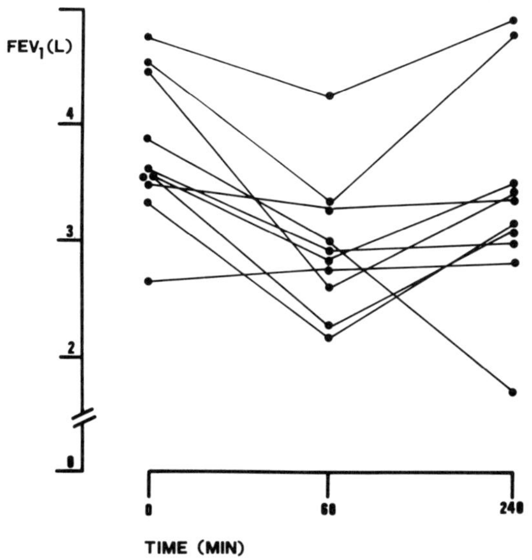

Fig. 2.: Time course of the lung function values (FEV_1) at the time points of blood collection following inhalative bronchial allergen challenge in 10 atopic patients.

Conclusions

We may conclude, that:

1. *The desactivation of the threshold synergism between PAF and collagen as an indicator of endogenous PAF release is lacking the sensitivity necessary to detect endogenous PAF release in a human anaphylactic model of bronchoconstriction.*

2. *PAF is released and acts locally. Only local PAF-induced events may be important in human bronchial asthma. Inspite of the experimental*

predictions in the anaphylactic human model chosen there are no changes in platelet function detectable when platelets leave the lungs after allergen-induced bronchoconstriction.

3. *There may be no major involvement of PAF-acether in the presented model of inhalative allergen provocation in man. However, one must emphasize that inhalative provocation procedures are of experimental nature. They do not necessarily reflect the natural bronchial antigen burden in spontaneous allergic bronchial asthma neither by the antigen dose nor by the time of the antigen influx. All experiments have been carried out under allergen free conditions and complete allergen avoidance. Thus, we can only speculate about the occurrence and the relevance of the PAF-induced platelet activation in allergic bronchial asthma in man.*

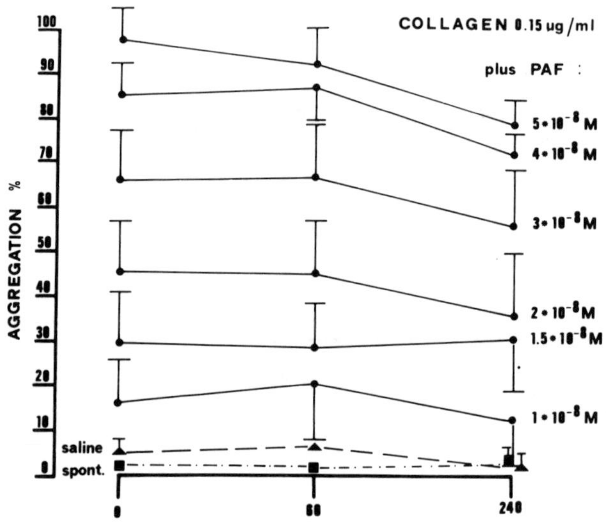

Fig. 3.: Time course of the threshold synergism of PAF and collagen in 10 atopic patients who underwent inhalative bronchial allergen challenge.

References

1.) *Beer, H.-J., and von Felten A. (1984) Wirkungen des Platelet-activating Factor (PAF) auf die Thrombozyten des Menschen. Arch. Diss. Med. Zürich*

2.) *Cuss, F.M., Dixon, C.M.S, and Barnes P.J. (1986) Effects of inhaled platelet-activating factor on pulmonary function and bronchial responsiveness in man. Lancet, ii, 189-192.*

3.) *Durham, S.R., Dawes, J., and Kay A.B.(1985) Platelets in asthma. Lancet, ii, 36.*

4.) *Henson, P.M. (1976) Activation and desensitization of platelets by platelet-activating factor (PAF) derived from IgE sensitized basophils. J Exptl Med 143:937-952.*

5.) *Henson, P.M., and Pinckard R.N. (1977) Basophil-derived platelet-activating factor (PAF) as an in vivo mediator of acute allergic reactions: Demonstration of specific desensitization of platelets to PAF during IgE-induced anaphylaxis. J Immunol 119(6):2179-2184.*

6.) *Kaplan K.L., and Owen J. (1981) Plasma levels of beta-thromboglobulin and platelet factor 4 as indices of platelet activation in vivo. Blood 57:199-202.*

7.) *Knauer K.A., Lichtenstein L.M., Adkinson N.F. Jr., and Fish J. (1981) Platelet activation during antigen-induced airway reactions in asthmatic subjects. N. Engl. J. Med. 304:1404-1407.*

8.) *Morley J., Page C.P., and Sanjar S. (1984) The platelet in asthma. Lancet ii:1142-1144.*

9.) *Pinckard R.N., Farr R.S., and Hanahan D. (1979) Physicochemical and functional identity of rabbit platelet-activating factor (PAF) released in vivo during IgE anaphylaxis with PAF released in vitro from IgE sensitized basophils. J. Immunol. 123:1847-1857.*

10.) *Schmitz-Schumann M., Menz G., Schäufele A., von Felten A., de Souza V., Matthys H., and Virchow Chr. (1987). Evidence of PAF release and platelet activation in analgesics-asthma-syndrome. Cf. in this issue.*

11.) Vargaftig B., Lefort J., Chignard M., and Benveniste J. (1982) Platelet-activating factor induces a platelet-dependent bronchoconstriction unrelated to the formation of prostaglandin derivatives. Europ. J. Pharmacol. 65:185-192.

BLEEDING TIME AND PAF-ACETHER-INDUCED PLATELET AGGREGATION IN ATOPY

A. Szczeklik, M. Krzanowski, E. Nizankowska and J. Musial

Department of Allergy and Clinical Immunology, Copernicus Academy of Medicine, Cracow, Poland.

Abstract

In a double-blind cross-over study 20 mg of aspirin or placebo were administered to 18 patients with respiratory atopy without eczema and to 12 healthy controls. Mean bleeding time before administration of either aspirin or placebo was on average about 1 min. longer in atopics than in the controls, and this difference was significant (p 0.05). Atopics' platelets also aggregated less well in response to arachidonic acid in comparison to controls. On the contrary, no difference in platelet aggregability was detected in response to either PAF-acether alone or to combination of subthreshold, synergistic concentrations of PAF-acether and collagen. Aspirin at a dose used did not affect either bleeding time or platelet aggregability. Thus, in respiratory atopy there exists a moderate hemostatic imbalance, the reason of which remains to be established.

Introduction

Platelet activation may be important in pathogenesis of asthma (8,10,11). It could be triggered through the action of platelet activating factor (PAF), a phospholipid mediator released by many of the inflammatory cells in asthmatic airways (3). There is growing evidence to suggest that platelet activation may occur in allergic and exercise-induced bronchoconstriction (6), and platelet products have been detected in the bronchial lavage fluid of asthmatic subjects (9). PAF is produced by alveolar macrophages obtained from asthmatic patients (2), and may contribute to the pathogenesis of bronchial hyperresponsiveness, which is the most characteristic abnormality in asthma (4). Bleeding time is a physiological measure of platelet function. We have, therefore, measured bleeding time and aggregability of platelets to PAF-acether at rest and following ingestion of a low dose of aspirin in a group of patients with respiratory atopy.

Patients and methods

Eighteen patients (11 men, 7 women; aged 19-46 years) suffering from asthma (n=10), or hay fever (n=8) or both (n=7) were recruited from the atopics without eczema, attending the out-patient clinic. The diagnosis was made by personal and family history, physical examination, skin tests to common airborne allergens and serum IgE determinations (IgE Fast, Allergenetics, USA). During the period of the study patients were free of symptoms of asthma or hay fever or eczema. Two atopics were on prolonged therapy with beclomethasone, one was taking clemastine. Twelve healthy individuals (8 men, 4 women; aged 21-44 years) without history of hay fever, asthma, eczema or epistaxis/bruising constituted the control group.

Studies were performed between 8 and 12 a.m. The subjects were fasting and had not taken aspirin or any other drugs known to affect platelet function during the previous ten days. They received in a randomized, double-blind cross-over manner placebo or 20 mg aspirin separated by at least 7 days. Bleeding time was measured and blood was drawn before administration of aspirin/placebo, and 2 hours later.

The bleeding time was measured using Simplate II devices (General Diagnostics, Morris Plains, N.J.). Two separate horizontal incisions were made 5 cm from the antecubital crease on the lateral aspect of the forearm. Venostasis was maintained at 40 mm Hg for 30 seconds before the first incision to the arrest of bleeding. All bleeding time measurements were performed by the same investigator, and the results were expressed as the mean of 2 readings.

Platelet-rich plasma (PRP) was prepared by centrifugation of citrated blood at 200 g for 15 min. The platelet count was adjusted to 250 x 10^9*/l with autologous platelet poor plasma (PPP). Platelet aggregation was measured turbidometrically in the aggregotometer adjusted so that PRP gave 10%, and PRP 90% light transmission. Arachidonic acid (AA) was prepared as described previously (12) and used in two concentrations: 450 and 900 uM. Stock solution of PAF (Sigma Chemical Co., 1 ng/ml methanol) was diluted immediately before use with Tyrode's buffer containing bovine* *serum albumin. PAF was used in 3 concentrations: 50, 500 and 2.000 nM. In addition, in all subjects, aggregability to cooperating, synergistic effects of combination of agonists used simultaneously at the subthreshold concentrations (1), was studied. To this aim, collagen at a constant dose of 0.1 ug/ml and PAF-acether at increasing doses of 10, 15 and 30 nM were simultaneously used.*

Student's t-test served for statistical evaluation of the results.

Results

The atopics's mean IgE was greatly increased, and averaged 324 IU/ml; the controls' IgE was in the normal range at 51 IU/ml ($p < 0.005$).

Table I - Bleeding time results (in seconds)

	Atopics		Controls	
	mean	S.E.	mean	S.E.
Before placebo	331.3	16.1	278.2	17.9
After placebo	361.1	30.4	286.4	32.3
Before aspirin	323.8	14.7	263.6	17.7
After aspirin	347.3	21.9	399.2	77.3

Both before placebo and before aspirin administration atopics' mean bleeding time was 53 and 75 seconds longer than that of the controls and this difference was significant ($0.02 < p < 0.05$ and $p = 0.01$, respectively). Neither administration of placebo nor 20 mg aspirin had any significant effect ($p < 0.05$) on mean bleeding time in the groups studied. Platelet aggregability to arachidonic acid was impaired in the patients. Thus, in 5 of 18 atopics 900 uM AA failed to produce irreversible aggregation as compared to only 1 of 12 controls. On the contrary, no such differences could be detected in response to PAF-acether. Thus, in 4 atopics and 3 controls, the highest PAF-acether concentration used, i.e. 2000 nM did not produce irreversible aggregation. Analysis of cases responding with irreversible aggregation did not reveal differences in the extent of aggregation between the two groups. Subthreshold doses of collagen + PAF-acether produced effective irreversible aggregation in all the *subjects of the two groups studied; the extent of the aggregation was similar in both groups.*

Aspirin at the dose used had no significant effect on the extent of aggregation in either AA or PAF-stimulated PRP.

Discussion

Appreciation of moderate differences in bleeding time became only recently feasible due to introduction of more accurate methods. Mean bleeding time in our patients with atopic asthma and/or hay fever was significantly longer than in the controls, thus confirming a recent report on prolongation of bleeding time in respiratory atopy (13). The difference was not great, and amounted on average to about one minute, but was present when tested on two different occasions (before placebo and before aspirin). Furthermore, the aggregability of platelets to arachidonic acid was depressed as compared to controls.

Previous studies of platelet aggregation in atopy have produced conflicting results (10). However, Maccia (7) examined a well defined group of atopics and found platelet aggregation depressed using adrenaline, thrombin, collagen and ADP as agonists. When a population of British patients with respiratory atopy was compared to controls (13), platelets of the former aggregated less well to ADP and collagen, but not to PAF-acether used in concentrations up to 400 nM. In this study we used much higher range of PAF-acether concentrations (up to 2000 nM), and similarly, have not observed differences in response of atopic platelets as compared to controls. Aggregability of platelets to combined, subthreshold concentrations of PAF-acether + collagen was also unchanged. Our subjects were in complete clinical remission; in acute severe asthma platelets may become less sensitive to effects of PAF, possibly as a result of tachyphylaxis to its endogenous release (14). The very low dose of aspirin, demonstrated recently to inhibit TxA_2 *generation and 12-lipoxygenase activity (5) failed to unmask any further differences in either bleeding time or platelet aggregability between the groups studied. In conclusion, our study points to moderate imbalance in hemostatic mechanism in respiratory atopy. The hypothetic reasons for this phenomenon have been recently discussed (13), and remain to be established.*

References

1. *Altman, R., Scazzio, T.A., Rouvier, J. and Cacchione, R. (1986) Synergistic actions of PAF-acether and sodium arachidonate in human platelet aggregation. Thromb. Res., 43, 103-111.*

2. *Arnoux, B., Simoes-Caeioro, M.H., Landes, A., Mathieu, M., Duroux P., and Benveniste, J. (1982) Alveolar macrophages from asthmatics release PAF-acether and lyso-PAF-acether when stimulated with specific antigen. Am. Rev. Resp. Dis., 125, A70*

3. *Benveniste, J., Henson, P.M., and Cochran, C.G. (1982) Leukocyte-dependent histamine release from rabbit platelets: the role of IgE, basophils and a platelet-activating factor. J. Exp. Med., 136, 1356-1362.*

4. *Cuss, F.M., Dixon, C. and Barnes, P.J. (1986) Effects of inhaled platelet activating factor on pulmonary function and bronchial responsiveness in man. Lancet., 2, 189-191.*

5. *Eynard, A.R., Galli, G., Tremoli, E., Maderna, P., Magni, F. and Paoletti, R. (1986) Aspirin inhibits platelet 12-hydroxyeicosatetraenoic acid formation. J. Lab. Clin. Med. 107, 73-78.*

6. *Knauer, K.A., Lichtenstein, L.M., Adkinson, N. Jr. and Fish, J.E. (1981) Platelet activation during antigen-induced reactions in asthmatic subjects. N. Engl. J. Med., 304, 1404-1407.*

7. *Maccia, C.A., Gallagher, J.A., Ataman, G., Glueck, H.J., Brooks, S.M. and Bernstein, H. (1977) Platelet thrombopathy in asthmatic patients with elevated immunoglobulin E. J. Allergy Clin. Immunol. 59, 101-108.*

8. *Martin, J.F., Slater, D.N., and Trowbridge, E.A. (1983) Abnormal intrapulmonary platelet production: a possible cause of vascular and lung disease. Lancet, 2, 793-796.*

9. *Metzger, W.J., Hunninghake, G.W., and Richerson, H.B. (1985) Late asthmatic responses: Inquiry into mechanisms and significance. Clin. Rev. Allergy, 3, 145-165.*

10. *Morley, J., Page, C.P., and Sanjar, S. (1984) The platelet in asthma. Lancet, 2, 1142-1144.*

11. *Page, C.P., Paul, W., and Morley, J. (1984) Platelets and bronchospasm. Int. Arch. Allergy Appl. Immunol. 74, 347-356.*

12. *Szczeklik, A., Gryglewski, R.J., Domagala, B., Dworski, R. and Basista, M. (1985) Dietary supplementation with vitamin E in hyperlipoproteinemias: effects on plasma lipid peroxides, antioxidants activity, prostacyclin generation and platelet aggregability. Thromb. Haemost. 54, 425-430.*

13. *Szczeklik, A., Milner, P.C., Birch, J., Watkins, J. and Martin, J.F Prolonged bleeding time, reduced platelet aggregation, altered PAF-acether sensitivity and increased platelet mass are a trait of asthma and*

hay fever. Thromb. Haemost. (In press)

14. *Thompson, P.J., Hanson, J.M., Bilani, H., Turner-Warwick, M. and Morley, J. (1984) Platelets, platelet activating factor and asthma. Am. Rev. Resp. Dis., 129, A3.*

Prof. A. Szczeklik M.D., Instytut Medcyny Wewtrznej AM, Klinika Alergii Immunologii, 31-066 Krakow, ul Skawinska 8, Poland

PLATELETS IN BRONCHOALVEOLAR LAVAGE FROM ASTHMATIC PATIENTS AND ALLERGIC RABBITS WITH ALLERGEN-INDUCED LATE PHASE RESPONSES

W. James Metzger, M.D.,* Kathleen Sjoerdsma, B.A.,* Hal B. Richerson, M.D.,** Pope Moseley, M.D.,** Donald Zavala, M.D.,** Marti Monick,** and Gary W. Hunninghake, M.D.**

*East Carolina University School of Medicine, Department of Medicine, Greenville, NC, Pitt. **The University of Iowa, Department of Internal Medicine, Iowa City, IA, Johnson.

Introduction

Our understanding of chronic allergic asthma has been enhanced by recent studies of the late asthmatic response (LAR). These studies have identified a significant degree of cellular inflammation as a consequence of allergen inhalation and IgE mediated responses to specific allergen [1]. Both animal studies [2,3] and human models [4-6] have been used to investigate the cells and inflammatory mediators required to produce late responses, and the bronchial airway hyperreactivity (BHR) that may result. Most LARs follow an immediate airway response, which is predominantly airway narrowing from mucosal edema and central airways bronchospasm [7], whereas the LAR results in persistent airway inflammation [1] and a more peripheral obstructive airways response [7].

For the most part, these studies of chronic allergic asthma have examined the peripheral effects of allergen inhalation; in order to directly assess the local response to allergen challenge in the airway, we initially evaluated the bronchoalveolar lavage (BAL) of mild allergic asthmatic patients after bronchoprovocation (BPC), and later developed a methodology for BAL following local allergen challenge (LAC) in subsegmental airways. Further in vivo and in vitro studies of the local inflammatory effects of allergen inhalation have been carried out using the allergic rabbit model, whereby neonatal rabbits were immunized from the day of birth intraperitoneally with antigen-in-alum to preferentially produce allergen-specific IgE antibody [2,3] or, more recently, using adult rabbits which were similarly immunized for two weeks following a single dose of cyclophosphamide (150 mg/ml). At the age of three months, these rabbits, after immunization to produce high titer allergen specific IgE antibodies, have hyperreactive airways ($PC_{35}Cdyn$ histamine = 8.7 mg/ml) compared to age-matched normal rabbits ($PC_{35}Cdyn$ = 43 mg/ml), and respond to aero-allergen challenge with early and late phase obstructive airway responses characterized by persistent cellular inflammation.

Human Studies

For human studies, allergic asthmatic patients volunteered and were selected by rigorous criteria. They were young, had mild seasonal allergic asthma, a positive allergen challenge, and had stable pulmonary function for three weeks prior to BAL [5]. Each individual was challenged with the appropriate allergen "out of season," and was off all medications. Patients returned for bronchoalveolar lavage 2, 4, or 24 hours after the immediate response to aeroallergen challenge. BAL was performed at these times through a "wedged" bronchoscope with 5 x 20 ml aliquots of warmed (37°C) saline, and the cells were cytocentrifuged and stained with Giemsa. Normal volunteers were lavaged 6 hours after an aerosol challenge of _Alternaria_ antigen (10,000 PNU/ml). Following BPC, there was a significant increase in the number of neutrophils and eosinophils in BAL of asthmatics ≤4 hours, but by 24 hours, only eosinophils remained elevated [6]. These fluxes in cell populations in BAL corresponded to the presence of neutrophil and eosinophil chemotactic activity in peripheral blood [8] and neutrophil chemotactic activity in BAL [9]. We also found significant elevations in β-thromboglobulin (β-TG) and fibrinopeptide-A (FPA) and a strong trend for an increase in platelet factor 4 (PF_4) in peripheral blood during early and late responses suggesting activation of platelets and generation of thrombin [10].

Local antigen challenge was performed following lavage of a baseline site by instilling increasing concentrations of allergen into a subsegmental airway through the "wedged" fiberoptic bronchoscope at intervals of 3 minutes until there was a visible airway response which was estimated as at least a 30% narrowing of the airway. The site was immediately lavaged and the cells were cytocentrifuged and stained. The initial dose of antigen was determined by end-point skin titration. Later, at 48 hours or 96 hours after the local airway response, the patient returned for bronchoscopy and the same segmental airway was re-lavaged.

Following LAC in subsegmental airways similar findings of eosinophil and neutrophil inflammation were obtained following installation of antigen. Here, the immediate visible response of the airway was blanching, reactive erythema, edema, and airway narrowing. Later, at 48 or 96 hours after the airway challenge, the airway remained edematous and narrowed, presumably as a result of a late response, since all of these patients demonstrated an LAR when challenged by BPC [11]. The amount of antigen required to produce an immediate airway response was highly correlated with that required to produce an immediate skin test, but was one-hundreth the concentration, so that the local immediate response resembled a very sensitive "skin test" of the lung. In asthmatic airways, 48 hours post challenge, total cells, macrophages, neutrophils, eosinophils, and lymphocytes were significantly elevated. Lymphocytes and eosinophils remained elevated at 96 hours, but neutrophils were at normal levels. Peroxidase-staining cells were significantly elevated at 48 hours, suggesting an influx of new monocytes, and helper T-cells were increased 5-fold. These appeared to be an influx of helper T-cells from peripheral blood, as suggested by previous studies using BPC [1], and was not seen in normals challenged with allergen. Gerblich and co-authors have recently confirmed this shift of helper T-cells following allergen BPC [12,13] from peripheral blood to the lung. Mast cells, although few in number, were found by Casale and co-workers to be elevated in asthmatic lungs compared to normals, concordant with an increase in lavage histamine levels [14]. These findings of cellular inflammation are summarized in table I.

Table I. Cellular inflammation of BAL in asthmatic and allergic rabbit airways

BAL After Challenge	Macrophage	Lymphocyte	Neutrophil	Eosinophil	Platelet
BPC					
≤ 4 hrs	NC	NC	↑	↑	+
24 hrs	↑*	NC	NC	↑	++
LAC					
Immediate	NC	NC	NC	NC	+++
48 hrs	↑	↑†	↑	↑	++
96 hrs	↑	↑	NC	↑*	+
Rabbit					blood BAL
EAR (30 secs)	↑	↑	↑	↑	↑ ↑↑
LAR (6 hrs)	↑	↑	↑	↑	↑ ↓

Abbreviations: BAL, bronchoalveolar lavage; BPC, bronchoprovocation; LAC, local antigen challenge; EAR, early phase asthmatic response; LAR, late phase asthmatic response; NC, no change from baseline levels; *, increased but not statistically different; ↑, significantly increased from baseline; †, helper T-cells were increased 5-fold.

Transmission electron microscopy of these inflammatory cells revealed evidence for piecemeal degranulation of mast cells and eosinophils. The eosinophil core material was released immediately into vesicles in the cytoplasm and carried to the cell membrane, where granule contents appeared to be released by fusion of these vesicles with the cell membranes [6]. This could explain the presence of major basic protein in the sputum of asthmatics [15] and deposits in asthmatic airways [16] described by Gleich and co-workers. Macrophages were activated as suggested by prominent ruffling of membranes, the accumulation of intracellular vesicles, and the ingestion of mast cell and eosinophil granules [6]. During these studies, we also noted the presence of platelets in BAL from asthmatic lungs following BPC and LAC. These platelets appeared to be of normal size (1-3 μ) and shape (Fig. 1A), but often granular material was lost (Fig. 1B). Platelets appeared most prominently during the immediate response in humans and were easily visible as single platelets (Fig. 2a) or in groups (Fig. 2b) by light microscopy. They were also seen in fewer numbers as late as 48 or 96 hours after challenge.

Finally, most macrophages obtained during the immediate response to LAC or ≤4 to 24 hours after BPC showed evidence of several to many lipid containing lamellar structures appearing as surfactant from Type II alveolar lining cells or as platelet membranes phagocytized by these macrophages (Fig. 3A, see also Fig. 2B). These cells, with their lamellar structures, were similar to "foamy macrophages" described by Ishihara et al. [17]. Platelets were also found in close approximation to macrophages (Fig. 3B), and in some cases to eosinophils. In a few cases, platelets appeared to be in communication with these cells through junctions in their membranes.

Rabbit Studies

In rabbits, platelets were seen by light and electron microscopy during both

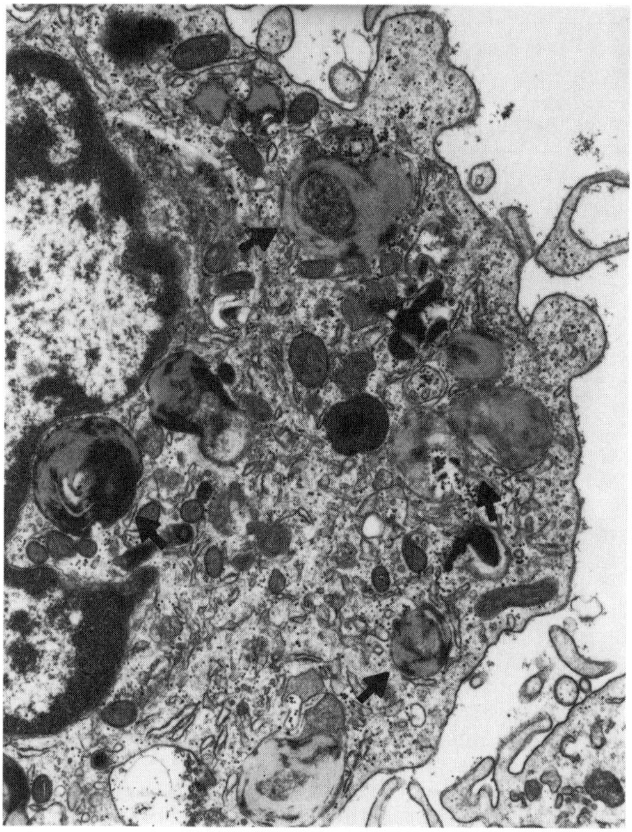

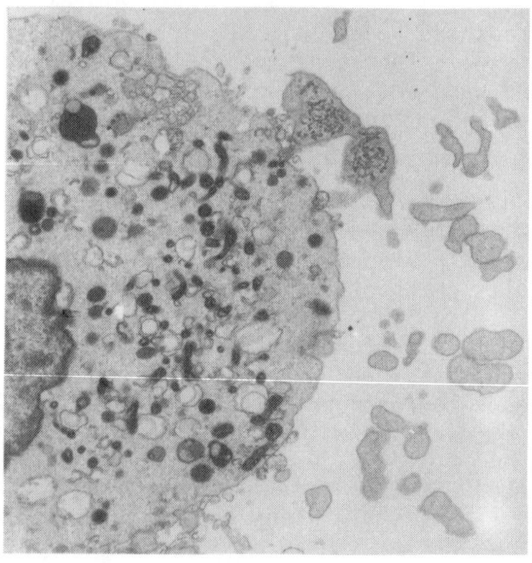

Fig. 3A. (Above) Electron photomicrograph of a "foamy macrophage" containing multiple lamellar bodies (arrows) and a mast cell granule, obtained immediately after local challenge. (x15,000)

Fig. 3B. (Right) Macrophage with adjacent platelets touching cell membrane from immediate response to local antigen challenge. (x6,750)

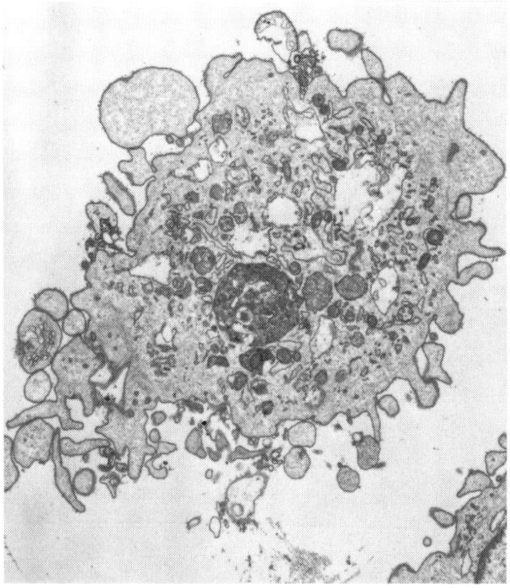

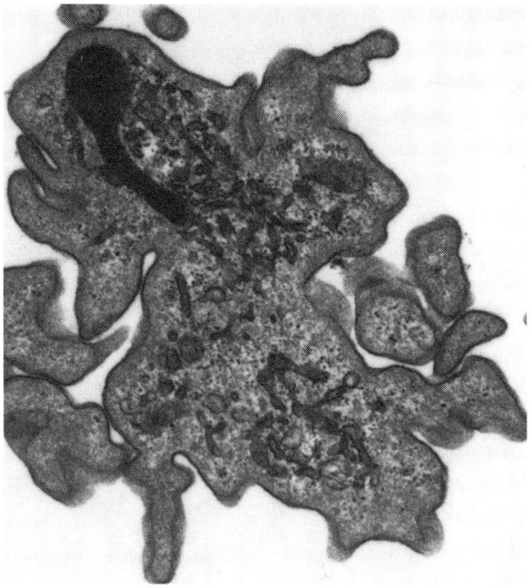

Fig. 1A. Platelet with granules and open canalicular system (48 hrs after local antigen challenge). (x6,750)

Fig. 1B. Platelet from bronchoalveolar lavage obtained immediately after local antigen challenge showing dense body and open canalicular system, but no granules. (x22,500)

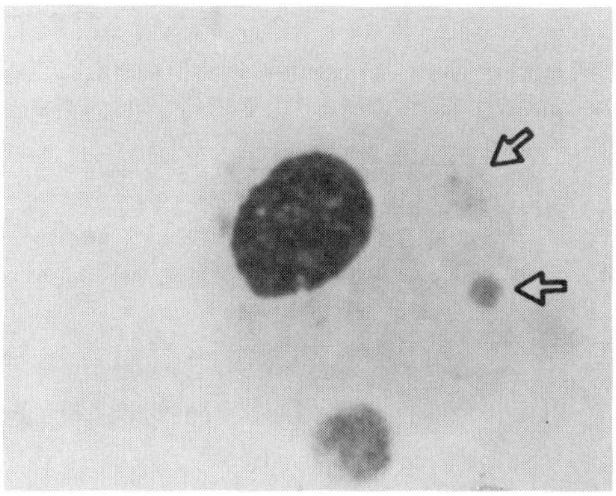

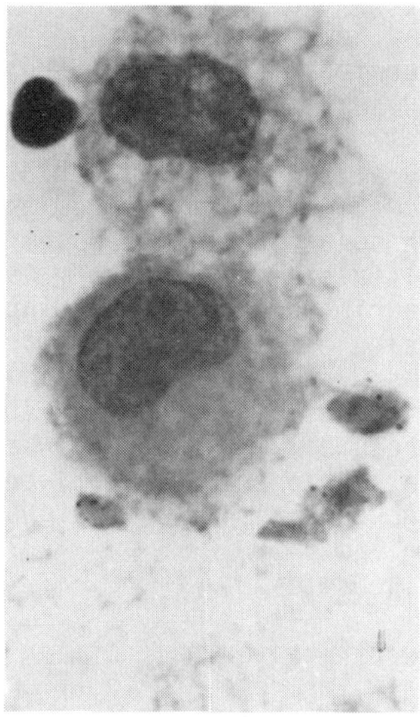

Fig. 2A. (Above) Macrophage with adjacent platelet indenting its membrane. Possible ingested platelets (arrows). (x400,oil)

Fig. 2B. (Right) Macrophage with a group of platelets surrounding it. An adjacent "foamy" macrophage and lymphocyte are also seen. (x400,oil)

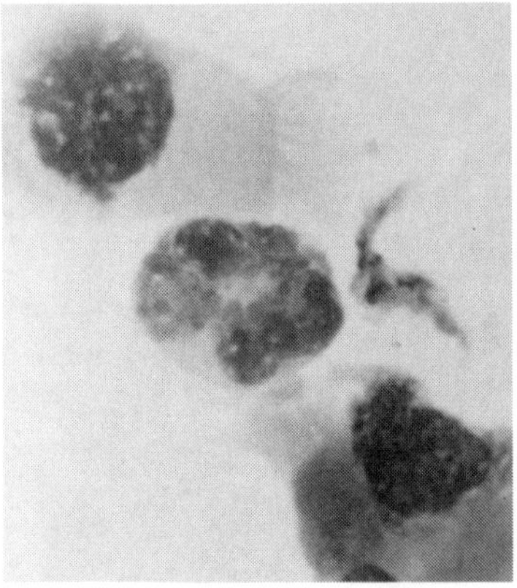

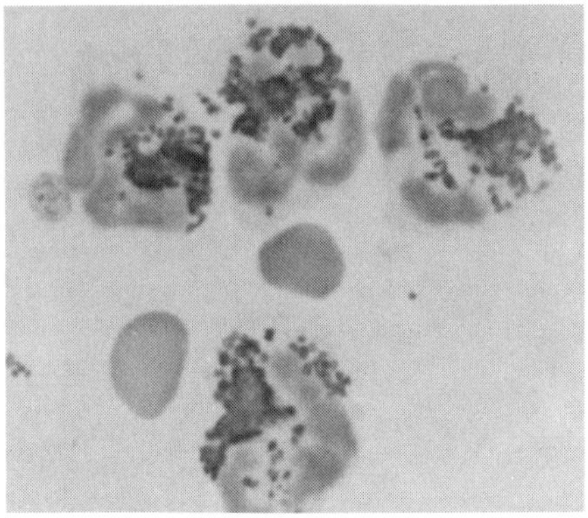

Fig. 4A. (Upper left) Platelet found between ciliated epithelial cells and eosinophil during early response (x 400,oil).
Fig. 4B. (Upper right) Single round platelet with granules adjacent to neutrophil during late phase response (x400,oil).
Fig. 4C. (Lower right) Platelet indenting eosinophil membrane during late phase response (x 400,oil).

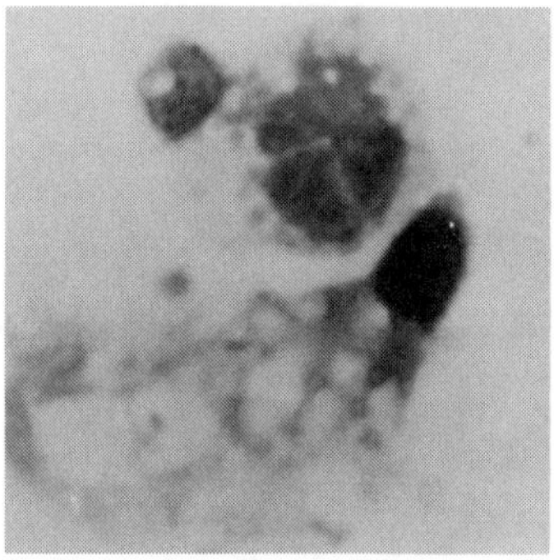

early and late phase responses (Fig. 4a, 4b, and 4c). In a group of seven rabbits, we counted platelets in peripheral blood and BAL during early and late phase asthmatic responses with a Coulter counter and found an immediate increase in platelets in BAL following aero-allergen challenge, and fluctuations in peripheral blood corresponding in time to early and late phase asthmatic responses (Fig. 5). There was a significant decrease of platelets in BAL during the LAR to levels below baseline. These data were confirmed by counting platelets in plasma and BAL with light microscopy using Unopett (Beckton-Dickinson, Rutherford, NJ). Inflammatory cells were observed "breaking through" openings created in the bronchial epithelium with cells passing from the capillaries into the alveolar space. Presumably, platelets, when they are elevated in peripheral blood, could pass into the bronchoalveolar space in a similar manner and be detected in BAL during the early airway response.

Discussion

Pertinent to the question of whether platelets might constitute part of the cellular response to allergen challenge in allergic asthma following early and late phase airway responses, we observed concordant elevations in peripheral blood of PF_4 and β-TG, products of platelet activation, and fibronopeptide-A, a product of thrombin generation, in a group of carefully selected seasonal, mildly asthmatic patients. Further, with the use of BAL following BPC or LAC, we found cellular inflammation, including the presence of platelets, occurring locally subsequent to allergen-induced early and

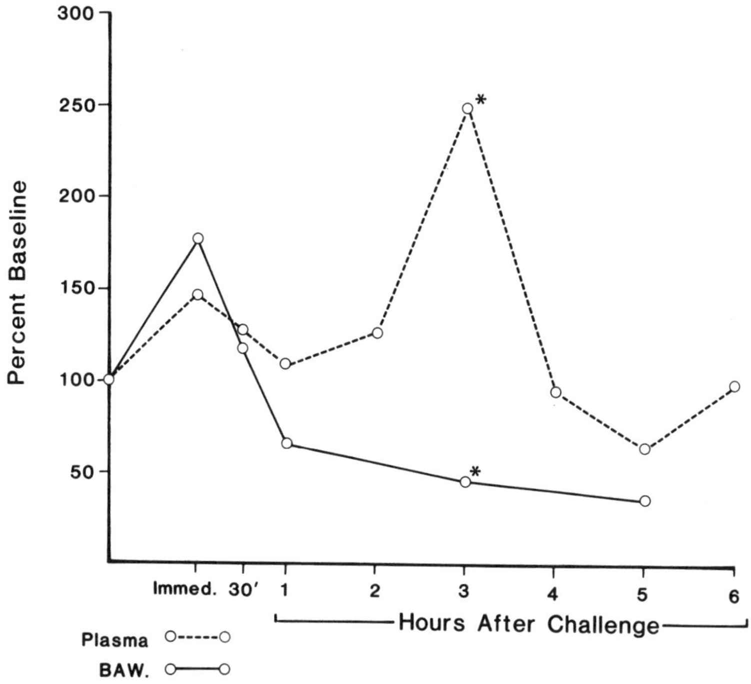

Fig. 5. Ragweed challenge in allergic rabbit showing a biphasic platelet response (dashed line) in peripheral blood, but an isolated rise in lavage fluids (solid line) during the early response, and a decrease below baseline during the late phase response.

late phase responses. Some platelets appeared to be activated, some in communication with eosinophils and macrophages, and some ingested by macrophages. In the allergic rabbit model, a biphasic rise in platelets in peripheral blood was consistent with the early and late phase of the IgE mediated airway response. Their numbers in BAL rose during the early response. The observation of certain cells "breaking through" tracheal epithelium suggests a mechanism for the presence of increased platelets in BAL. Recently, Page and Morley have shown an accumulation of platelets in the lungs from peripheral circulation in guinea pigs challenged with antigen [18]. The finding here of platelets in BAL is consistent with their observation and suggests a role for platelets in allergic asthma. Transmission electron microscopic studies suggest that platelets may be degranulated in BAL and their membranes ingested by macrophages.

Phagocytosis of platelet membranes by activated macrophages could further stimulate macrophages to secrete mediators of inflammation. The contribution of platelet mediators such as PF_4 [19] to the early and late response, as well as the potential for macrophages to secrete mediators such as platelet activating factor (PAF) suggests an explanation for the persistence of late phase responses characterized by cellular inflammation in bronchial asthma and an increase in BHR [20]. The observations of Morley, Page, and Sanjar [21] indicate that PAF can increase airway hyperreactivity and cause inflammatory responses in bronchial airways. A second IgE receptor on platelets, macrophages, and eosinophils [22] that is responsive to IgE-immune complexes may provide an explanation for direct activation of platelets in asthma [1]. The models of BAL following LAC or BPC in humans, and the allergic rabbit model for the LAR are useful for investigating the mechanisms of bronchial hyperreactivity and cellular inflammation as a result of IgE-initiated early and late phase airway responses. The information presented here indicates the presence of platelets at local sites of allergen challenge and a potential role for platelets in the inflammatory response to antigen in allergic asthma.

References

1. Metzger, W.J., Hunninghake, G.W., and Richerson, H.B. (1985) Late asthmatic responses: Inquiry into mechanisms and significance. Clin Allergy 3, 145-165.
2. Richerson, H.B., Metzger, W.J., and Hunninghake, G.W. (1986) Experimental models of bronchial asthma in man and rabbit. Kay, A.B. (Editor) Asthma: Clinical pharmacology and therapeutic progress. (Blackwell, London) pp. 23-32.
3. Shampain, M.P., Behrens, B.L., Larsen, G.L., and Henson, P.M. (1982) An animal model of late pulmonary responses to Alternaria challenge. Amer Rev Resp Dis 126, 493-498.
4. Durham, S.R., and Kay, A.B. (1985) Eosinophils, bronchial hypersensitivity, and late-phase asthma reactions. Clin Allergy 15, 411-418.
5. Metzger, W.J., Nugent, K., Richerson, H.B., Moseley, P., Lakin, R., Zavala, D., and Hunninghake, G.W. (1985) Methods for bronchoalveolar lavage in asthmatic patients following bronchoprovocation and local antigen challenge. Chest 87, 16s-19s.
6. Metzger, W.J., Richerson, H.B., Worden, K., Monick, M., and Hunninghake, G.W. (1986) Bronchoalveolar lavage of allergic asthmatic patients following allergen bronchoprovovation. Chest 89, 477-483.
7. Metzger, W.J., Nugent, K., and Richerson, H.B. (1985) Site of airflow obstruction during early and late phase asthmatic responses to allergen bronchoprovocation. Chest 88, 369-375.
8. Metzger, W.J., Richerson, H.B., and Wasserman, S.I. (1986) Generation and partial characterization of eosinophil chemotactic activity and neutrophil chemotactic activity during early and late-phase airway responses. J Allergy Clin Immunol 78, 282-290.
9. Metzger, W.J., Moseley, P., Wasserman, S.I., Nugent, K., Richerson, H.B., Zavala, D., and Hunninghake, G.W. (1985) Local antigen challenge of allergic asthmatic airways. Clin Res 33, 516A.
10. Metzger, W.J., Henriksen, R.A., Zaleski, A., and Donnelley, A. (1983) Evidence for platelet release and thrombin generation in early and late asthmatic responses. Clin Res 33, 164.
11. Metzger, W.J., Moseley, P., Nugent, K., Richerson, H.B., and Hunninghake, G.W. (1986) Local allergen challenge and bronchoalveolar lavage of allergic asthmatic lungs. Chest 87, 155s-156s.
12. Gerblich, A.A., Campbell, A.E., and Schuyler, M.R. (1984) Changes in

T-lymphocytes populations after antigenic bronchial provocation in asthmatics. New Eng J Med 310, 1349-1352.
13. Gerblich, A.A., Salik, H., and Schuyler, M.R. (1986) T-lymphocyte migration following antigen bronchoprovocation: A model of cellular events in bronchial asthma. Amer Rev Resp Dis 133, 134.
14. Casale, T.B., Wood, D., Trapps, S., Richerson, H.B., Metzger, W.J., Zavala, D., and Hunninghake, G.W. (1986) Elevated bronchoalveolar lavage (BAL) fluid histamine levels in allergic asthmatics are associated with methacholine bronchial hyperresponsiveness. J Clin Investig (submitted).
15. Frigas, E., Loergering, D.A., Solley, G.O., Farrow, G.M., and Gleich, G.J. (1981) Elevated levels of the eosinophil granule major basic protein in the sputum of patients with bronchial asthma. Mayo Clin Proc 56, 345-353.
16. Filley, W.V., Holley, K.E., Kephart, G.M., and Gleich, G.J. (1982) Identification by immunofluorescence of eosinophil major basic protein in lung tissues of patients with bronchial asthma. Lancet ii: 11-15.
17. Ishihara, T., Akizuki, S., Yokota, T., Takahasi, M., Uchino, F., and Matsumoto, N. (1984) Foamy cells associated with platelet phagocytosis. Am J Path 114, 104-111.
18. Page, C.P., Paul, W., and Morley, J. (1984) Platelets and bronchospasm. Int Arch Allergy Appl Immuno 74, 347-350.
19. Brindlay, L.L., Sweet, J.M, and Goetzl, E.J. (1983) Stimulation of histamine release from human basophils by human platelet factor 4. J Clin Investig 72, 1218-1223.
20. Cartier, A., Thomson, N.C., Frith, P.A., Roberts, R., and Hargreave, F.E. (1982) Allergen-induced increase in bronchial responsiveness to histamine: Relationship to the late asthmatic response and change in airway caliber. J Allergy Clin Immunol 70, 170-177.
21. Morley, J., Page C.P., and Sanjar, S. (1985) Pulmonary response to platelet-activating factor. Prog Resp Res 19, 117-123.
22. Capron, A., Dessaint, J.P., Capron, M., Joseph, M., Ameisen, J.C., and Tonnel, A.B. (1986) From parasites to allergy: A second receptor for IgE. Immunology Today 7, 15-18.

Dr. W. James Metzger, Department of Medicine, East Carolina University School of Medicine, Greenville, North Carolina 27834-4354, USA.

PLATELET KINETICS IN STABLE ASTHMATIC PATIENTS. -

A. Taytard*, M.D., L. Vuillemin**, ph.D.
* Clinique de Pneumologie, Hôpital Xavier-Arnozan, Centre Hospitalo-Universitaire de Bordeaux, 33600 Pessac - France
** Service de Médecine Nucléaire, Hôpital du Haut-Levêque, 33600 Pessac, France.

Introduction

Recent clinical and experimental investigations have shown that platelets could play a role in the pathophysiology of asthma (1, 2). So, repeated bronchial stimulation, commonly experienced by asthmatic patients, would be expected to lead to long term alterations of the platelets.
Two investigations were undertaken to see whether the so called "hyper activity" of the platelets of asthmatic patients might change their kinetic patterns, and if some drugs were able to act on this phenomenon.

Patients, materials, and methods

In a first study (3) we involved 20 stable non corticosteroid dependant asthmatic patients 10 of them receiving a short term corticosteroid treatment (0.5 mg/kg/day of prednisone) (AC), 10 of them without any corticosteroids (ANC).

In a second study (4) we tested 9 subjects, non-smokers and light smokers (5 women, 4 men ; < 5 cigarettes/day) suffering from atopic asthma (clinical history, skin testing, bronchial challenge, and IgE).
All these patients were in the asymptomatic phase and at least 2 weeks had expired since their last asthma attack. Usual treatment consisted in the administration of bronchodilator (theophyline ; MDI beta-2-agonists). No patient received delayed corticotherapy less than two months, antihistaminic, ketotifen or cromoglycate less than one month, or immediate corticotherapy less than one week prior to the study ; this excludes corticosteroid dependant patients. Any systemic treatment was stopped at least 48 hours before the test. The patient was advised to take only as needed MDI beta-adrenergic. 13 healthy non-smoker and non-atopic subjects served as controls.

A - Platelet kinetics

a/ Labelling technique.

A total of 40 ml of blood was extracted on ACD form A on day 0. Erythrocytes separation was achieved by slow centrifugation (200 g) for 20 minutes. The platelet-rich plasma was removed and re-centrifuged (600 g) for 10 minutes. The platelet pellet was then resuspended in 1.5 ml of autologous, acidified plasma and labelled with ^{111}Indium (Ox)3. The platelets were then washed with autologous platelet-poor plasma to eliminate any free Indium. The labelling efficiency was approximately 90 %. Such a preparation contains no more than 5 to 6 % white blood cells, principally lymphocytes (82 %) and monocytes (11 %), and 1 to 2 % red blood cells. The final procedure involved re-administering of the platelets to the subject at noon.

b/ Measurement of platelet survival.

Blood samples were taken at 5 min, 1, 2, 4, 6, 10, 24, 48 and 72 hours after re-injection of the platelets and the platelet bound radioactivity measured with a gamma counter ; the percentage of circulating platelets (defined as the ratio of radioactivity measured at a given time over the radioactivity measured at 5 minutes) was then calculated at each of the above times. Thus we could plot arithmetically and logarithmically the platelet survival curve, which was extrapolated beyond the 3 rd day.

c/ Study of pulmonary transit.
Pulmonary fields were viewed with the help of a large-field gamma camera (type CGR acti-camera) interfaced to a CGR MAC 7630 computer in a 128 x 128 acquisition matrix. The heart area and the two pulmonary fields were examined via an anterior view. Indium radioactivity was measured at equilibrium, 15 minutes, 1, 4 and 20 hours after injection. Correction was made for the physical decay of the radioisotope, and the progression in time of pulmonary radioactivity was plotted on semilogarithmic coordinates. Thus, the pulmonary half-life was determined.

d/ Determination of hepatic and splenic uptake and sequestration.
Initial uptake in each organ at equilibrium (10 minutes after injection of labelled platelets) was calculated from the ratio of the radioactivity measured in the organ to the radioactivity measured in the precordial area. The same measurement was repeated each time and was compared to the equilibrium radioactivity of each of the organs after correcting for the physical decay of the radioisotope. A curve was plotted as a function of time in which only the measurement at 48 hours was used to express sequestration ; the upper limit of normal sequestration was 1.5.

B - Statistical analysis.
Mean values (m $\pm$ SD) for each group (patients and healthy subjects) were compared using the Student's t test for unpaired values.

Results

A - Platelet kinetics.

a/ Platelet survival.

In healthy subjects platelet survival was 8.9 ± 1 days ; platelet survival curves of healthy subjects were monoexponential (slope : $\lambda = 0.010 \pm 0.002$ % d^{-1}).
In ANC platelet survival was 4.8 ± 1 days ; the platelet survival curves were biexponential.
In AC platelet survival was 6.3 ± 0.7 days ; the platelet survival curves were biexponential in 7 out of 10.
In atopic asthmatics platelet survival was 4.7 ± 1.3 days ; platelet survival curves displayed a biexponential decay pattern (slopes : $\lambda_1 = 0.134 \pm 0.044$ % d^{-1} ; $\lambda_2 = 0.013 \pm 0.003$ % d^{-1}). One population showing short survival (< 24 h) represented 30 to 50 % of the total platelet population.
There was a highly significant difference between the platelet survival of healthy subjects and of each group of asthmatics. The difference between the value of the single slope of healthy patients and the second slope of asthmatic patients was not significant.

b/ Pulmonary transit.

No difference was seen between the lung images of healthy subjects and those of asthmatic subjects. The difference in the pulmonary half-life of platelets between asthmatic patients (18 ± 5 hours) and healthy subjects (15 ± 4 hours) was not statistically significant.

c/ Hepatic and splenic sequestration.

Hepatic and splenic sequestration of platelets measured in 8 patients in the second trial remained in the range of normal values (spleen = 1.12 ± 0.23 ; liver = 1.24 ± 0.16).

Discussion

In most of the examined asthmatic patients, the platelet decay curve showed a bi-exponential decay pattern whereas, in normal subjects, the curve was monoexponential.

30 to 50 % of the platelet population in asthma patients was affected by the occurence of accelerated destruction ; the remaining platelets displayed a normal survival curve. The cause of this reduced survival time is not clear and some hypotheses can be postulated. Shortened platelet survival corresponding to a monoexponential curve is found in chronic respiratory deficiency and attributed to hypoxia. Indeed, severe hypoxia is required to obtain such a condition, and it is not the case for the patients tested. Independently of this, using the same conditions as in the present study, we studied at stable periods between acute episodes, nine patients, all smokers, suffering from chronic bronchitics (paO^2 = 8.1 $\pm$ 0.6 kPa ; $paCO^2$ = 6 $\pm$ 1.1 kPa ; pH = 7.38 $\pm$ 0.03). We only found one slope and the mean platelet survival (8.5 $\pm$ 1 days) did not differ from that of healthy subjects.

The hypothesis of a platelet sequestration, or vascular marginalisation in the lungs, was not confirmed. Nevertheless, the pulmonary transit time was slightly longer, although not significantly, in asthmatic subjects. The insignificant difference was possibly due to the small sample size. Similarly, no preferential sequestration in the spleen or in the liver was observed, suggesting that platelet destruction is not specific to one structure but that the whole reticulo-endothelial system participates.

The decay curves show that there are two very different populations of platelets. A first rapidly decreasing population and a second one whose curve is identical to that of the normal subjects. The same observation has already been reported in auto-immune thrombocytopenic purpura (ATP), in which platelet destruction is related to the presence of membrane IgG's. The shortened survival time was not so considerable as in ATP, but the platelet count of the patients of the second study was abnormal ($295 \pm 71 \cdot 10^3$) and statistically different from control subjects ($p < 0.05$). In this case an immunological process could account for the destruction of antibody labelled platelets ; IgE receptors have been found on platelet membranes and thus it is probable that they could have found circulating IgE's in asthmatic subjects. Although the IgE blood level was high in this group of atopic patients (821 ± 822 IU/ml), an immunoperoxydase assay did not reveal any IgG or IgE bound to the platelets of these patients, but this method is perhaps not sensible enough for this purpose.

One must also consider both the aspecific lesions of the platelet membrane due to repeated aggregations and the release caused by bronchial stimulation. All these elements could lead to an accelerated, non immuno-dependant, phagocytosis of platelets by the reticulo-endothelial cells.

The fact that the corticosteroid treated patients have a significantly longer platelet life span seems an evidence for the immunologic hypothesis, but that may also mean that an unstimulated platelet is able to normalize its function.

In conclusion, it appears that the functional capacity of a substantial fraction of circulating platelets is modified in asthmatic patients. The causes and functional consequences of this perturbation remain to be clarified.

Bibliography

1. Knauer KA, Lichtenstein LM, Adkinson NF, et al. Platelet activation during antigen-induced airway reactions in asthmatic subjects. N. Engl. J. Med., 1981 ; 304 : 1404-7.

2. Page CP, Paul W, Basraan GS, et al. Platelet activation in asthma. N. Engl. J. Med. 1982 ; 306 : 251-2.

3. Taytard A, Guenard H, Vuillemin L, et al. Platelet kinetics in stable asthmatic patients. Effect of corticosteroid therapy (abstract). Am. Rev. Respir. Dis. 1985 ; 131 : A285.

4. Taytard A, Guenard H, Vuillemin L, et al. Platelet kinetics in stable atopic asthmatic patients. Am. Rev. Respir. Dis. 1986 ; 134 : 983-985.

PLATELET ACTIVATION BY IgE AND ASPIRIN

M. Joseph, A. Capron, A. Tsicopoulos, J.C. Ameisen, J.B. Martinot, and A.B. Tonnel

Centre d'Immunologie et de Biologie Parasitaire
(Unité mixte INSERM 167-CNRS 624)
Institut Pasteur Lille, France

The involvement of platelets in allergic disorders, and more particularly asthma, has been suggested by direct and indirect evidence (8). In this context, the activation of platelets during antigen-induced asthma has been reported (10,16), together with the IgE-mediated accumulation of thrombocytes in the lung of rabbits (20). Some recent aspects of this debated question are summarized elsewhere in this issue (cf. C. Page, and P. Gresele). The interaction of platelets with various other cell types and tissues, through an increasing number of mediators, has strengthened the hypothesis of the participation of thrombocytes to immunopathological and inflammatory reactions (18). The results have led to the suggestion that platelets could play a role in bronchial hyperreactivity in asthma and in delayed skin reactions to allergen in atopic subjects.

The identification of a specific receptor for IgE on the platelet surface (14) has opened new perspectives on their direct participation in immediate hypersensitivity and allergic asthma, and has allowed the demonstration of a new mechanism of platelet activation in allergic and pseudoallergic disorders (3).

1. The IgE-dependent activation of platelets

1.1. The receptor of IgE. The presence of IgE on blood platelets from rat and man was evidenced by flow cytofluorometry with fluorescein-labelled anti-IgE, showing that only 10% of the washed platelet population exhibited a specific fluorescence for IgE in normal individuals.

In man, this percentage was increased to 20% by a preincubation with myeloma IgE prior to the fluorescent labelling (14). In patients with high level of circulating IgE (i.e. helminth infections or IgE-dependent allergy), the subpopulation of IgE-positive platelets was twice that observed in normal subjects, before, as well as after, a preincubation with IgE. In some cases, the fluorescence specific for IgE even reached or exceeded 50% of the thrombocyte preparation. Similarly, Schistosoma mansoni-infected rats had 4 times platelets able to bind IgE than normal rats.

The IgE specificity of the binding was demonstrated with radiolabelled IgE or IgG, which was only inhibited by an excess of unlabelled immunoglobulins of the same isotype (14). Polyclonal and monoclonal anti-IgE receptor antibodies, prepared against lymphocyte or eosinophil receptors, specifically inhibited the binding of radiolabelled IgE but not of IgG (7,14). The Scatchard analysis of the binding of radioiodinated IgE indicated the presence of about 1,000 binding sites per platelet with an affinity constant of 3×10^{7} $L.M^{-1}$*, i.e. in the range previously reported for the specific receptor of IgE on the other inflammatory cells on which it has been described (4).*

These results evidenced, therefore, the reality of a Fc_E *receptor on a subpopulation of blood platelets, independent from the* Fc_G *receptor, and showing antigenic and physicochemical similarities with the IgE receptor already described on lymphocytes, eosinophils, or mononuclear phagocytes, distinct from that on basophils and mast cells, and, thus, proposed as the second class of receptor for IgE* (Fc_ER_2)*(4).*

1.2. The role of the IgE receptor

1.2.1 Anti-parasite effector functions. As already observed with mononuclear phagocytes (9) and eosinophils (6), the presence of the Fc_ER_2 *on blood platelets allowed the expression of cytotoxic functions in vitro an in vivo against the larval stages of various helminths inducing infections associated with increased levels of IgE (11,12). These effector functions were induced by the binding of parasite specific IgE antibodies into the epsilon receptor, and expressed by the excretion of cytocidal mediators as a consequence of the cross-linking of occupied receptors with specific ligands of IgE antibodies (i.e. parasitic antigens, or, possibly, anti-IgE antibody). In contrast with mononuclear phagocytes and eosinophils, which normally required a close contact with the target parasites, platelets could express their cytotoxic properties across filters by the release of soluble mediators (15). However, to an immunological point of view, the most interesting consequence of this IgE-dependent activation was its demonstration in IgE-mediated allergic disorders.*

1.2.2 Allergen-specific activation. With platelets from patients with IgE-dependent allergies (allergen-induced asthma, and wasp- or bee-venom hypersensitivity), it was possible to demonstrate that, whatever the specificity of the IgE bound to the platelet membrane, the addition of the antigen of the corresponding specificity - but not of unrelated antigens - or, alternatively, of anti-IgE - but not of anti-IgG - induced the activation of the platelets, leading to the killing of the parasites, a parameter which was taken here as a probe of the thrombocyte activity (14). In this context, platelets from patients with mite- or grass pollen-induced asthma could be activated against parasite targets by a simultaneous incubation with Dermatophagoides or mixed grass pollen allergens, respectively. Platelets from patients hypersensitive to Hymenoptera venom also expressed anti-parasite cytotoxic properties in vitro by the addition of venom allergen (13). Whereas this effect could be obtained directly with platelets isolated from allergic individuals, similar results were observed with platelets isolated from healthy donors, if they had been preincubated with the IgE-rich serum from asthmatic or hypersensitive patients. The narrow IgE-dependency of this mechanism was clearly demonstrated, in these conditions of passive sensitization, by its abolition after the immunoadsorption of the activating sera on anti-IgE immunosorbents(14).

Another parameter of platelet activation was associated with the IgE interaction, and could be used for the detection of the platelet sensitivity to various allergens: the generation of oxygen metabolites, expressed by a chemiluminescence in the presence of luminol, luciferin, and peroxidase (15,23). With this second criterion, the platelet reactivity could be observed in the very conditions inducing the parasite killing, i.e. with parasitic antigens on platelets from patients with schistosomiasis or filariasis, and with specific allergens, or venoms, on platelets from patients with asthma, or venom hypersensitivity.

The two in vitro parameters of activation described above (cytotoxicity and chemiluminescence) were abolished after specific desensitization of the patients: as soon as the desensitization was obtained, platelets became inactive, both against parasites and in the chemiluminescent assay, and they remained in the same state for several months (22). The favourite hypothesis associated with desensitization mechanisms is the involvement of blocking IgG antibodies, produced in the course of the immunotherapy. In fact, an increase of the IgG isotypes could actually be observed in most of the patients studied here. However, an alternative and interesting suggestion could be formulated, based on the observation of an inhibition of the platelet-dependent parasite killing and of the chemiluminescence by a lymphokine produced by mitogen- or the antigen-stimulation of T lymphocytes.

2. A platelet activity suppressive lymphokine

In man and in rat, Con A- and antigen-stimulated T cell supernatants have been demonstrated to contain a factor able to inhibit, in a dose-dependent manner, the platelet cytotoxicity towards the parasite larvae (19). This platelet activity suppressive lymphokine (PASL) also strongly inhibited the IgE-mediated generation of oxygen-dependent luminescence by platelets stimulated with anti-IgE or with the specific antigen. In man, the subpopulation producing the PASL was identified as $CD8^+$ lymphocytes. The lymphokine had a molecular weight of 15,000 to 20,000 and an isoelectric point of 4.6. It was heat- and acid-stable, sensitive to trypsin and to proteinase K, but was insensitive to neuraminidase. Finally, PASL was specifically absorbed by the platelet membrane, suggesting its action through the binding to a receptor. The involvement of PASL in vivo could be related with the observation that the cytotoxic properties expressed by platelets from S. mansoni -infected rats rapidly decreased after 8 weeks of infection, just after reaching a maximum, in spite of the presence of IgE antibodies in the serum of these animals (13). Therefore the participation of T cell factors, such as PASL, produced by the stimulation of T suppressor lymphocytes with S. mansoni circulating antigens, should be considered in such a decline and this mechanism would appear as a feadback regulation of the platelet immune functions in parasitic *infections. The same PASL also inhibited the reactivity of platelets from asthmatic or hypersensitive patients, demonstrated by the abolition of the killing properties and of the light production. In both situations, PASL has opened the possibility of a potential regulation of immunopathological disorders. It is too early to assert the participation of this lymphokine in allergic patient desensitization. PASL could at least represent an immunopharmacological substance of great interest in the management of allergic diseases where platelets are possibly involved.*

3. Aspirin-induced asthma

3.1 A platelet abnormality. In the analysis of the IgE-dependent cytotoxicity, aspirin was demonstrated to inhibit very significantly the lethal effect of platelets against parasite larvae. When using platelets from aspirin-sensitive asthmatics (ASA), aspirin appeared totally inefficient to inhibit the IgE-mediated cytotoxic process, and even increased the killing mechanism. In fact, the platelets from these patients exhibited anti-parasitic properties - and generated chemiluminescence - by the only addition of aspirin or other cyclooxygenase-inhibiting non-steroidal anti-inflammatory drugs (NSAIDs), auch as indomethacin or flurbiprofen (2). The involvement of an IgE-dependent mechanism was ruled out by the absence of inhibitory effect of anti-Fc_ER_2 *antibodies, and by the inability of serum from such patients to passively sensitize platelets from healthy donors. This abnormal responsiveness to NSAIDs was restricted, among inflammatory cells, to platelets: indeed, the patient leukocytes, which could kill parasites and generate chemiluminescence when triggered by IgE-dependent stimuli, did not express any cytocidal properties nor generate chemiluminescence in the presence of NSAIDs.*

Besides the possible development of a diagnostic test in vitro for this disorder, the above observations suggested a possible involvement of platelets in the asthmatic attacks of the ASA-patients, and raised the question of the mechanism of this abnormal platelet response to NSAIDs.

3.2 The mechanism of the abnormal response. It was shown that sodium salicylate and salicylamide, which are structurally related to aspirin but have no cyclooxygenase-inhibiting activity, had no activating effect on platelets from ASA-patients. Furthermore, when platelets from patients with aspirin-induced asthma were incubated with salicylate before the addition of the analgesics, a highly significant inhibition of the activation induced by the drugs was observed. The preventive effect of salicylate was selective, since it did not affect the IgE-dependent triggering of the platelets. The abnormal platelet activation appeared therefore related to the inhibition of cyclooxygenase. This enzyme transforms arachidonic acid into prostaglandin (PG) endoperoxides, which are further processed into PG or into thromboxane A_2 *(*TxA_2*). Since imidazole, a selective blocker of the thromboxane synthetase, did not activate the patient platelets, the reduction of* TxA_2 *production was not directly involved in the abnormal response of the platelets. Further experiments pointed to the reduced synthesis of* PGH_2 *endoperoxide as a cause of the platelet stimulation, and more particularly to a reduced binding of endogenous* PGH_2 *endoperoxide to its platelet receptor. In fact, the addition of exogenous* PGH_2*, or of its non metabolizable analogue* U_{44069} *, almost completely inhibited the platelet-mediated cytotoxicity induced by NSAIDs, while being inactive on the IgE-induced activation of these ASA platelets (1). Finally, trimetoquinol, a selective antagonist of the* PGH_2*-receptor, triggered the abnormal response of such platelets. This implies that endoperoxides play a regulatory role in the platelets of ASA-patients, which NSAIDs would disrupt. However, the lipoxygenase pathway of arachidonic acid seems also involved in the activating process of the ASA-platelets: ETYA and* BW_{755c}*, which inhibit cyclooxygenase and lipoxygenase pathways, not only were unable to induce the abnormal response of ASA-platelets but also impaired the NSAIDs induced activation. Similarly, NDGA and esculetin, which are more specific inhibitors of lipoxygenase, abolished the activating effect of NSAIDs on these platelets. The precise role of lipoxygenase metabolites of arachidonic acid in this process is presently under investigation. Its determination will enlight the biochemical mechanisms of the abnormal response of ASA-platelets to cyclooxygenase blocking agents (21).*

Conclusion

Altogether, the observations reported above bring new insights into the possible involvement of platelets in the physiopathology of allergy (17). The demonstration of a specific receptor for IgE on the surface of a platelet subpopulation on one hand, and the description of an abnormal response, apparently restricted to platelets, in patients with aspirin-induced asthma on the other hand, both raise the question of a direct platelet activation in some pathological situations. The analysis of the triggering mechanisms in these models and the identification of the mediators produced will define the precise specificity of the described stimulations, compared to the classical concepts of the platelet activation in haematology. In this optic, aggregation and thrombopenia could be unreliable parameters for evidencing the participation of platelets in allergy and inflammation. One aim of the present report was thus to open new perspectives in this field and to suggest original tracks for the exploration of the biological role of these blood elements in allergic and pseudoallergic disorders.

References

1. Ameisen, J.C., Capron, A., Joseph, M. and Tonnel A.B. (1986) Platelets and aspirin-induced asthma. in "Asthma. Clinical, Pharmacology and Therapeutic Progress", Kay, A.B. ed., pp 226-236, Blackwell, Oxford.

2. Ameisen, J.C., Capron, A., Joseph, M., Maclouf, J., Vorng, H., Pancré, V., Fournier, E., Wallaert, B. and Tonnel, A.B. (1985) Aspirin-sensitive asthma: abnormal platelet response to drugs inducing asthmatic attacks; diagnostic and physiopathological implications. Int. Archs. Allergy appl. Immun., 78, 438-448.

3. Capron, A., Ameisen, J.C., Joseph, M., Auriault, C., Tonnel, A.B. and Caen, J.P. (1985) New functions for platelets and their pathological implications. Int. Archs. Allergy appl. Immun., 77, 107-114.

4. Capron, A., Dessaint, J.P., Capron, M., Joseph, M., Ameisen, J.C. and Tonnel A.B. (1986) From parasites to allergy: a second receptor for IgE. Immunology Today, 7, 15-18.

5. Capron, A., Dessaint, J.P., Spiegelberg, H.L., Melewicz, F.M., Ferreri, N.R., Rakin, J.A., Tonnel, A.B., Capron, M., Jouault, T. and Joseph, M. (1986) IgE receptors on inflammatory cells. Ann. Immunol., 137c, 353-381

6. Capron, M., Spiegelberg, H.L., Prin, L., Bennich, H., Butterworth, A.E., Pierce, R.J., Ouaissi, M.A. and Capron, A. (1984) Role of IgE receptors in effector function of human eosinophils. J. Immunol., 132, 462-468.

7. Capron, M., Jcuault, T., Prin, L., Joseph, M., Ameisen, J.C., Butterworth, A.E., Papin, J.P., Kusnierz, J.P. and Capron, A. (1986) Functional study of a monoclonal antibody to IgE Fc receptor (Fc_ER_2) of eosinophils, platelets and macrophages. J. exp. Med., 164, 72-89.

8. *Day, R.P., Behrmann, S., Dolovich, J. and Hargreave, F.E. (1975) Inflammatory effects of leukocytes and platelets. J. Allergy Clin. Immunol., 55, 87-92.*

9. *Dessaint, J.P., Capron, A., Joseph, M., Auriault, C. and Prestel, J. (1983) Macrophage-mediated IgE ADCC to helminth parasites and IgE-dependent macrophage activation. in "Macrophage-mediated antibody-dependent cellular cytotoxicity", Koren, H.S. ed., pp 315-338, Marcel Dekker Inc., New York.*

10. *Gresele, P., Todisco, T., Merante, F. and Nenci, G.G. (1982) Platelet activation and allergic asthma. New Engl. J. Med., 306, 549.*

11. *Haque, A., Cuna, W., Bonnel, B., Capron, A. and Joseph, M. (1985) Platelet-mediated killing of larvae from different filarial species in the presence of Dipetalonema viteae stimulated IgE antibodies. Parasite Immunol., 7, 517-526.*

12. *Joseph, M., Auriault, C., Capron, A., Vorng, H. and Viens, P. (1983) A new function for platelets: IgE-dependent killing of schistosomes. Nature, 303, 810-812.*

13. *Joseph, M., Capron, A., Ameisen, J.C., Caen, J.P., Tsicopoulos, A. and Tonnel, A.B. (1986) The IgE-dependent participation of platelets to cellular mechanisms in allergy. Proceedings of the XII International Congress of Allergology and Clinical Immunology, Washington, Oct. 1985, J. Allergy Clin. Immunol., pp 135-139.*

14. *Joseph, M., Capron, A., Ameisen, J.C., Capron, M., Vorng, H., Pancré, V., Kusnierz, J.P. and Auriault, C. (1986) The receptor for IgE on blood platelets. Eur. J. Immunol., 16, 306-312.*

15. *Joseph, M., Auriault, C., Capron, M., Ameisen, J.C., Pancré, V., Torpier, G., Kusnierz, J.P., Ovlaque, G. and Capron, A. (1985) IgE-dependent platelet cytotoxicity against helminths. Adv. Exp. Med. Biol., 184, 23-31.*

16. *Knauer, K.A., Lichtenstein, L.M., Adkinson, N.F. and Fisch, J.E. (1981) Platelet activation during antigen-induced airway reactions in asthmatic subjects. New Engl. J. Med., 304, 1404-1407.*

17. *Morley, J., Page, C.P. and Sanjar, S. (1984) The platelet in asthma. Lancet, ii, 1142-1144.*

18. *Oxholm, P. and Winther, K. (1986) Thrombocyte involvement in immune inflammatory reactions. Allergy, 41, 1-10.*

19. *Pancré, V., Auriault, C., Joseph, M., Cesbron, J.Y., Kusnierz, J.P. and Capron, A. (1986) A suppressive lymphokine of platelet cytotoxic functions. J. Immunol., 137, 585-591.*

20. *Pinckard, R.M., Halonen, M., Palmer, J.D., Butler, C., Shaw, J.P. and Henson, P.M. (1977) Intravascular aggregation and pulmonary sequestration of platelets during IgE-induced systemic anaphylaxis in*

the rabbit: abrogation of lethal anaphylactic shock by platelet depletion. J. Immunol., 119, 2185-2193.

21. *Szczeklik, A., Gryglewski, R.J. and Cerniawska-Mysik, G. (1975) Relationship of inhibition of prostaglandin biosynthesis by analgesics to asthma attacks in aspirin-senitive patients. Br. Med. J., i, 67-69.*

22. *Tsicopoulos, A., Tonnel, A.B., Wallaert, B., Joseph, M., Ameisen, J.C. and Capron, A. (1986) IgE-dependent platelet activation in hymenoptera hypersensitivity decreases after specific desensitization. J. Allergy Clin. Immunol., 77 (1), 233a.*

23. *Whitehead, T.P., Thorpe, G.H.G., Carter, T.J.N., Groucutt, C. and Kricka, J.L. (1983) Enhanced luminescence procedure for sensitive determination of peroxidase-labelled conjugates in immunoassay. Nature, 305, 158-159.*

Dr. Michel Joseph, Centre d'Immunologie et de Biologie Parasitaire, Institut Pasteur, B.P.245, 59019 Lille, France

METABOLITES OF ARACHIDONIC ACID IN THE LUNG

RYSZARD J. GRYGLEWSKI

*Department of Pharmacology, Copernicus Academy of Medicine,
Cracow, Poland*

Apart from its main function, i.e.gas exchange, the lung performs also two other functions: firstly, the metabolic function by activating and inactivating various biogenic substances which pass with blood through the lung, e.g.angiotensin I, bradykinin, prostaglandin E_2, 5-hydroxytryptamine, adenosine etc. (74) and, secondly, the endocrine function by secreting biologically active substances which are biosynthetized in the lung, e.g.prostacyclin (29).

The oxidative metabolism of arachidonic acid (AA) in the lung is one of the most versatile mechanisms in the body. Permanent and temporary cell-residents in the lung convert AA via the cyclo-oxygenase (COX) pathway to primary prostaglandins (PGE_2, PGF_{2alpha}, PGD_2), to thromboxane A_2 (TXA_2), to prostacyclin (PGI_2), and via the lipoxygenase (LOX) pathway to monohydroperoxy- and monohydroxy-eicosatetraenoic acids (HPETEs, HETEs), to leukotrienes (LTs), to trihydroxy-eicosatetraenoic acids - lipoxins (LXs) and to trihydroxy-eicosatrienoic acid (THETA). PAF-acether is another biologically active lipid that is likely to be released from the lung (22,56). In vivo the lung of humans and cats, on the contrary to the lung of dogs and rabbits, hardly metabolizes exogenous AA during its passage across the pulmonary circulation (53) whereas in vitro perfused or chopped lungs effectively convert exogenous AA to PGI_2 and TXA_2. The ratio of TXA_2/PGI_2 increases with an increase in a dose of AA that is infused into the pulmonary circulation (3,63). On the other hand, endogenous AA is a good substrate for pulmonary enzymes both in vivo and in vitro.

Many of chemical, immunological and mechanical stimuli have been known which liberate endogenous AA and expose it to the available enzymes in the lung, e.g. bradykinin preferentially stimulates the release of PGI_2 from the perfused lung (63) whereas calcium ionophore A 23 187 stimulates predominantly the release of TXA_2 and LTs (18).

The methodological approach to this kind of studies is of the utmost importance. The most common in vitro methods comprise using in experiments isolated lungs perfused via pulmonary artery or via trachea (61,18), superfused tracheal, arterial and parenchymal strips of the lung (17,27,64,77), incubated chopped lungs (33,63), incubated lung homogenates (49) or stimulated cultured lung cells (38,42). The results obtained in vitro, though valuable, must not be directly applied to an in vivo situation. In vivo the intact lung cells interact with platelets, leukocytes, mastocytes and macrophages which are efficient factories of the AA metabolism by themselves as well as they might be suppliers of intermediates.

We believe that various AA metabolites are generated in different cellular compartments of the lung. Although the methodological traps just mentioned hinder the final solution of this problem, however, we have been the first to propose a conception of the compartmentalization of the AA metabolism in the lung (27). The hypothesis was based on the following data. Superfused strips of guinea pig trachea contracted by histamine released a PGE_2-like substance and no TXA_2 was detected, while contracted by histamine lung parenchymal strips released a TXA_2 - like substance but no PGE_2. Moreover, pretreatment of isolated strips with a COX inhibitor (indomethacin) not only abolished the release of COX products but also it potentiated the histamine-induced contraction of tracheal strips and attenuated histamine-induced contractions of parenchymal strips. A hypothesis has been put forward that, when contracted, smooth muscle of large airways generates a bronchodilator PGE_2 as an expression of a self-defensive negative feedback mechanism whereas contractile elements of parenchyma when stimulated by a constrictor generate another contractile substance, i.e. TXA_2 as an expression of a positive feedback mechanism that operates in peripheral airways. Recently our findings have been confirmed in a series of experiments similar to ours. In those experiments, instead of histamine, LTC_4, LTD_4 and LTE_4 were used as contractile agents and, *instead of the bioassay of PGE_2 and TXA_2, a radioimmunoassay of TXB_2 was employed (77). It has been also found that TXB_2 is produced by a line of cultured fibroblasts from human lung parenchyma (36). Following the discovery of PGI_2 (51) we have subsequently discovered that the lung is a powerful generator of PGI_2 and that the pulmonary endothelium is responsible for this activity (25,28,29). This proposal was based on in vivo data which were obtained in experiments on anaesthetized cats, the lung of which had been stimulated by activated platelets (25,28). Presently our hypothesis is that the pulmonary endothelium when triggered by the releasers of endogenous AA such as angiotensin II, bradykinin, muscarinic receptor agonists (25,53), P_2 purinoceptor agonists (35), chemoreceptor agonists or hydrodynamic forces (73), or when the pulmonary endothelium interacts with the PG endoperoxide donors such as activated platelets and leukocytes - then it secretes PGI_2 into blood stream (26). In a way this secretion of PGI_2 might be considered as the endocrine function of the pulmonary endothelium. In humans PGI_2 has little effect on airway resistance (70) and it hardly affects the tone of isolated airway smooth muscle (52,59).Therefore, the primary function of PGI_2 is rather to be sought for in the circulatory system. Most of all pulmonary, coronary and cerebral vascular beds are likely to benefit from vasodilatory and antithrombotic properties of PGI_2 (28,29).*

Since 1978 we have proposed that smooth muscle of large airways, contractile elements of lung parenchyma and the pulmonary endothelium generate PGE_2, TXA_2 and PGI_2, respectively (27,29). Whereas PGE_2 and TXA_2 are local hormones in the lung, PGI_2 apart from its vasodilatory effect on the pulmonary artery (40) is also a circulating hormone (29). Evidence for the pulmonary endothelium as a source of PGI_2 is indirect, steming from the fact that similar agents (muscarinic receptor agonists, angiotensin II, bradykinin) release PGI_2 from the lung in vivo (26,53) and from cultured endothelial cells in vitro (78). The role of so called "circulating PGI_2" has been frequently misinterpreted. We do not consider the lung as a reservoir being filled with PGI_2 from which it is continuously and at random outflowing into blood stream. Our conception is that the pulmonary endothelium releases PGI_2 in response to a strong, frequently pathological stimulus such as bradykinin, angiotensin II, muscarinic receptor agonists, ADP, endotoxin, chemoreceptor stimulants, activated platelets or *leukocytes, hydrodynamic changes in pulmonary circulation and, last not least, some of pharmacological agents. A shot of the released* PGI_2 *at its peak plasma concentration might be biologically active outside the lung, e.g. in cerebral and cardiac circulation. The compartmentalization of the AA metabolism within the lung must not be treated too strictly, e.g. pulmonary endothelial cells release mainly* PGE_2*, much less of* PGI_2 *(62) and a trace of* TXA_2 *(16), although in cultured human pulmonary endothelial cells basic release of* PGI_2 *surpasses by a factor of 5 the generation of* PGE_2 *(38). On the other hand, rabbit intrapulmonary arterial strips generate not only* PGI_2 *but also* TXA_2 *(64). Species differences may contribute to those discrepancies. Little is known about the compartmentalization of the AA metabolism by the human lung.*

The lung not only generates eicosanoids but it is also capable of rapid uptake and metabolism of the primary prostaglandins (7,8). Chemically unstable PGI_2 *is the only prostanoid that is not actively removed by the lung (19).*

Knowledge on the generation and biological actions of the COX products in the lung is well established and has been thoroughly reviewed (7, 21). Within the pulmonary circulation all of the primary prostaglandins (PGF_2*alpha,* PGD_2*,* PGE_2*) increase the pulmonary vascular resistance as it has been shown in several animal species (40). 11,9-Epoxymethano analogue of* PGH_2 *(U 46619), a recognized agonist of* TXA_2/PGH_2 *receptors, is more potent than any of naturally occurring primary prostaglandins in constricting of the canine pulmonary vascular bed (39). It might be expected that* TXA_2 *is a powerful vasoconstrictor in pulmonary circulation. Indeed,* TXA_2 *was proposed to play a pathognomonic role in pulmonary vasoconstriction induced by intoxication with oxygen metabolites, endotoxin and during pulmonary embolism, whereas a hypoxic increase in pulmonary arterial resistance does not seem to be mediated by the COX products (11).* PGI_2 *is the only COX product which is vasodilatory in the pulmonary circulation of humans (70) and laboratory animals (40) and effictively counteracts pulmonary vasoconstriction (75).* PGI_2 *was tried for the treatment of patients with primary and secondary pulmonary hypertension. As said before* PGI_2 *has little effect on the human airway resistance either being infused intravenously or inhaled by volunteers and patients with bronchial asthma (70). The main bronchodilator among the COX products is*

PGE_2, although owing to its local irritating properties PGE_2 precipitates cough when administered by inhalation. Other primary prostaglandins and TXA_2 cause bronchoconstriction. Among the LOX products only LTs are known to exert a significant effect on the lung function. Biological role of other LOX products is not clear, although it has been shown that LXA stimulates superoxide anion generation by human neutrophils (68) and LXB inhibits natural killer cell cytotoxicity against K 562 target cells (67). LTs are generated not only by neutrophil leukocytes (2) and mastocytes (66) but also by stimulated chopped human lungs (33), by chopped lungs of sensitized guinea-pigs when stimulated by an antigen (43) and by perfused guinea-pig lungs challenged by ionophore A 23187 or by ovalbumin (18). The inhibition of the COX activity by indomethacin potentiates the release of LTs (43, 13, 18). Lipidopeptide LTs (LTC_4, LTD_4 and LTE_4) represent the biological activity of slow-reacting substance of anaphylaxis (SRS-A)(12, 17, 41, 66), whereas a dihydroxy-eicosatetraenoic acid - LTB_4 is a potent chemotactic and chemokinetic factor for polymorphonuclear leukocytes.

Lipidopeptide LTs are bronchoconstrictors and promote plasma exudation from precapillary venules, being in both respects more potent than histamine by two to three orders of magnitude. Unlike histamine, lipidopeptide LTs preferentially decrease pulmonary dynamic compliance rather than increase the upper airway resistance (34).

Lipidopeptide LTs exert direct and indirect bronchoconstrictory action. Indirect bronchoconstrictory action of LTs seems to be associated with the release of TXA_2 from the lungs (9, 59, 72, 77), although not all of the scientists share this point of view (4). PAF-acether also induces a similar indirect bronchoconstriction via the release of TXA_2 from the lung (45). In vivo indirect action of LTC_4 and LTD_4 has been following intravenous route of their administration into guinea pigs. Drugs which are inhibitors of either COX or TXA_2 synthetase largely diminish bronchoconstrictory effect of LTs (72). When lipidopeptide LTs are administered through the intratracheal route then only a direct bronchoconstrictory effect is observed. In vitro LTs exert a direct contractile effect on human bronchial and parenchymal strips (65), whereas their indirect action has been demonstrated in perfused guinea-pig lungs and in superfused tracheal and parenchymal strips of guinea-pig lungs (59, 65, 77). In those preparations LTB_4 also elicits a contractile response *that is mostly mediated through the release of TXA_2 (65). Indirect action of lipidopeptide LTs may also involve the release from the lung tissue of another COX product - PGI_2 (9, 24). Indeed, in the perfused rat lung LTC_4 releases both TXA_2 and PGI_2, although in this preparation LTC_4-induced constriction of pulmonary vasculature is mainly completed through a direct LTC_4 mechanism (37). It may well be that in vivo PGI_2, though ineffective per se as a bronchodilator (61, 70) still modulates contractile action of LTs. LTs-induced generation of PGI_2 in the lung might be responsible for desensitization or tachyphylaxis to LTs induced contractile responses of parenchymal strips (52). Direct bronchoconstrictory and vasoconstrictory responses to LTs are mediated via a receptor mechanism. Receptors for LTB_4, LTC_4, LTD_4 and LTE_4 are likely to be heterogenous (23, 44, 69). Lipidopeptide LTs, LTB_4 along with HETEs and the COX products are released by a variety of stimuli from leukocytes, mastocytes, macrophages and other migrating cells, however, the lung tissue itself or pulmonary artery adventitia cannot be excluded as the source of LTs (33, 65). LTs constrict pulmonary vasculature and are not rapidly degraded in pulmonary circulation (37). Only a half of the biological activity of LTD_4 disappears during one passage through the pulmonary circulation, most likely owing to the biotransformation of LTD_4 to less active LTE_4 (57) whereas the biological activity of LTC_4 is enhanced in the pulmonary circulation due to its conversion to the biologically more active LTD_4 (46).*

A combined direct and indirect action of LTC_4 and LTD_4 on airway smooth muscle, contractile elements of pulmonary parenchyma and pulmonary microvessels along with stimulation of mucus release (50) and recruitment of leukocytes by LTB_4 may lead to the obstruction of airway via constriction of airways and inflammation of mucosa. This pulmonary production of LTs may contribute to pathogenesis of bronchial asthma (34) Interestingly, beta-receptor agonists inhibit (81) while beta-receptor antagonists potentiate (10) direct bronchoconstrictory effect of LTC_4 in the guinea-pig. This last group of drugs also stimulates generation of TXA_2 (9). Calcium antagonists (verapamil and nicardipine) and disodium cromoglycate partially inhibit the effect of LTD_4 on the pulmonary airway resistance in the guinea-pig (1). Platelet-activating factor (PAF-acether) seems to be a direct releaser of LTC_4 and LTD_4 from the rat lung parenchyma (76).

Since the LOX products play an important role in pathophysiology of the lung it is most urgent to find a precise site of their generation in the lung, to elucidate a mode of their interaction with the COX products and other endogenous mediators and, finally, to look for inhibitors of their biosynthesis and antagonists of their receptor action.

Presently our working hypothesis on the compartmentalization of the AA metabolism in the lung is as follows. The main site for the generation of PGE_2 *is smooth muscle of large airways; for the generation of* PGI_2 *the pulmonary endothelium; for the generation of* TXA_2 *contractile elements of the lung parenchyma (27); for the generation of* PGD_2 *mastocytes residing in the lung (47) and for the generation of LTs alveolar macrophages (49) LTs may be also generated by infiltrating neutrophils, by one or another type of the stationary lung cells (33) or by pulmonary artery adventitia (55, 65).*

Interrelation of the COX and LOX pathways in the lung is poorly understood. Infusion of AA into pulmonary artery of isolated, perfused guinea-pig lungs triggers primarily the COX pathway. With increasing concentrations of AA, PGI_2*, PGs and* TXA_2 *will subsequently appear in the effluent. Immunological challenge of perfused (preferably through trachea) guinea-pig lungs (61) or chopped human lungs (33) releases a mixture of the LOX and COX products. Pharmacological blockade by aspirin-like drugs of the COX pathway in the lung has been found to be responsible for precipitation of bronchoconstriction in patients with aspirin-sensitive asthma (71). One of the proposed mechanisms of this phenomenon is the diversion of the pulmonary AA metabolism from the COX to the LOX products. This conception lacks experimental evidence and also it is unlikely to be valid if our hypothesis concerning the compartmentalization of the AA metabolism in the lung were true. A transfer of AA which was not utilized by COX in bronchial smooth muscle or pulmonary endothelium to macrophages or mastocytes would be difficult to accept. Alternatively, the COX products such as* PGD_2 *(18),* PGE_2 *or* PGI_2 *(32) (released from various pulmonary compartments) may interact with alveolar macrophages, infiltrating leukocytes and mastocytes leading to the suppression of the release of LTs by those cells. Still another possibility is that* PGE_2 *and* PGI_2 *decrease the responsiveness of specific receptors to LTs in the lung. Indeed,* PGI_2 *relaxes the guinea-pig tracheal strips which are maximally contracted by* LTD_4 *(60).* PGI_2

antagonizes also LT-induced contractions of parenchymal strips of the guinea-pig lung (52). PGI_2 activates adenylate cyclase in the guinea-pig lung homogenates (49) and in perfused dog lungs (48). On the other hand, TXA_2 shows a synergistic action with LTs (58).

In summary, it is feasible that the LOX and COX products of the AA metabolism interact in the lung. PGE_2 and PGI_2 seem to play a defensive role against the bronchoconstrictory action of LTs (52) and a promoting role towards the inflammatory action of LTs (80), while TXA_2 is a mediator of an indirect bronchoconstrictory action of LTs (59).

A search for inhibitors of the biosynthesis of LTs and for their receptor antagonists is a promising approach to the therapy of bronchial asthma (5). Dual LOC/COX inhibitors like BW 755 C are not a right answer to the problem. Antioxidants (e.g.nordehydroguaiaretic acid), nafazatrom, flavonoids (quercetin, cirsiliol), caffeic acid are inhibitors of plant and animal lipoxygenases in vitro *and, similarly to specific 5-LOX inhibitors such as 5-6-methano leukotriene A_4 (42) or some of disulfide aromatic compounds (20) are better candidates for erasing the activitiy of LTs from the map of eicosanoid turnover in the lung. A prostacyclin analogue , 6,9-deepoxy-6,9-(phenylimino)-6,8- prostaglandin I_2 (U-60257) inhibits biosynthesis of LTC_4 and LTD_4 in intact cells and it seems to antagonize biological action of LTs as well (5, 6). A polyphloretin derivative FPL 55712 is in a common laboratory use as a receptor antagonist for LTs, however, it can be hardly considered as a specific antagonist of SRS-A since it inhibits also the release of histamine, TXA_2 synthetase (79) COX (14) and phosphodiesterase activities (15).*

In conclusion, the products of both cyclo-oxygenation and lipoxygenation of arachidonic acid are formed in the lung and/or by cells which abide in the lung. Airway resistance, pulmonary circulation as well as the function of epithelial and connective tissue are influenced by AA metabolites. TXA_2, $PGF_{2\ alpha}$ and LTs increase airway resistance. PGE_2 is a bronchodilator. All of AA metabolites with an important exception of PGI_2 increase the pulmonary vascular resistance. The lung is a powerful generator of PGI_2 that is released into circulation from the lung by a number of stimuli. Inflammatory response in the lung is promoted by most of AA metabolites. A hypothesis on the compartmentalization of the AA metabolism in the lung may help to understand a pathophysiological role and *interrelation between the COX and LOX products. Biologically active metabolites of AA arise from enzymic introduction of molecular oxygen to a molecule of AA and, therefore, the gas-exchange function of the lung may influence its metabolic and endocrine functions. Indeed, chronic hyperoxia (via oxygen-mediated damage to the pulmonary endothelium) or the intoxication with paraquat (via oxygen-mediated damage to the pulmonary epithelium) both produce profound, though different disturbances in the AA metabolism in the lung (18). The superoxide anion-sensitive EDRF (31) is generated along with PGI_2 (30) by cultured aortic endothelial cells. It is most likely that EDRF is also generated by the pulmonary endothelium and, then, its biological action would be controlled by oxygen free radicals available in the lung.*

References

1. *Advenier, C., Cerrina, J., Duroux, O., Floch, A., Pradel, J. and Rennier, A. (1983) Sodiumchromoglycate, verapamil and nicardipine antagonism to leukotriene D_4 bronchoconstriction. Br. J. Pharmacol. 78: 301.*

2. *Aehringhaus, U., Wolbling, R.H., Konig, W., Patrono, C., Peskar, B.M. and Peskar, B.A. (1982) Release of leukotriene C_4 from human polymorphonuclear leukocytes as determined by radioimmunoassay. FEBS Letts. 146: 111.*

3. *Alabaster, V.A. and Hawkeswood, E. (1978) Detection and bioassay of pharmacologically active substances released by arachidonic acid from guinea-pig lungs. J. Pharmacol. Meth. 1: 341.*

4. *Austen, K.F., Corey, E.J., Drazen, J.M. and Leitch, A.G. (1983) The effect of indomethacin on the contractile response of the guinea pig lung parenchymal strip to leukotrienes B_4, C_4, E_4. Br. J. Pharmacol. 80: 47.*

5. *Bach, M.K.(1984) Prospects for the inhibition of leukotriene synthesis. Biochem. Pharmacol. 33: 515.*

6. *Bach, M.K., Brashler, J.R. and Fitzpatrick, F.A. (1983) In vivo and in vitro actions of a new selective inhibitor of leukotriene C and D synthesis. In Advances in Prostaglandin, Thromboxane and Leukotriene Research. (Eds. B. Samuelsson, R. Paoletti and P.W. Ramwell) Raven Press, New York p.39.*

7. *Bakhle, Y.S. (1981) Biosynthesis of prostaglandins and thromboxanes in lung. Bull. Europ. Physiopath. Resp. 17: 491.*

8. *Bakhle Y.S. and Vane, J.R. (1974) Pharmacokinetic function of the pul-*

monary circulation. Physiol. Rev. 54*: 1007.*

9. *Berti, F., Folco, G.C. and Omini, C. (1981) Pharmacological control of thromboxane* A_2 *in lung. Bull. Europ. Physiopath. Resp.* 17*: 509.*

10. *Bougrani, S., Razzetti, R., Folco, G.C. and Schiantarelli, P. (1983) Potentiation of leukotriene* C_4 *bronchoconstriction by beta-adrenoceptor antagonists in the guinea pig. In Advances in Prostaglandin, Thromboxane and Leukotriene Research, (Eds. B. Samuelsson, R. Paoletti and P. Ramwell) Raven Press, New York. p. 143.*

11. *Brigham, K.L., Newman, J.H., Snapper, J.R. and Ogletree, M.L. (1982) Metabolites of arachidonic acid in the pathophysiology of pulmonary circulation. In Advances in Prostaglandin, Thromboxane and Leukotriene Research. (Ed. J. Oates) Raven Press, New York, vol.* 10*: p. 357.*

12. *Brocklehurst, W.E. (1960) The release of histamine and formation of a slow-reacting substance (SRS-A) during anaphylactic shock. J. Physiol.* 151*: 416.*

13. *Burka, J. and Saad, M. (1983) Mediators of arachidonic acid induced contractions of indomethacin-treated guinea-pig airways: leukotrienes* C_4 *and* D_4*. Br. J. Pharmacol.* 81*: 464.*

14. *Casey, F.B., Appleby, B.J. and Buck, D.C. (1983) Selective inhibition of the lipoxygenase metabolic pathway of arachidonic acid by the SRS-A antagonist FPL 55712. Prostaglandins* 25*: 1.*

15. *Chasin, M. and Scott, C. (1978) Inhibition of cyclic nucleotide phosphosdiesterase by FLP 55712, an SRS-A antagonist. Biochem. Pharmacol.* 27*: 2065.*

16. *Crutchley, D.J., Ryan, J.W., Ryan, U.S. and Fischer, G.H. (1983) Bradykinin-induced release of prostacyclin and thromboxanes from bovine pulmonary endothelial cells. Biochem. Biophys. Acta* 751*: 99.*

17. *Dahlen, S.E., Hedquist, P. and Hammarström, S. (1983) Contractile activity of several cysteine-containing leukotrienes in the guinea pig lung strip. Europ. J. Pharmacol.* 86*: 207.*

18. *De Nucci, G. (1986) Lung injury and eicosanoid release from guinea-pig isolated lungs. A thesis for the degree of Doctor of Philisophy, presented at the Institute of Basic Medical Sciences. Royal College of Surgeons, University of London.*

19. *Dustings, G.J., Moncada, S. and Mullane, K.M. (1978) Biotransformation of arachidonic acid in the circulation of the dog. Br. J. Pharmacol.* 63*: 359.*

20. *Egan, R.W., Tischler, A.M., Baptista, E.M., Ham, E.A., Soderman, D.D. and Gale, P.H. (1983) Specific inhibition of oxidative regulation of 5-lipoxygenase. In Advances of Prostaglandin, Thromboxane and Leukotriene Research. (Eds. B. Samuelsson, R. Paoletti and P.W. Ramwell) Raven Press, New York,* 11*:151.*

21. *Eling, T.E. and Ally, A.I. (1984) Pulmonary biosynthesis and metabolism of prostaglandins and related substances. Environmental Health Prospects 55: 159.*

22. *Fitzgerald, M., Moncada, S. and Parente, L. (1985) The release of PAF-acether and lyso-PAF from sensitized guinea-pig lungs. Br. J. Pharmacol. 86: 573P.*

23. *Fleisch, J.J., Rinkema, L.E. and Baker, S.R. (1982) Evidence for multiple leukotriene D_4 receptors in smooth muscle. Life Sci. 31: 577.*

24. *Falco, G.C., Omini, C., Vigano, T., Brunelli, G., Rossoni, G. and Berti, F. (1982) Biological activity of leukotriene C_4 in guinea pigs. In Leukotrienes and Other Lipoxygenase Products. (Eds. B. Samuelsson and Paoletti, R.) Raven Press, New York, p. 153.*

25. *Gryglewski, R.J. (1980) The lung as a generator of prostacyclin. In Metabolic Activities of the Lung. Ciba Found. Symposium 78, Excerpta Medica, Amsterdam p. 147.*

26. *Gryglewski, R.J. (1982) Regulation of prostacyclin release into circulation. In Advances in Pharmacology and Therapeutics, (Eds. H. Yoshida, Y. Hagihara and S. Ebashi) Pergamon Press, Oxford. vol. 4, p. 235*

27. *Gryglewski, R.J., Dembinska-Jiec, A., Grodzinska, L. and Panczenko, B. (1976) Differential generation of substances with prostaglandin-like and thromboxane-like activities by guinea-pig trachea and lung strips. In Lung Cells in Disease, (Ed. A. Bouhuys) Elsevier, Amsterdam, p. 289.*

28. *Gryglewski, R.J., Korbut, R. and Ocetkiewicz, A. (1978a) Generation of prostacyclin by lungs in vivo and its release into arterial circulation. Nature: 273:765 (1987a).*

29. *Gryglewski, R.J., Korbut, R., Ocetkiewicz, A., Splawinski, J., Wojtaszek, B. and Swies, J. (1978b) Lungs as a generator of prostacyclin - a hypothesis on physiological significance. Naunyn Schmiedeberg's Arch. Pharmacol. 304: 45.*

30. *Gryglewski, R.J., Moncada, S. and Palmer, R.M.J. (1986a) Bioassay of prostacyclin and endothelium-derived relaxing factor (EDRF) from porcine aortic endothelial cells. Br. J. Pharmacol. 87: 685.*

31. *Gryglewski, R.J., Palmer, R.M.J. and Moncada, S. (1986b) Superoxide anion is involved in the breakdown of endothelium-derived vascular relaxing factor. Nature 320:454.*

32. *Ham, E.A., Soderman, D.D., Zanetti, M.E., Dougherty, H.W., McCauley, E. and Kuehl, F. (1983) Inhibition by prostaglandins of leukotriene B_4 release from activated neutrophils. Proc. Natl. Acad. Sci. USA 80:, 4349.*

33. *Hansson, G., Bjorck, T., Dahlen, S.E., Hedquist, P., Grandström, E. and Dahlen, B. (1983) Specific allergen induces contraction of bronchi and leukotrienes C_4, D_4 and E_4 in human asthmatic lung. In Advances in Pro-*

staglandin, Thromboxane and Leukotriene Research, (Eds. B. Samuelsson, R. Paoletti and P.W. Ramwell) Raven Press, New York, 12: p. 153 .

34. *Hedquist, P. and Dahlen, S.E. (1983) Pulmonary and vascular effects of leukotrienes imply involvement in asthma and inflammation. In Advances in Prostaglandin, Thromboxane and Leukotriene Research, (Eds. B. Samuelsson, R. Paoletti and P.W. Ramwll) Raven Press, New York, 11:27.*

35. *Hellewell, P.G. and Pearson, J.D. (1984) Purinoceptor mediated stimulation of prostacyclin release in the porcine pulmonary vasculature. Br. J. Pharmacol. 83, 457.*

36. *Hopkins, N.K., Sun, F.F. and Gorman, R.R. (1978) Thromboxane A_2 biosynthesis in human lung fibroblasts WI-38. Biochem. Biophys. Res. Commun. 85: 827.*

37. *Iocopino, V.J., Compton, S., Fitzpatrick, T., Ramwell, P., Rose, J. and Kot, P. (1984) Response to leukotriene C_4 in rat perfused lung. J. Pharmacol. Exp. Ther. 229: 654.*

38. *Johnson, A.R., Callahan, K.S., Tsai, S.C. and Campbell, W.B. (1981) Prostacyclin and prostaglandin biosynthesis in human pulmonary endothelial cells. Bull. Europ. Physiopath. Resp. 17: 531.*

39. *Kadowitz, P.J. and Hyman, A.L. (1977) Influence of a prostaglandin endoperoxide analogue on the canine pulmonary vascular bed. Circ. Res. 40: 282.*

40. *Kadowitz, P.J., Lippton, H.L., McNamara, D.B., Spannhake, E.E. and Hyman A.L. (1982) Action and metabolism of prostaglandins in pulmonary circulation. In Advances in Prostaglandin, Thromboxane and Leukotriene Research, (Ed. J. Oates) Raven Press, New York, 10:333.*

41. *Kellaway, C.H. and Trethewie, E.R. (1940) The liberation of a slow-reacting smooth muscle-stimulating substance in anaphylaxis. Q. J. Exp. Physiol. 30: 121.*

42. *Koshihara, Y., Murota, A. and Nicolau, K.C.(1983) 5,6-Methano Leukotriene A_4. A potent specific inhibitor for 5-lipoxygenase. In Advances in Prostaglandin, Thromboxane and Leukotriene Research, (Eds. B. Samuelsson, R. Paoletti and P.W. Ramwell) Raven Press, New York, 11: 163.*

43. *Krell, R.D. and Kusner, E.J. (1984) Differential effect of cyclooxygenase inhibition on antigen- and ionophore-induced release of slow reacting substance from fragmented guinea-pig lung. Br. J. Pharmacol. 82: 871.*

44. *Krell, R.D., Tsai, B.S., Berdoilay, A., Barone, M. and Giles, R.E. (1983) Heterogeneity of leukotriene receptors in guinea pig trachea. Prostaglandins 25: 171.*

45. *Lefort, J., Rotilio, D. and Vargaftig, B.B. (1984) The platelet-independent release of thromboxane A_2 by PAF-acether from guinea-pig lungs*

involves mechanisms distinct from those for leukotriene. Br. J. Pharmacol. 82: 565.

46. *Letts, L.G., Plamer, M.A. and Piper, P.J. The fate of leukotrienes C_4 and D_4 in the pulmonary and (1982) coronary circulations in vitro. Br. J. Pharmacol. 75: 5P.*

47. *Lewis, R.A., Soter, N.A., Diamond, P.T., Austin, K.F., Oates, J.A. and Roberts, L.J. (1982) II Prostaglandin D_2 generation after activation of rat and human mast cells with anti-IgE. J. Immunol. 129: 1627.*

48. *Littner, M.R., Kazmi, G.I. and Lott, F.D. (1982) The effects of arachidonic acid, PGI_2 and 6-keto-PGF_1 alpha on cyclic nucleotide concentrations in a ventilated and artificially perfused isolated dog lungs. Prostaglandins, Leukotrienes and Medicine 9: 257.*

49. *MacDermont, J. and Barnes, P.J. (1980) Activation of guinea pig pulmonary adenylate cyclase by prostacyclin. Europ. J. Pharmacol. 67: 419.*

50. *Marom, Z., Shelhamer, J.H., Bach, M.K., Morton, D.R. and Kaliner, M. (1982) Slow-reacting substances, leukotrienes C_4 and D_4 increase the release of mucus from human airways in vitro. Am. Rev. Respir. Dis. 126: 449.*

51. *Moncada, S., Gryglewski, R.J., Bunting, S. and Vane, J.R. (1976) An enzyme isolated from arteries transforms prostaglandin endoperoxides into unstable compound that inhibits platelet aggregation. Nature 263:663.*

52. *Mugridge, K.G., Higgs, G.A. and Moncada, S. (1984) Prostacyclin modulates the responses to leukotrienes C_4 and D_4 of guinea pig airway smooth muscle. Europ. J. Pharmacol. 104:1.*

53. *Nowak, J., Brandt, R., Dembinska-Kiec, A., Gryglewski, R.J. and Korbut, R. (1985) Carbaminoilcholine stimulates release of prostacyclin from the human pulmonary vascular bed. In Prostacyclin - Clinical Trials, p. 95 (Eds. R. J. Gryglewski, A. Szczeklik and J.C. McGiff) Raven Press, New York, p. 95.*

54. *Nowak, J., Radomski, M., Kaijser, L. and Gryglewski, R.J. (1981) Conversion of exogenous arachidonic acid to prostaglandins in the pulmonary circulation: a human and animal study. Acta Physiol. Scand. 112: 405.*

55. *Omini, C., Moncada, S. and Vane, J.R. (1977) The effect of prostacyclin (IGI_2) on tissues which detect prostaglandins (PGs). Prostaglandins 14:625.*

56. *Parente, L., Fitzgerald, M., De Nucci, G. and Moncada, S. (1985) The release of lyso-PAF from guinea-pig lungs. Europ. J. Pharmacol. 112: 281.*

57. *Piper, P.J., Tippins, J.R., Samhoun, M.N., Morris, H.R., Taylor, G.W. and Jones, C.M. (1981) SRS-A and its formation by the lung.*

Bull. Europ. Physiopath. Resp. 17:571.

58. *Piper, P.J., Letts, L.G. and Galton, S.A. (1983) Generation of a leukotriene-like substance from porcine vascular and other tissues. Prostaglandins* 25:591.

59. *Piper, P.J. and Samhoun, M.N. (1983) Comparison of the actions of leukotriene* E_4 *with those of leukotrienes* B_4, C_4 *and* D_4 *on guinea pig lung and ileal smooth muscle in vitro. In Advances in Prostaglandin, Thromboxane and Leukotriene Research, (Eds. B. Samuelsson, R. Paoletti and P.W. Ramwell) Raven Press, New York,* 12:127.

60. *Piper, P.J. and Tippins, M. (1982) Interaction of leukotrienes with cyclooxygenase products in guinea pig isolated trachea. In Leukotrienes and Other Lipoxygenase Products, (Eds. B. Samuelsson and R. Paoletti) Raven Press, New York, p. 183.*

61. *Piper, P.J. and Vane, J.R. (1969) Release of additional factors in anaphylaxis and its antagonism by anti-inflammatory drugs. Nature* 223: 29.

62. *Ryan, J.W. and Ryan, U.S. (1977) Synthesis of prostaglandins by endothelial cells. Fed. Proc.* 36: 2683.

63. *Saldeen, P. and Saldeen T. (1983) 6-Keto prostaglandin* F_1 *alpha/thromboxane* B_2 *ratio in vascular and lung tissue. Thromb. Res.* 30: 643.

64. *Salzman, P.M., Salmon, J.A. and Moncada, S. (1980) Prostacyclin and thromboxane* A_2 *synthesis by rabbit pulmonary artery. J. Pharmacol. Exp. Ther.* 215: 240.

65. *Samhoun, M.N. and Piper, P.J. (1984) Actions and interactions of lipoxygenase and cyclooxygenase products in respiratory and vascular tissues. Prostaglandins, Leukotrienes and Medicine* 13: 79.

66. *Samuelsson, B. (1983) Leukotrienes: a new class of mediators of immediate hypersensitivity reactions and inflammation. In Advances in Prostaglandin, Thromboxane and Leukotriene Research, (Eds. B. Samuelsson, R. Paoletti and P.W. Ramwell) Raven Press, New York,* 11:1.

67. *Samuelsson, B. (1985) Leukotrienes and related compounds. In Advances in Prostaglandin, Thromboxane and Leukotriene Research, (Eds. O. Hayashi and S. Yamamoto) Raven Press, New York,* 15: 1.

68. *Serhan, C.N., Hamberg, M. and Samuelsson, B. (1984) Lipoxins: novel series of biologically active compounds of arachidonic acid in human leukocytes. Proc. Natl. Acad. Sci. USA* 81: 5335.

69. *Sirois, P., Roy, S. and Borgeat, P. (1983) Specificity of receptors for leukotrienes* A_4, B_4, C_4, D_4, E_4 *and histamine on the guinea pig parenchyma. Prostaglandins* 26: 91.

70. *Szczeklik, A., Gryglewski, R.J., Nizankowska, E. and Musial, J. (1978) Pulmonary and anti-platelet effects of intravenous and inhaled prosta-*

cyclin in man. Prostaglandins 16: 651.

71. *Szczeklik, A. and Gryglewski, R.J. (1983) Asthma and anti-inflammatory drugs: mechanisms and clinical patterns. Drugs 25: 533.*

72. *Ueno, A., Tanaka, K., Hirota, R., Shishido, M. and Katori, M. (1983) Possible involvement of thromboxane in hypertensive and bronchoconstrictor effects of leukotrienes C_4 and D_4. In Advances in Prostaglandin, Thromboxane and Leukotriene Research, (Eds. B. Samuelsson, R. Paoletti and P.W. Ramwell) Raven Press, New York, 12: 139.*

73. *Van Grondelle, A., Worthen, G.S., Ellis, D., Mathias, M., Murphy, R.C., Strife, R.J., Reeves, J.T. and Voeklel, F. (1984) Altering hydrodynamic variabilities influences PGI_2 production by isolated lungs and endothelial cells. J. Appl. Physiol.: Environ. Exercise Physiol. 57: 388.*

74. *Vane, J.R. (1980) Metabolic activities of the lung. In Symposium on Metabolic Functions of the Lung. Excerpta Medica, Amsterdam, p.1.*

75. *Voelkel, N.F., Gerber, J.G., McMurtry, I.F., Nies, A.S. and Reeves, J.T. (1981) Release of vasodilator prostaglandin PGI_2 from isolated rat lung during vasoconstriction. Circ. Res. 48:207.*

76. *Voelkel, N.F., Simpson, J., Worthen, S., Reeves, J.T., Henson, P.M. and Murphy, R.C. (1983) Platelet activating factor cause pulmonary vasoconstriction and oedema via platelet-independent leukotriene formation. In Advances in Prostaglandin, Thromboxane and Leukotriene Research, (Eds. B. Samuelsson, R. Paoletti and P.W. Ramwell) Raven Press, New York, 12: 179.*

77. *Wasserman, M.A., Weichman, B.M., Woodward, D.F., Muccitelli, R.M. and Gleason, J.G. (1983) Differentiation of the tracheal and lung parenchymal effects of synthetic leukotrienes in the guinea pig. In Advances in Prostaglandin, Thromboxane and Leukotriene Research, (Eds. S. Samuelsson, Paoletti, R. and P.W. Ramwell) Raven Press, New York, 12: 133.*

78. *Weksler, B.B., Markus, A.J. and Jaffe, E.A. (1977) Synthesis of prostaglandin I_2 (Prostacyclin) by cultured human and bovine endothelial cells. Proc. Natl. Acad. Sci. USA 74: 9322.*

79. *Welton, A., Hope, C.W., Tobias, L.D. and Hamilton, J.G. (1981) Inhibition of antigen-induced histamine release and thromboxane synthase by FPL 55712, a specific SRS-A antagonist. Biochem. Pharmacol. 30: 1378.*

80. *Williams, T.J. (1983) Interaction between prostaglandins, leukotrienes and other mediators of inflammation. Brit. Med. Bull. 39: 239.*

81. *Zijlstra, E., Bonta, I.L. and Vincent, J.E. (1983) Tachyphylaxis of leukotriene C_4-induced release of thromboxane A_2 from guinea pig lung parenchyma and isoproterenol inhibition of this release. In Advances in Prostaglandin, Thromboxane and Leukotriene Research, (Eds. B. Samuelsson, R. Paoletti and P.W. Ramwell) Raven Press, New York, 12: 167.*

EICOSANOIDS AND ASPIRIN-SENSITIVE ASTHMA

A. Szczeklik

Department of Allergy and Clinical Immunology, Copernicus Academy of Medicine, Cracow, Poland.

Introduction

In most patients with asthma aspirin has no clear effect on either symptoms of bronchial obturation or pulmonary function tests. There are, however, two distinct exceptions. One, patients who develop bronchoconstriction following aspirin ingestion, and two, patients whose asthma improves on aspirin. First are relatively common, second are rare. These two opposite types of reaction to aspirin have been recently well characterized which justifies their distinction as separate clinical syndromes. Here we discuss the evidence that in both syndromes eicosanoids play a vital role. We also point briefly to the possible modulatory role of eicosanoids in late--asthmatic reactions.

1. Aspirin-induced Asthma

In about 10% of adult patients with asthma, but rarely in children, aspirin precipitates asthmatic attacks accompanied by rhinorrhea and conjunctival injection. Often, scarlet flush over head and neck appears, but urticaria is unusual. Aspirin-provoked attacks are a hallmark of this type of asthma which has a characteristic sequence of symptoms and natural history (12,20, 22,24,30).

Aspirin is not the only analgesic aggravating asthma. In the same patients, several other, though not all, nonsteroidal anti-inflammatory drugs (NSAID) produce very similar reactions. We have suggested (25) that a common principle which distinguishes NSAID precipitating asthmatic attacks is their ability to inhibit cyclooxygenase. We also proposed (25) that it is this pharmacological action of the drugs, i.e. inhibition of a specific enzyme, and not immunological reaction which accounts for the attacks. Indeed, as more and more analgesics were discovered to induce asthma in the sensitive patients, it became apparent that their chemical structures differed enormously. This made their immunological cross-reactivity most unlikely. On the other hand, all these drugs were cyclooxygenase inhibitors. NSAID not affecting cyclooxygenase are devoid of bronchospastic properties (table). There is also a positive correlation between the potency of NSAID

Table. Tolerance of anti-inflammatory drugs in aspirin- induced asthma

Precipitate attacks of asthma	Well tolerated (cause no bronchoconstriction)
Aspirin	Sodium salicylate
Indomethacin	Choline salicylate
Ibuprofen	Salicylamide
Fenoprofen	Dextropropoxyphene
Ketoprofen	Benzydamine
Amidopyrine	Chloroquine
Sulfinpyrazone	Paracetamol (see text)
Phenylbutazone	
Mefenamic acid	
Flufenamic acid	
Cyclofenamic acid	
Piroxicam	
Sulindac	
Tioprofenic acid	
Zomepirac	
Tolmetin	
Naproxen	
Diclofenac	

in inhibiting cyclooxygenase in vitro and their potency in inducing asthmatic attacks in sensitive patients (24). Tartrazine, a yellow azo-dye which does not inhibit cyclooxygenase in vitro, is not exception to this rule. Contrary to older reports, recent controlled studies indicate that intolerance to tartrazine is rare among aspirin-sensitive asthmatics, well below 3 per cent (2, 21).

What happens when we intervene pharmacologically with function of other enzymes catalyzing arachidonic acid transformation? Under experimental conditions, steroids reduce prostaglandin generation (9) through release of antiphospholipase proteins (19). Intravenous hydrocortisone may sporadically provoke bronchoconstriction in patients with aspirin-sensitive asthma. In 31 such patients the mean FEV_1 fell significantly 5 min. after an intravenous bolus of 300 mg of hydrocortisone, but not after the solvent, and returned to initial values 1 hour later (28). At this time, only 3 of 31 patients displayed clinical signs of impairment of airflow, which resolved spontaneously. Since betamethasone, dexamethasone and methylprednisone are well tolerated by AIA patients, it remains to be seen whether adverse reaction to hydrocortisone is related to its capacity to interfere with prostaglandin generation.

A more precise pharmacological intervention can be achieved with specific thromboxane A_2 (TXA_2) synthetase inhibitors. Such drugs have only recently became available for clinical studies. Inhibition of TXA_2 generation might be of special interest in AIA, because: 1) The synthetase converts cyclic endoperoxides produced by cyclooxygenase into TXA_2, and 2) because TXA_2 is a potent bronchoconstrictor. Administration of high dose of a specific TXA_2 synthetase inhibitor to 16 patients with AIA, blocked TXA_2 generation in their platelets, but had no effect on either clinical symptoms or pulmonary function test (29). Thus, blocking an enzyme, located in close vicinity to cyclooxygenase along the pathway of arachidonic acid biotransformation, does not produce the same reaction as the blockade of cyclooxygenase itself. This finding points again to special role of cyclooxygenase in AIA.

It would be of value to study eicosanoid metabolism in tissues of respiratory tract, but there are great technical difficulties. Nasal polyps, which develop frequently in patients with AIA, offer an interesting possibility. Patients suffering from nasal polyps and bronchial hyperreactivity independently of aspirin-intolerance have an elevated TXA_2 formation in polyp tissues (16), whereas PGE_2 is within the range of control group (16, 26). When slices or homogenates of nasal polyps obtained from aspirin--sensitive patients with asthma were compared with those from patients without aspirin intolerance, an increased sensitivity of cyclooxygenase to aspirin was observed in the former as compared to the latter (26). Another interesting tissue specimen can be obtained by bronchial lavage. Stimulated alveolar macrophages from aspirin-intolerant asthma patients release smaller quantities of PGE_2, $PGF_{2\alpha}$ and TXB_2 than do alveolar macrophages from normal subjects (6), which points to an intrinsic defect of arachidonate metabolism in the respiratory tract of aspirin-intolerant donors.

Interesting observations on altered cyclooxygenase function in platelets of AIA-patients were recently described by Capron et al. (1, 3). In vitro, addition of aspirin, indomethacin or flurbiprofen to platelets from these patients led to platelets strong activation as expressed by release of cytotoxic mediators killing Schistosoma mansoni larvae. In contrast, these drugs, even at high concentrations, had no activating effect on platelets from controls, whether healthy donors or extrinsic asthmatics. The authors were able to rule out an IgE-dependent mechanism. They, furthermore, could show that sodium salicylate, which is structurally related to aspirin but has no cyclooxygenase inhibiting activity, did not activate platelets from asthmatic patients with aspirin intolerance. These results raise the question of the possible involvement of blood platelets in asthmatic attacks precipitated by aspirin. It is worth noting that a strong case has been made recently for causal participation of platelets in other types of bronchial asthma (14).

It is not yet known whether similar abnormalities are shared by other blood cell elements. In contrast to platelets, neither basophils nor monocytes from aspirin-sensitive asthmatics expressed cytotoxic properties nor any chemiluminescence burst in presence of aspirin (1). On the other hand, Goetzl et al. (7) reported that in vitro, aspirin (but not sodium salicylate) modified differently oxygenation of arachidonic acid in basophil--enriched suspensions of mononuclear leukocytes from patients with aspirin--induced asthma than from the controls. Thus, the inhibitory effect of aspirin on PGE_2 generation by anti-IgE stimulated leukocytes was significantly greater for the aspirin-sensitive patients than either the aspirin-

-tolerant patients with asthma or the normal subjects. In view of these results it is worth mentioning that a role for superoxide radicals generated by leukocytes has been suggested in aspirin-induced asthma (13).

All these recent data support the hypothesis (25) put forward over 13 years ago which stated that inhibition of cyclooxygenase triggers attacks of asthma in the sensitive patients. What follows, however, at the biochemical level, remains a mystery. For reasons explained elsewhere (23), we do not favor the popular concept of shunting of arachidonic acid from the relatively more inhibited cyclooxygenase to 5-lipoxygenase pathway. We rather think that cyclooxygenase products might play a special regulatory role in the bronchi of aspirin-intolerant asthmatics. Important interactions were observed to occur between prostaglandins and leukotrienes (11), e.g. PGE_2 inhibited directly initiation of leukotriene synthesis. F. Kuehl (11) reasoned that aspirin-like drugs, by causing a local deficiency of PGE_2 and PGI_2 may remove damping mechanism controlling leukotriene production; release of leukotrienes would lead to asthma attacks. Though in the patients, infusions of prostacyclin do not prevent attacks of asthma precipitated by aspirin (17) this does not falsify definitely Kuehl's concept since PGE_2 and PGI_2 actions are not always the same in man.

2. Asthma improved by aspirin

A single dose of aspirin may relieve some patients with asthma of shortness of breath and improve objective parameters of their ventilatory function. When we administered 600 mg aspirin to 98 consecutive adult patients with asthma who attended the clinic at our Department, only in 3 FEV_1 increased by more than 15%, and in only 1 of these 3 patients could we consistently reproduce this improvement in a double-blind way. The practicing physicians have long been aware of such patients, and cases of asthma responding favorably not only to aspirin, but also to indomethacin, mefenamic acid, amidopyrine and dipyrone have been reported (for ref. see: 15, 24). Based on study of 6 cases of asthma improved by aspirin we have demonstrated (27) characteristic features of this syndrome, which to us constitute a distinct type of asthma. Last clinical reports (18) confirm this conclusion.

In patients whose pulmonary function improve on aspirin, similar improvement can be obtained with other NSAID which block cyclooxygenase. Analgesics deprived of this property, e.g. salicylamide, benzydamine or dextropropoxyphene do not affect lung function in these patients. We have, therefore, suggested (27) that pharmacological removal of a product of arachidonic acid cyclooxygenation from the respiratory tract of patients responding favorably to aspirin-like drugs help them to overcome their airways obstruction.

3. Possible participation of eicosanoids in the late asthmatic reactions

Late phase of asthmatic response might be more representative of clinically severe asthma than early reactions. Fairfax et al. (5) demonstrated in 4 patients partial inhibition of late asthmatic reaction with a single dose of 3 NSAID prior to allergen challenge. In 8 of 11 delayed asthmatic responders, Joubert et al. (10) effectively suppressed the delayed response by pretreatment with indomethacin 72 hours before the antigen challenge. The IgE-mediated delayed inflammatory skin reactions in which thromboxane appears to participate as a mediator, may represent an analogue pathogenesis to events which cause delayed airways obstruction (4). Such reactions can to a large extent be attenuated by indomethacin and other cyclooxygenase agents (4, 8). These observations suggest participation of cyclooxygenase products in late-phase allergic reactions.

References

1. Ameisen, J.C., Capron, A., Joseph, M. and Tonnel, A.B. (1986) Platelets and aspirin-induced asthma. In: Asthma. Clinical Pharmacology and Therapeutic Progress, ed. by A.B. Kay.(Blackwell,London), pp. 226-236.

2. Bianco, S., Schmitz-Schumann, M., Virchow, Chr., Juhl, E., Robuschi, M., Damonte, C., Menz, G. and Kamburoff-Prime, P. (1986) Tartrazinintoleranz bei Patienten mit Analgetika-Asthma Syndrom. Eine Multizenterstudie (Davos-Krakau-Mainland). Medidact. Hosp. 6,49-52.

3. Capron, A., Ameisen, J.C., Joseph, M., Auriault, C., Tonnel, A.B., Caen, J. (1985) New functions for platelets and their pathological implications. Int. Arch. Allergy appl. Immunol. 77, 107-114.

4. Dorsch, W., Ring, J., Reimann, H.J. and Geiger, R. (1982) Mediator studies in skin blister fluid from patients with dual skin reactions and intradermal allergen injection. J. Allergy Clin. Immunol. 70, 236-242.

5. Fairfax, A.J., Hanson, J.M. and Morley, J. (1983) The late reaction following bronchial provocation with house dust mite allergen. Dependence on arachidonic acid metabolism. Clin. Exp. Immunol. 52, 393-398.

6. Godard, P., Chantreuil, J., Damon, M., Coupe, M., Flandre, O., Crastes de Paulet, A., Michel, F.B. (1982) Functional assessment of alveolar macrophages: comparison of cells from asthmatic and normal subjects. J Allergy Clin. Immunol. 70, 88-94.

7. Goetzl, E.J., Valacer, D.J., Payan, D.G. and Wong, M.Y.S. (1986) Abnormal responses to leukocyte oxygenation of arachidonic acid in adults with aspirin intolerance. J Allergy Clin. Immunol 77, 693-698.

8. Grönnenberg, R., and Zetterström,O. (1985) Inhibition of the late phase response to anti-IgE in humans by indomethacin. Allergy 40, 36-41.

9. Gryglewski, R.J., Panczenko, B., Korbut, R., Grodzinska, L., Ocetkiewicz, A. (1975) Corticosteroids inhibit prostaglandin release from perfused mesenteric blood vessels of rabbit and from perfused lungs of sensitized guinea pig. Prostaglandins 10, 343-355.

10. Joubert, J.R., Shephard, E., Mouton, W., Van Zyl, L. and Viljoen, I. (1985) Non-steroidal anti-inflammatory drugs in asthma: dangerous or useful therapy? Allergy 40, 202-207.

11. Kuehl, F.A., Dougherty, H.W., Ham, E.A. (1984) Interactions between prostaglandins and leukotrienes. Biochem. Pharmacol. 33, 1-5.

12. Migueres, J., Migueres, M. (1986) L'asthme à l'aspirine. Allergie Immunol. 18, 4-11.

13. Moneret-Vautrin, D.A., Martin, R. (1985) Intolerance to aspirin: a role for free radicals. Lancet 1, 929.

14. Morley, J., Sanjar, S., Page, C. (1984) The platelet in asthma. Lancet 2, 1142-1144.

15. Nelson, R.P., Stablein, J.J., Lockey, R.F. (1986) Asthma improved by acetylsalicylic acid and other nonsteroidal anti-inflammatory agents. N.Engl.Reg.Allergy Proc. 7, 117-121.

16. Nigam, S., Kunkel, G., Herold, D., Baumer, F.E., Jusuf, L. (1986) Nasal polyps and their content of arachidonic acid. N.Engl. Reg. Allergy Proc. 7, 109-112.

17. Nizankowska, E., Czerniawska-Mysik, G., Szczeklik, A. (1986) Lack of effect of prostacyclin in aspirin-induced asthma. Eur. J. Resp. Dis. in press.

18. Resta, O., Foschino-Barbaro, M.P., Carnimeo, N., Bavoso, P., Picca, V.

(1984) Asthma relieved by acetylsalicylic acid and nonsteroidal anti-inflammatory drugs. Respiration 46, 121-127.

19. Di Rosa, M., Flower, R.J., Hirata, F., Parente, L., Russo-Marie, F. (1984) Anti-phospholipase proteins. Prostaglandins 28, 441-442.

20. Schmitz-Schumann, M., Juhl, E., Costabel, U., Rühle, K-H., Menz, G., Virchow, C., Matthys, H. (1985) Analgetikaprovokationsproben bei Analgetika-Asthma Sydrom. Atemw. Lungenkrkh. 11, 479-486.

21. Simon, R.A. (1984) Adverse reactions to drug additives. J. Allergy Clin. Immunol. 74, 623-630.

22. Stevenson, D.L. (1984) Diagnosis prevention and treatment of adverse reactions to aspirin and nonsteroidal anti-inflammatory drugs. J. Allergy Clin. Immunol. 74, 617-622.

23. Szczeklik, A. (1986) Adverse reactions to aspirin and nonsteroidal anti-inflammatory drugs. Ann Allergy - in press.

24. Szczeklik, A., Gryglewski, R.J. (1983) Asthma and anti-inflammatory drugs. Mechanisms and clinical patterns. Drugs 25, 533-543.

25. Szczeklik, A., Gryglewski, R.J., Czerniawska-Mysik, G. (1975) Relationship of inhibition of prostaglandin biosynthesis by analgesics to asthma attacks in aspirin-sensitive patients. Br. Med. J. 1, 67-69.

26. Szczeklik, A., Gryglewski, R.J., Olszewski, E., Dembinska-Kiec, A., Czerniawska-Mysik, G. (1977) Aspirin sensitive asthma: The effect of aspirin on the release of prostaglandins from nasal polyps. Pharmacol. Res. Commun. 9, 415-425.

27. Szczeklik, A., Nizankowska, E. (1983) Asthma improved by aspirin-like drugs. Br. J. Dis. Chest 77, 153-158.

28. Szczeklik, A., Nizankowska, E., Czerniawska-Mysik, G., Sek, S. (1985) Hydrocortisone and airflow impairment in aspirin-induced asthma. J.Allergy Clin. Immunol. 76, 530-536.

29. Szczeklik, A., Nizankowska, E., Splawinski, J., Dworski, R., Gajewski, P. (1986) Effects of inhibition of thromboxane A_2 synthetase in aspirin--induced asthma. J. Allergy Clin. Immunol. - submitted for publication.

30. Virchow, C. (1976) Analgetika-Intoleranz bei Asthmatikern (Analgetika--Asthma-Syndrom). Prax. Klin. Pneumol. 30, 642-692.

Prof. Andrew Szczeklik, M.D., Department of Allergy and Clinical Immunology, Copernicus Academy of Medicine, Skawinska 8, 31-066 Cracow, Poland.

PHARMACOLOGICAL ATTEMPTS TO MODULATE LEUKOTRIENE SYNTHESIS IN ASPIRIN-INDUCED ASTHMA

E. Nizankowska, A.Q. Sheridan, M.H. Maile, C.J. Cross, G. Czerniawska-Mysik and A. Szczeklik

Department of Allergy and Clinical Immunology, Copernicus Academy of Medicine, Cracow, Poland, and The Upjohn Company, Kalamazoo, MI, USA

Introduction

The idiosyncrasy to aspirin which affects 5-10% of adult asthmatics, has been thought since several decades to be of allergic origin while, in fact, numerous extensive immunological studies have ruled out typical IgE-mediated allergic mechanisms for aspirin-induced asthma. In 1974, a novel hypothesis was put forward (26) stating that in sensitive patients, the precipitation of asthmatic attacks by aspirin and by certain nonsteroidal antiinflammatory drugs (NSAID) results from inhibition of cyclooxygenase in the bronchi, leading to an imbalance of prostanoids in the respiratory tract. The precise nature of the mechanism of this idiosyncrasy remains unknown. Attacks of asthma, following aspirin ingestion, may develop either because the synthesis of bronchodilatory prostanoids, e.g. PGE_2 ceases suddenly or because more arachidonic acid becomes available for the production of bronchoconstrictor leukotrienes, lipoxins or, yet unknown, metabolites of arachidonic acid.

We attempted to reduce leukotriene generation in two ways: 1) via inhibition of leukotriene synthesis from arachidonic acid by Piriprost (U-60,257) - a selective inhibitor of 5-lipoxygenase, and 2) via action of prostacyclin (PGI_2) which in vitro has an inhibitory effect on initial stages of leukotriene formation.

1. The effect of Piriprost on aspirin-induced asthma

Aspirin-like drugs, by blocking cyclooxygenase, might thus divert, might "shunt" arachidonic acid metabolism from cyclooxygenase to lipoxygenase pathway. Leukotrienes synthetized in large amounts could then induce symptoms of asthma (12, 16, 32). Obviously, if the "shunting" concept is right, then specific inhibitors of leukotriene synthesis or leukotriene antagonists at the receptor level should prevent the asthmatic attack provoked by aspirin.

We, therefore, attempted to reduce the leukotriene formation in patients with aspirin-induced asthma by using a highly specific inhibitor of leukotriene synthesis - Piriprost (U-60,257). This synthetic compound from The Upjohn Co. (Kalamazoo, MI) is a pyrrole analog of prostacyclin with the chemical structure of 6,9-deepoxy-6,9-(phenylimino)-$\Delta^{6,8}$*-prostaglandin* I_1 *(24). Piriprost is a selective inhibitor of 5-lipoxygenase without significant effect on 12- or 15-lipoxygenase, or cyclooxygenase (4, 23, 25). It does not affect histamine release in anaphylaxis models in vitro (2).*

Piriprost has inhibited leukotriene formation in ionophore-stimulated rat peritoneal mononuclear cells and in passively sensitized human lung fragments during a challenge with antigen E in vitro (2). It has also inhibited the synthesis of leukotrienes in lung fragments obtained from birch pollen allergic asthmatics and challenged in vitro with birch pollen (6).

In vivo, Piriprost inhibited the bronchopulmonary sequelae of anaphylaxis in ovalbumin-sensitized guinea-pigs (3) and given intravenously or by inhalation to Ascaris-sensitive monkeys produced significant, long lasting protection from challenges with aerosolized Ascaris antigen (10).

The aforementioned significant pharmacological activity in animal experiments prompted us to examine the effect of Piriprost on aspirin challenge in aspirin-sensitive asthmatics.

In a pilot double-blind placebo controlled study, we established that in 16 healthy subjects and 16 atopic asthmatic patients, there was good tolerance of Piriprost and no significant changes in spirometric parameters occurred after inhalation of its increasing (0.001, 0.01, 0.1, 1.0 mg) doses (Fig. 1). Similarly, 10 patients with aspirin-induced asthma showed good tolerance of the inhaltion of 1 mg of Piriprost.

In all of these ten patients hypersensitivity to aspirin was confirmed by oral challenge test (26, 27, 30). The threshold dose of aspirin which provoked 20% decrease of FEV_1 was established 4 - 8 weeks

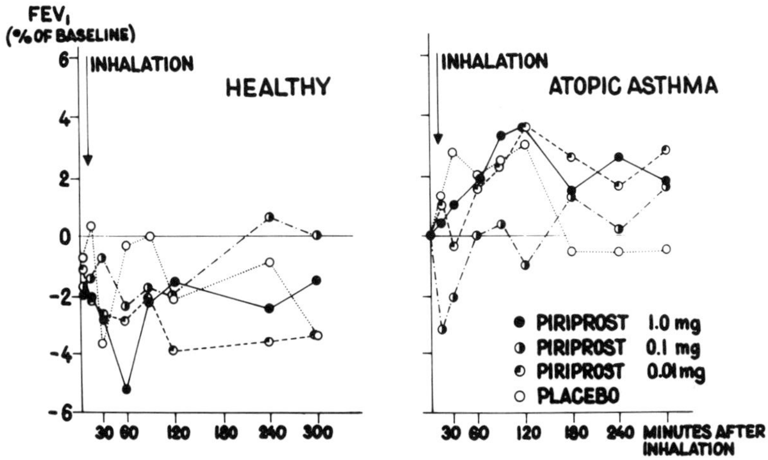

Fig. 1. Mean FEV_1 values following the inhalation of increasing doses of Piriprost or placebo in healthy subjects (n=16) and patients with atopic asthma (n=16).

before the experiment proper. In eight of these patients we then performed two oral challenges with the threshold dose of aspirin: first - after inhalation of 1 mg of Piriprost, and the second - after inhalation of placebo. The study was double-blind and randomized.

FEV_1 values following the challenges with the threshold dose of aspirin are shown on figure 2. Although the mean values were slightly lower following the challenge preceded by placebo inhalation, the differences were not statistically significant.

Similarly, the lowest individual FEV_1 values during aspirin challenge and the time at which FEV_1 dropped below 80% of baseline did not differ in the two challenges. Thus, a single dose of Piriprost was not able to block the bronchiconstriction induced by aspirin.

As the peak clinical reaction following aspirin challenge occurred about two hours following aspirin ingestion, one might thus suppose that the duration of pharmacological action of Piriprost could have been insufficient to block this reaction.

To rule out this possibility, in six patients we performed the challenges with aspirin during repeated 4 inhalations of 1 mg of Piriprost or placebo (Fig. 3). By this procedure, the total dose of Piriprost inhaled

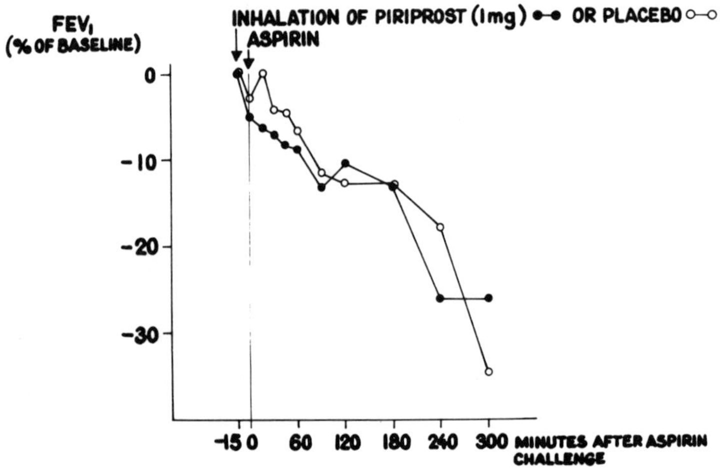

Fig. 2. Mean FEV_1 values following the oral challenge with threshold dose of aspirin, performed after inhalation of 1 mg of Piriprost (U-60, 257) or placebo in patients with aspirin-induced asthma (n=8).

by the patients was four times higher.

Nevertheless, even four inhalations of Piriprost did not have protective effect against aspirin-induced attacks of asthma. The higher doses of Piriprost (10 mg) given by inhalation were highly irritative to the throat and bronchi, making examination of its effects on aspirin challenge impossible (19)

We are well aware of the limitations of our clinical study. There are no data on the pharmacokinetics of Piriprost in man available. We do not know whether the amounts given by inhalation, although applied in the range which were active in monkey models (10), were sufficient to block leukotriene production in human bronchi and lungs.

Prostacyclin, administered similarly by inhalation reaches the bronchial tree and lungs, does absorb to the blood, as may be judged from its significant effects on platelets (37). One may suppose that inhibition of the synthesis of leukotrienes in human polymorphonuclear leukocytes in vitro by Piriprost (25) might not necessarily apply to mast cells, eosinophils, platelets, macrophages and monocytes in the lung (17, 22I9.

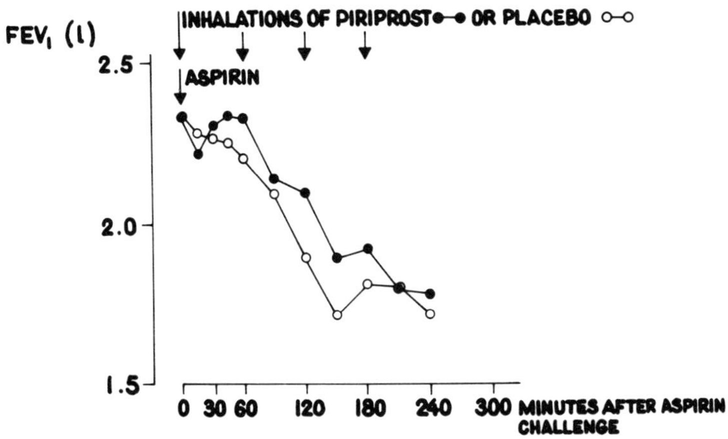

Fig. 3. Mean FEV_1 values following the oral challenge with threshold dose of aspirin, performed during the series of four inhalation of 1 mg of Piriprost or placebo in patients with aspirin-induced asthma (n=6).

Such outcome may suggest that either the leukotrienes are not responsible for bronchoconstriction induced by aspirin, or Piriprost has not been a strong enough inhibitor of leukotriene synthesis.

2. The effect of prostacyclin on aspirin-induced asthma.

Recently, Kuehl and others (11) have suggested a new explanation for mechanism of bronchospasm following aspirin ingestion in aspirin-sensitive patients. They found that there are different pools of arachidonic acid for production of prostaglandins and leukotrienes in rat peritoneal macrophages and human neutrophiles. Furthermore, they did not observe the increased synthesis of leukotrienes after inhibition of cycloocygenase by indomethacine. This observation goes against the notion of the direct mechanistic "shunting" of arachidonic acid from cycloocygenase to lipoxygenase pathway.

Kuehl's hypothesis of bronchospasm mechanism in aspirin-induced asthma is based on the finding that PGE_2 *and* PGI_2 *exert in vitro inhibitory effects on the initial stages in the formation of leukotrienes. Thus, aspirin-like drugs, by causing a local deficiency of* PGE_2 *and* PGI_2*, may eliminate one of the inhibitory mechanisms controlling leukotriene synthesis and release.*

We decided to test this hypothesis in a separate study (18) by observing whether PGI_2 *infusion could prevent or alleviate attacks of asthma precipitated by a threshold dose of aspirin.*

There were two additional reasons for expecting that prostacyclin infusion will prevent asthmatic attacks induced by aspirin. 1) As we know from the in vitro studies of Mugridge et al. (15) PGI_2 *opposes the bronchoconstrictive action of leukotriene on guinea-pig airway smooth muscle. Even small amounts of* PGE_2*, as released from isolated challenged guinea-pig lungs, are sufficient to modulate the myotropic responses to leukotrienes (7). Those results led us to assume that modulation of leukotriene responses by prostacyclin might take place in the airways in vivo. 2) Moreover,* PGI_2 *is the most potent antiplatelet agent (8, 9, 31) and the activation of platelets might be instrumental in attacks of asthma (13, 14, 21).*

Thus, we studied nine patients with asthma, sensitive to aspirin, who underwent oral challenges with pre-determined dose of aspirin while they were receiving a continuous 8 h i.v. infusion of prostacyclin (Flolan, Wellcome Res. Labs., Beckenham, U.K.) or placebo (glycine buffer). The study was double-blind and infusions randomized, separated by a minimum period of two weeks. The dose of PGI_2 *was 2.5 ng/kg/min during the first hour and 5.0 ng/kg/min for the remaining 7 hours. Aspirin oral challenges commenced at the end of third hour of the infusion. Blood pressure, pulse rate, pulmonary function tests were recorded before the infusion and then repeated at hourly intervals for the first 3 hours and then every 30 minutes for the next 5 hours.*

Any blockade and watery discharge from the nose were recorded by the patients themselves, rated using 4-point scale and a final score was then obtained. The FEV_1 *changes during the challenges with aspirin are given in figure 4.*

We did not observe any changes in spirometric parameters during the *first 3 h of infusion of PGI_2 or its placebo. Bronchoconstriction occured following challenge with threshold dose of aspirin. In three patients the bronchial reaction provoked by aspirin was exactly the same during infusions of either PGI_2 or placebo. In 5 patients the reactions seemed slightly more accentuated during PGI_2 infusion, while in one patient during administration of placebo.*

Statistical analysis of spirometric parameters revealed no differences between the two regimens at any time after aspirin challenge.

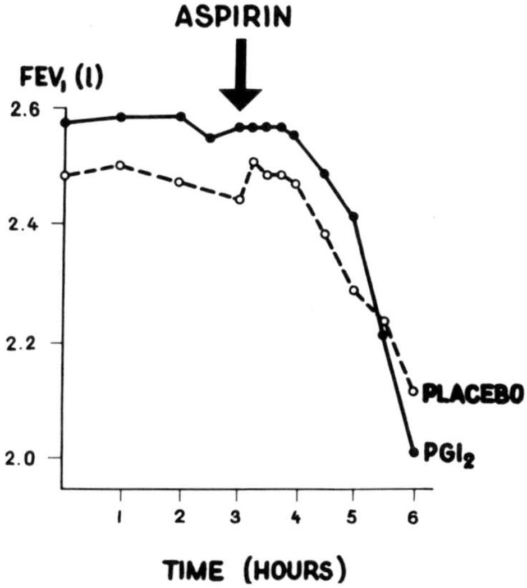

Fig. 4. Mean FEV_1 values following the oral challenge with aspirin, performed with simultaneous i.v. infusion of prostacyclin (PGI_2) or placebo in patients with aspirin-induced asthma (n=9).

In four patients nasal discharge was more intense while they were receiving PGI_2 rather than placebo, while in one patient the opposite phenomenon was observed.

The effects of PGI_2 in man have been studied extensively for the last decade (9, 29, 31) and there were many reasons, indeed, for expecting prevention by prostacyclin of aspirin-induced attacks (11). The 5 ng/kg/min dose of prostacyclin that we administered to our patients, proved to have worked as a potent inhibitor of platelet activation. This has been already well substantiated by our previous research (29). Nevertheless, contrary to the theoretical expectations, PGI_2 did not offer any protection against *aspirin-induced bronchoconstriction. Our results do not support the hypothesis on the regulatory role of PGI_2 in bronchi of the asthmatic patients with aspirin idiosyncrasy. For a definite rejection of this hypothesis, one would have to prove that i.v. administered PGI_2 leaves the vascular compartment in quantities adequate to influence leukotriene synthesis in bronchopulmonary tissue.*

Certain other prostaglandins, however, do cross the vascular wall and influence the pulmonary parenchyma, e.g. $PGF_{2\alpha}$ produces moderate airway constriction in man, when given intravenously (20).

The possibility of endogenous activation of platelets during attacks of asthma has lately raised a great interest (14, 21). Moreover, Capron et al. (5) and Ameisen et al. (1) have recently suggested that blood platelets might be involved in the asthmatic attacks in aspirin-intolerant patients. Our results raise some doubts about participation of platelets in this special type of asthma, since PGI_2 is a powerfull inhibitor of platelet activation.

Conclusions

Still bearing in mind the limitations of clinical studies our results can be briefly summarized as follows: 1) The specific inhibitor of 5-lipoxygenase - Piriprost - in the dose of 1 and 4 mg did not block the bronchospasm induced by a threshold dose of aspirin in aspirin-sensitive patients. 2) the inhibitory effect of PGI_2 on aspirin challenge has not been confirmed.

Our results suggest that either the inhibitory effects of Piriprost and PGI_2 on leukotriene generation described in vitro do not apply in vivo, or the importance of leukotrienes has been overestimated in this type of asthma.

References

1. *Ameisen, J.C., Capron, A., Joseph, M. and Tonnel, A.B. (1986) Platelets and aspirin-induced asthma. In: Asthma. Clinical Pharmacology and Therapeutic Progress, ed. by A.B. Kay (Blackwell, London), pp 226-236.*

2. *Bach, M.K., Brashler, J.K., Smith, H.W., Fitzpatrick, F.A., Sun, F.F., and McGuire, J.C.: (1982) 6,9-deepoxy-6,9-(phenylimino)-$\Delta^{6,8}$-prostaglandin I_2 (U-60,257) a new inhibitor of leukotriene C and*

D synthesis: in vitro studies. Prostaglandins 23, *759-771.*

3. *Bach, M.K., Brashler, J.R., Fitzpatrick, F.A., Griffin, R.L., Iden, S.S., Johnson, H.G., McNee, M.L., McGuire, J.C., Smith, H.W., Sun, F.F., and Wasserman, M.A. (1983) In vivo and in vitro actions of a new selective inhibitor of leukotriene C and D synthesis. Adv. Prostagl. Thrombox. Leukotr. Res.* 11, *39-44.*

4. *Bach, M.K., Brashler, J.R., Peck, R.E. and Morton, Jr., D.R. (1984) Leukotriene C synthetase, a special glutathione S-transferase: Properties of the enzyme and inhibition studies with special reference to the mode of action of U-60,257, a selective inhibitor of leukotriene synthesis. J. Allergy Clin. Immunol.* 74, *353-357.*

5. *Capron, A., Ameisen, J.C., Joseph, M., Auriault, C., Tonnel, A.B., and Caen,J.: (1985) New functions for platelets and their pathological implications. Int. Arch. Allergy Appl. Immunol.* 77, *107-114.*

6. *Dahlen, S.E., Hansson, G., Hedquist, P., Björck, T., Granström, E. and Dahlen, B.: (1983) Allergen challenge of lung tissue from asthmatics elicits bronchial contraction that correlates with the release of leukotrienes* C_4, D_4 *and* E_4. *Proc. Natl. Acad. Sci. USA* 80, *1712-1716.*

7. *Folco, G.C., Omini, C., Vigano, T., Brunelli, G., Rossni, G., and Berti, F. (1982) Biological activity of leukotriene* C_4 *in guinea pigs. In: Leukotrienes and Other Lipoxygenase Products, ed. by B. Samuelsson and R. Paoletti. (Raven Press, New York), p. 153.*

8. *Gryglewski, R.J., Bunting, S., Moncada, S., Flower, R.J. and Vane, J.R. (1976) Arterial walls are protected against deposition of platelets thrombi by a substance (Prostaglandin X) which they make from prostaglandin endoperoxides. Prostaglandins,* 12, *685-713.*

9. *Gryglewski, R.J., Szczeklik, A., and McGiff, J. (1985) Prostacyclin. Clinical Trials (Raven Press, New York).*

10. *Johnson, H.G., McNee, M.L., Bach, M.K., and Smith, H.W. (1983) The activity of a new, novel inhibitor of leukotriene synthesis in Rhesus monkey Ascaris reactors. Int. Arch. Allergy Appl. Immunol.* 70, *169-173.*

11. *Kuehl, F.A. Jr., Dougherty, H.W., and Ham, E.A. (1984) Interactions between prostaglandins and leukotrienes. Biochem. Pharmacol.* 33, *1-5.*

12. *Lewis, R.A.: (1985) Leukotrienes and other lipid mediators of asthma. Chest* 87, *suppl. 5S-10S.*

13. *Martin, J.F., Slater, D.N., and Trowbridge, E.A.: (1983) Abnormal intrapulmonary platelet production: a possible cause of vascular and lung disease. Lancet* 1, *793-796.*

14. *Morley, J., Page, C.P., and Sanjar, S. (1985) Platelets in asthma. Lancet* 2, *726-727.*

15. *Mugridge, K.G., Higgs, G.A., and Moncada, S. (1984) Prostacyclin*

modulates the responses to leukotrienes C_4 and D_4 of guinea pig airway smooth muscle. Eur. J. Pharmacol. 104, *1-5.*

16. *Murphy, R.C., Hammarström, S. and Samuelsson, B. (1979) Leukotriene C: a slow-reacting substance from murine mastocytoma cells. Proc. Natl. Acad. Sci. (Wash.)* 76, *4275-4279.*

17. *Murphy, R.C. and Henson, P.M. (1985) Mediator network. Bull. Inst. Pasteur (Immunol.)* 136D, *219-221.*

18. *Nizankowska, E., Czerniawska-Mysik, G., and Szczeklik, A. (1986) Lack of effect of prostacyclin in aspirin-induced asthma. Eur. J. Resp. Dis. (In press).*

19. *Nizankowska, E., and Szczeklik, A. (1977) Bronchial hyperreactivity in asthma (in Polish). Post. Hig. Med. Dosw.* 31, *853-874.*

20. *Nowak, J. (1985) Eicosanoids and the lung. Ann. Clin. Res.* 16, *269-286.*

21. *Page, C.P., Sanjar, S., and Morley, J. (1985) Platelets and asthma. Lancet* 1, *346-347.*

22. *Peters, S.P., Naclerio, R.M., Freeland, H.S., Togias, A., Schleimer, R.P., MacGlashan Jr., Kagey-Sobotka, A., Fox, C., Adkinson, Jr., N.F. and Lichtenstein, L.M. (1985) Mast cells and mast cell mediators in models of airways disease. In: Leukotrienes in Cardiovascular and Pulmonary Function. (Alan R. Liss, Inc.) pp 153-161.*

23. *Smith, R.J., Sun, F.F., Bowman, B.J., Smith, H.W., and McGuire, J.C. (1982) Effect of 6,9-deepoxy-6,9,(phenylimino)-$\Delta^{6,8}$- prostaglandin I_1 (U-60,257), an inhibitor of leukotriene synthesis, on human neutrophil function. Biochem. Biophys. Res. Commun.* 109, *943-949.*

24. *Smith, H.W., Bach, M.K., Harrison, A.W., Johnson, H.G., Major, N.J., and Wasserman, M.A. (1982) The synthesis of 6,9-deepoxy-N-phenylimino-$\Delta^{6,8}$-prostaglandin I_1, a novel inhibitor of leukotriene C and D synthesis. Prostaglandins* 24, *543-546.*

25. *Sun, F.F. and McGuire, J.C. (1983) Inhibition of human neutrophil arachidonate 5-lipoxygenase by 6,9-deepoxy-6,9-(phenylimino)-$\Delta^{6,8}$-prostaglandin I_1 (U-60,257). Prostaglandins* 26, *211-221.*

26. *Szczeklik, A., Gryglewski, R.J. and Czerniawska-Mysik, G. (1975) Relationship of inhibition of prostaglandin biosynthesis by analgesics to asthma attacks in aspirin-sensitive patients. Br. Med. J.* 1, *67-69.*

27. *Szczeklik, A., Gryglewski, R.J. and Czerniawska-Mysik, G. (1977) Clinical patterns of hypersensitivity to nonsteroidal anti-inflammatory drugs and their pathogenesis. J. Allergy Clin. Immunol.* 60, *276-284.*

28. *Szczeklik, A., Gryglewski, R.J., Nizankowska, E., Nizankowska, R. and Musial, J. (1978) Pulmonary and antiplatelet effects of intravenous and inhaled prostacyclin in man. Prostaglandins* 16, *651-660.*

29. *Szczeklik, A., and Gryglewski, R.J. (1985) Prostaglandins and therapy of cardiovascular disease. Adv. Prostagl. Thrombox. Leukotr. Res. 13, 345-354.*

30. *Szczeklik, A., Gryglewski, R.J., Czerniawska-Mysik, G. and Nizankowska, E. (1986) Aspirin-sensitive asthma and arachidonic acid transformation. N. Engl. Region. Allergy Proc. 7, 21-25.*

31. *Vane, J.R. (1982) Prostacyclin: a hormone with a therapeutic potential. J. Endocrinol. 95, 3P-105P.*

32. *Weiss, J.W., Drazen, J.M., Coles, N., McFadden, E.R., Corey, E.J., Lewis, R.A. and Austen, K.F. (1982) Bronchoconstrictor effects of leukotriene C in humans. Science 216, 196-198.*

Dr. med Ewa Nizankowska, Department of Allergy and Clinical Immunology, Copernicus Academy of Medicin, Skawinska 8, 31-066 Cracow, Poland

EVIDENCE OF PAF RELEASE AND PLATELET ACTIVATION IN ANALGESICS-ASTHMA-SYNDROME

M. Schmitz-Schumann (1), G. Menz (1), A. Schäufele (3), A. von Felten (2), H. Matthys (3), V. de Souza (1) and Chr. Virchow (1)

Hochgebirgsklinik (1), Davos-Wolfgang, Switzerland, Department of Internal Medicine, University Hospital Zürich (2),Switzerland, and Department of Pneumonology, Medizinische Universitätsklinik Freiburg (3), Germany

INTRODUCTION

The phenomenon of bronchial constriction induced by analgesics and anti-inflammatory drugs (analgesics-asthma-syndrome, syn.: aspirin-induced asthma,) has been known for decades (11,12). For a long time it was attributed almost exclusively to aspirin (acetylsalicylic acid, ASA). Later on, numerous analgesics, antipyretic and anti-inflammatory drugs of different chemical structure were found to induce bronchospasm in certain predisposed patients. Recent findings seem to indicate that the analgesics-induced-asthma syndrome can be attributed to a mode of action common to all these drugs, i.e. the inhibition of prostaglandin biosynthesis (cf. Szczeklik, 9). Platelet activation and platelet accumulation within the pulmonary vasculature have been reported to be associated with allergic bronchoconstriction in man (cf. Gresele et al.) Recently, Ameisen et al. (1) demonstrated an abnormal platelet response to aspirin *in vitro* in patients with aspirin-sensitive asthma (cf. Jospeh et al.). The present study has attempted to find evidence for *in vivo* platelet activation and endogenous PAF release following *in vivo* challenge with ASA in patients with analgesics-asthma-syndrome.

METHOD

21 patients with bronchial asthma and 28 healthy subjects have been studied. The bronchospastic response in analgesics-asthma syndrome was

induced by using the inhalative provocation test with lysine-acetylsalicylic acid (lys-ASA) as described previously (8,10). Lys-ASA inhalation challenges were carried out in a total of 11 patients with analgesics-asthma syndrome (n=6, no pretreatment except inhaled beta-2-agonists on demand; n=5, pretreatment including systemic or inhaled steroids, cromoglycate, ketotifen or methylxanthines). Treatment was withheld prior to provocation according to Chai et al. (4). The bronchospastic response pattern in a group of 25 male asthmatics with analgesics-induced asthma is depicted in Fig.1 (10). The lys-ASA-induced bronchoconstriction develops gradually within 30 to 45 minutes after inhalation of the individual lys-ASA threshold dose, remains unchanged between 45 to 90 minutes and diminishes slowly about 240 minutes without dual or late responses.

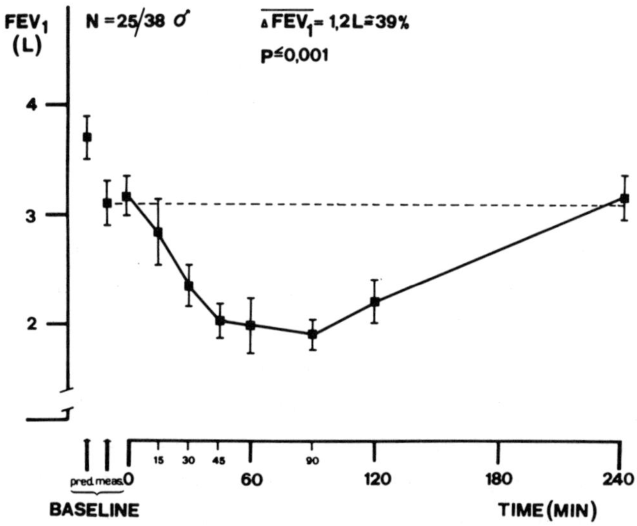

Fig.1.: The bronchospastic response pattern of the lys-ASA inhalation challenge in 25 male patients with analgesics-asthma-syndrome (FEV_1, mean $\pm$ SD). Mean threshold dose: 7.65 $\pm$ 5.6 mg of lys-ASA (10). Pred. - predicted. MEAS. - measured.

The inhibitory effect of a single oral dose of 25 mg of ASA on the threshold synergism of PAF and collagen was determined in a subgroup of 6 healthy volunteers.

The influence of a bronchospastic reaction on PAF & collagen-induced platelet aggregation was studied by an inhalative acetylcholine (n=6) or carbachol (n=4) provocation test in asthmatic subjects (7).

The threshold synergism between PAF-acether and collagen has been determined by utilising the bioassay technique described by Henson and Pinckard (5,6) and modified by Beer and von Felten (2,3). Citrated venous blood was collected by puncture of the cubital vein under a constant pressure of 40 mm Hg. Platelet rich plasma (PRP) was adjusted to 200.000 platelets/ul and total platelet count in the PRP was used to detect thrombocytopenia. The aggregation was induced by increasing doses of PAF-acether (1-o-octadecyl-2-acetyl-sn-glyceryl-3-phosphocholine, Bachem, Basle) in the presence of collagen, 0.15 ug/ml (Hormon Chemie, Munich, FRG). Synergistic doses that induce an increase in light transmission of 70% of the maximal aggregation amplitude induced by collagen (35 ug/ml) were defined as threshold synergism of PAF-acether and collagen (2,3), Fig.2.

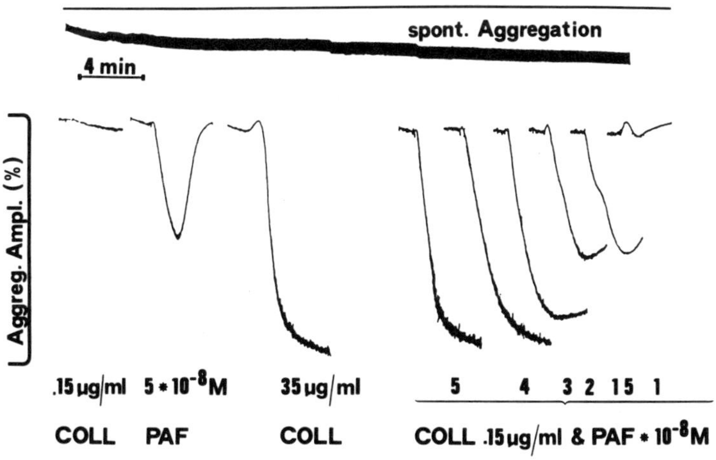

Fig.2.: The determination of the threshold synergism of PAF-acether and collagen. The maximal aggregation induced by 35 ug/ml of collagen corresponds to the 100% reading of the aggregation amplitude.

The desactivation of platelets by PAF in vitro was achieved by preincubation of samples of PRP (30 min, 20° C) with either increasing doses of PAF-acether (5 x 10^{-9}, x 10^{-10} and x 10^{-11} M) or saline (control). Thereafter PAF-acether and collagen are added in threshold concentrations individually determined in advance.

Aliquots of 450 ul of supernatant were deep frozen for beta-thromboglobulin (BTG) analysis (Amersham RIA-kit).

RESULTS

In healthy subjects threshold concentrations of PAF-acether vary between 1 and 4 x 10^{-8} M of PAF-acether. Threshold concentrations are easily determined and interindividually highly reproducible, Fig. 3. The in vitro desactivation of the threshold synergism of PAF and collagen by preincubation of PRP with increasing concentrations of PAF-acether is linear, dose dependent and specific, Fig. 4. Neither inhibitory nor activating influences of the solvent (saline) are present. Ingestion of a single oral dose of 25 mg of ASA is followed by a slight inhibition of the collagen part of the synergistic action indicating a spurious desactivation of the threshold synergism. However, inhaled lys-ASA in threshold concentrations (5-12.5 mg) which are sufficient to induce bronchoconstriction in ASA-sensitive patients do not affect the threshold synergism of PAF and collagen.

Although carbachol and acetylcholine elicited a significant bronchoconstriction ($p \leq 0.01$) in asthmatic patients neither platelet activation/desactivation nor changes in BTG levels have been found.

*In patients with analgesics-asthma-syndrome a specifically induced bronchoconstriction is accompanied by a platelet activation which parallels the lung function time course, Fig.5. Sixty minutes after inhalation of the individual threshold dose of lys-ASA (5 to 12.5 mg) there is an enhancement of the synergistic activity of PAF and collagen leading to an increase in the aggregation amplitude of 38% ($p \leq 0.05$). This activation corresponds to decreased numbers of platelets in PRP (n.s.) and to the maximal bronchospastic response as documented by a significant increase in specific total resistance of airways ($sRAW_{tot}$, kPa*sec), $p \leq 0.001$. Although in group data a reduced aggregation amplitude of the synergism of 24.6% was suggestive of a desactivation of the threshold synergism, p values did not reach*

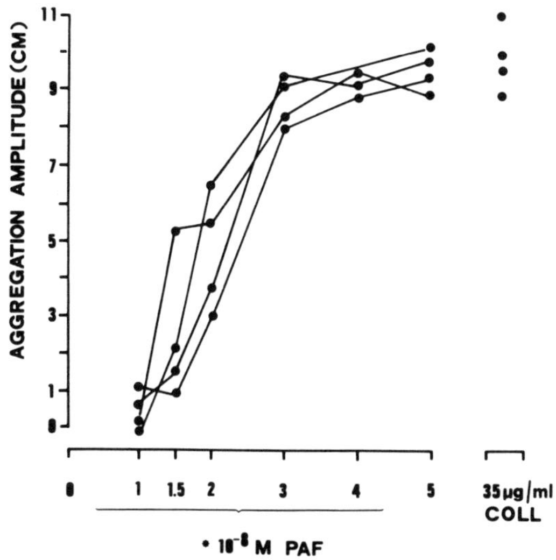

Fig.3.: Reproducibility of the dose-response curve of synergistic actions of PAF-acether and collagen in a healthy volunteer.

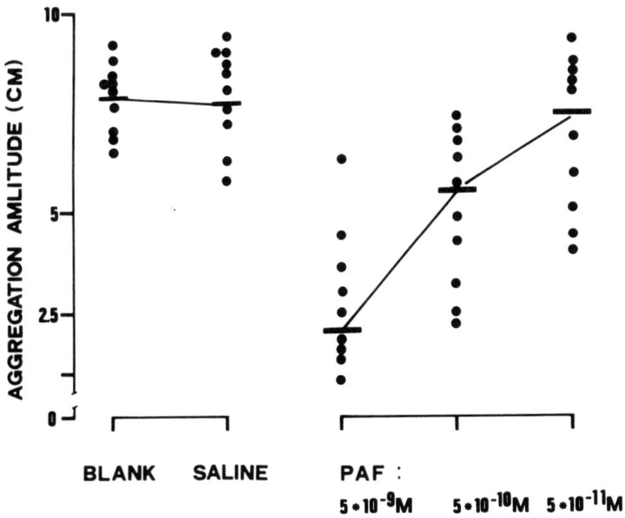

Fig.4.: The desactivation of the threshold synergism of PAF-acether and collagen after preincubation of platelets in PRP (200.000 / ul) with increasing concentrations of PAF-acether.

the level of significance, Fig.5. However, individual differences in the time course as well as the aggregatory response became evident. In a female patient (45 yrs., threshold dose of lys-ASA: 7.5 mg) a strong activation/desactivation response pattern was observed, Fig. 6. In a male patient the bronchospasm developped very rapidly after inhalation of 5 mg of lys-ASA and the desactivation of the threshold synergism of PAF and collagen was already detected 180 minutes after lys-ASA inhalation (⊙), Fig.5.

In ASA-sensitive patients who underwent pretreatment including systemic or inhaled steroids, cromoglycate, ketotifen or methylxanthines no changes in aggregation have been found following positive lys-ASA inhalation challenge. However, increases in BTG levels (2000 $\pm$ 500 to 4100 $\pm$ 800 ng/ml, $p \leq 0.05$) indicate a platelet activation in that group of patients.

CONCLUSIONS

We may conlude, that:

1.) *The desactivation of the threshold synergism of PAF-acether and collagen is sensitive and specific to detect PAF activity in vitro. The effect is linear, dose dependent and reproducible. There is no inhibition of the threshold synergism by 5 to 12.5 mg of ASA. However, amounts of ASA exceeding a single oral dose of 25 mg inhibit the synergistic activity of collagen in the concentration used.*

2.) *Unspecifically induced bronchoconstriction by carbachol or acetylcholine is neither followed by platelet activation nor endogenous PAF release in man.*

3.) *In patients with analgesics-asthma-syndrome the inhalation challenge with lys-ASA may lead to an activation of peripheral blood platelets. In some patients the desactivation of the threshold synergism of PAF-acether and collagen 180 or 240 minutes following challenge is suggestive of endogenous PAF release.*

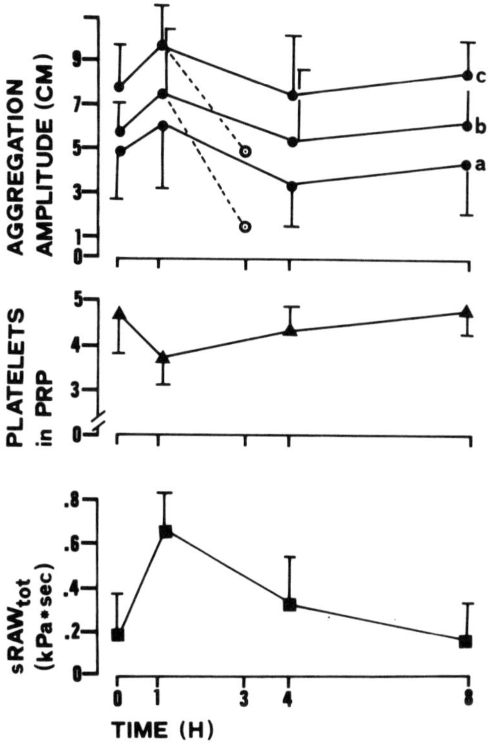

Fig.5.: Activation and desactivation of the threshold synergism of PAF-acether and collagen in patients with analgesics-asthma-syndrome (n=6) following lys-ASA inhalation challenge. Platelets in PRP - x 10^5/ul.

Fig.6.: Response pattern of total airway resistance ($sRAW_{tot}$), platelet count in PRP and aggregation amplitude of the threshold synergism of PAF-acether and collagen in a female asthmatic following lys-ASA inhalation challenge. A - 1.0, B - 1.5, C - 3.0 x 10^{-8} M PAF-acether & collagen 0.15 ug/ml. Platelets in PRP - x 10^5/ul.

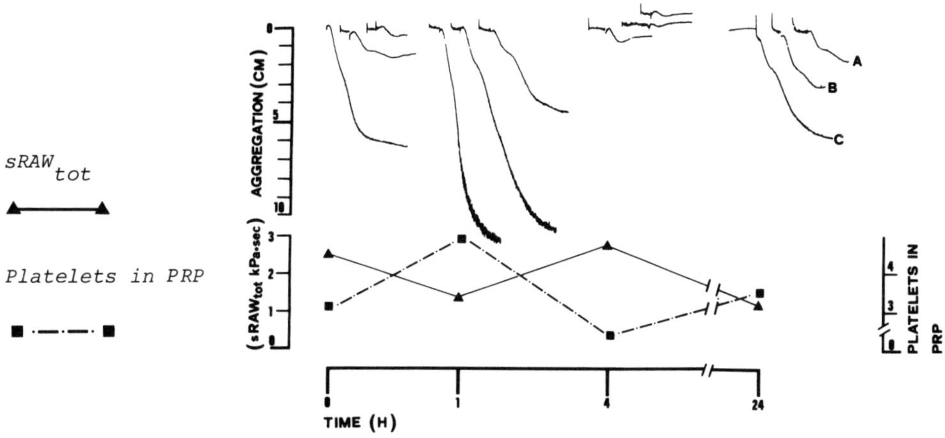

4.) *Since the activation of peripheral blood platelets parallels the time course of the bronchospastic reaction the activation step seems to occur within the lung vasculature either by direct action of ASA (1, cf. Joseph et al.) or by locally released, yet unknown mediators.*

5.) *In contrast to platelet activation the detection of endogenous PAF release is not a consistent finding in the patients studied. PAF release in analgesics-induced asthma syndrome appears to contribute partially to the pathophysiology of the syndrome. However, the ASA-induced bronchoconstriction seems not to be primarily based on the contracting properties of PAF. Since analgesics-induced asthma syndrome is self-limitating and refractory (8,11,12), it is not very likely that mediators which cause persistent inflammation of the airways and increase bronchial hyperreactivity play a predominant role in the pathophysiology of analgesics-asthma-syndrome.*

REFERENCES

1.) *Ameisen, J.C., Capron, A., Jospeh, M., Maclouf, J., Vorng, H., Pancré, V., Fournier, E., Wallaert, B., and Tonnel, A.B. (1985) Aspirin-sensitive asthma: Abnormal platelet response to drugs inducing asthmatic attacks. Diagnostic and physiopatholigical implications. Int. Archs Allergy appl. Immunol. 78: 438 - 448.*

2.) *Beer, H.-J., and von Felten, A. (1984) Wirkungen des Platelet-activating Factor auf die Thrombozyten des Menschen. Arch. Diss. Med. Zürich*

3.) *Beer, J., and von Felten, A. (1986) Reduced 'Threshold Synergism' between PAF-acether and collagen: sensitive test system to detect desensitization of human platelets to PAF-acether in vitro and ex vivo. In: Russo-Marie, F., Mencia Huerta, J.M., and Chignard, M. (edts), Advances in Inflammation research. (Raven Press, New York) 10: 323 - 325.*

4.) *Chai H., Farr R.S., Froehlich L.A., Mathison D.A., McLean J.A., Rosenthal R.R., Sheffer A.L., Spector Sh.L., and Townley R.G. (1975) Standardization of bronchial inhalation challenge procedures. J Allergy Clin Immunol 56(4):323-327.*

5.) *Henson P.M. (1976) Activation and desensitization of platelets by platelet-activating factor (PAF) derived from IgE sensitized basophils. J Exptl Med 143:937-952.*

6.) *Henson, P., and Pinckard R.N. (1977) Basophil-derived platelet-activating factor (PAF) as an in vivo mediator of acute allergic reactions: Demonstration of specific desensitization of platelets to PAF during IgE-induced anaphylaxis. J Immunol 119(9): 2179 - 2184.*

7.) *Klein G. and Matthys H. (1986) Bronchiale Hyperreagibilität. Nachweismethoden mit pharmakodynamischen Substanzen. Prax. Klin. Pneumol. 40:156-166.*

8.) *Schmitz-Schumann, M., Schaub, E., and Virchow, Chr. (1982) Inhalative Provokation mit Lysin-Azetylsalizylsäure bei Analgetika-Asthma-Syndrom. Prax. Klin. Pneumol 36: 17 - 21.*

9.) *Schmitz-Schumann, M. (1985) Asthma, analgesics and arachidonic acid metabolites. Triangle Suppl., 23(1): 8 - 10.*

10.) *Schmitz-Schumann M, Juhl E., Costabel G., Rühle K.-H., Menz G., Virchow Chr., Matthys H. (1985) Analgetikaprovokationsproben bei Analgetika-Asthma-Syndrom 11(10): 479-486.*

11.) *Szczeklik A. (1986) Analgesics, Allergy and Asthma. Drugs 32(Suppl.4):148-163.*

12.) *Virchow, Chr., Schmitz-Schumann, M., and Juhl- Schaub E. (1986) Pyrazolones and analgesics-induced asthma. In: ed. K. Brune, 100 years of Pyrazolone Drugs. Agents and Actions Supplements, 19: 291 - 301.*

NEW CONCEPTS IN THE PATHOGENESIS OF BRONCHIAL HYPERRESPONSIVENESS

Peter J Barnes, DM, FRCP. Department of Clinical Pharmacology, Cardiothoracic Institute, Brompton Hospital, LONDON, U.K.

Introduction

The pathogenesis of asthma is still elusive, although recently several advances have been made in our understanding of the disease. This should eventually lead to more effective therapy.

Airway obstruction in asthma is due to more than contraction of airway smooth mucle. Pathological studies suggest that inflammatory swelling of the airway wall and plugging of the lumen by viscous mucous secretions may also contribute and these phenomena may be more important than smooth muscle contraction in chronic asthma. Bronchial hyperresponsiveness, an exaggerated bronchoconstrictor response to many different stimuli, is a key feature of asthma, and relates more closely to the severity of asthma and the frequency of symptoms than does resting lung function (Juniper et al, 1981). To determine the cause of asthma it is necessary to understand the mechanisms for bronchial hyperresponsiveness, and effective control of asthma involves reducing bronchial responsiveness. Increased bronchial responsiveness can be induced by exposure to allergen, ozone, industrial chemicals or virus infections in animals and humans (Boushey et al, 1980).

Inflammation

There is now considerable experimental evidence that induced induced hyperresponsiveness is associated with inflammation in the airways (Chung, 1986). Histopathological studies from asthmatic patients who have died during asthma attacks show that there is marked inflammation in the airways, with infiltration of inflammatory cells, particularly eosinophils, disruption of airway epithelium and mucus hypersecretion (Dunnill, 1960). Similar pathological changes have also been found in bronchial biopsies from asthmatics who are relatively mild (Laitinen et al, 1985) and suggest that airway inflammation may underly bronchial hyperresponsiveness.

It now seems likely that several different cells are involved in the pathogenesis of asthma, and that these cells produce a variety of mediators which interact in a complex way to produce a number of pathological effects which, together, contribute to bronchial hyperresponsiveness. Recent advances have involved recognition of the different cells and inflammatory mediators involved in asthma, and of neural mechanisms which may contribute to or modify the inflammatory events.

Cells Involved in Asthma

Airway Smooth Muscle

Contraction of airway smooth muscle is believed to be the basis for rapid bronchospasm, and reversal of this contraction is likely to be the major action of bronchodilators. Contraction of airway smooth muscle depends on an increase in intracellular calcium ions which may result from movement of calcium into the cell or from release from internal stores. Contraction of airway smooth muscle is largely independent of extracellular calcium, and therefore calcium antagonists such as nfedipine which block calcium entry, are not effective in asthma (Barnes, 1985). It is more likely that spasmogens stimulate breakdown of membrane phosphoinositides which lead to intracellular calcium release (Grandordy et al, 1985).

It is still uncertain whether airway smooth muscle is abnormal in asthma. Studies of contractile responses of airways *in vitro* to various spasmogens show no relationship to the degree of airway reactivity shown to the spasmogens *in vivo* (Vincenc et al, 1983). However, few true asthmatics have been studied in this way and, in any case, it is likely that removal of airway smooth muscle from its inflammatory microenvironment will result in disappearance of any abnormality, such as receptor-linked abnormalities or altered gap junctions. Airway smooth muscle hyperplasia is present even in relatively mild asthmatics, possibly as a result of various growth factors released from inflammatory cells, such as platelet-derived and macrophage-derived growth factors. It seems likely that hyperplasia of airway smooth muscle would contribute to airway hyperresponsiveness, and may explain the persistence of bronchial hyperresponsiveness after inflammation has subsided.

Mast Cells

For many years mast cells have been assumed to play a central role in the pathogenesis of asthma, but recent evidence has argued strongly against their involvement in bronchial hyperresponsiveness. Cromoglycate was shown to stabilise rat mast cells and this seemed a reasonable explanation for its ability to prevent early and late responses to allergen. More potent mast cell stabilisers, such as lodoxamide and oxatomide, which were later developed, failed to show any clinically useful effect and, although some protected against early responses to allergen, none protected against late responses or reduced bronchial hyperresponsiveness. Furthermore, β2-agonists, which are potent stabilisers of human mast cells, fail to inhibit late responses or to reduce bronchial hyperreactivity (Kraan et al, 1985; Kerrebijn et al, 1987). Thus, although the mast cell may be involved in immediate responses to allergens (and possibly exercise), it is unlikely to be involved in bronchial hyperresponsiveness. Attention has therefore focussed on other inflammatory cells.

Macrophages

Macrophages are present throughout the respiratory tract, and the recent demonstration that they may be activated by IgE-dependent mechanisms has suggested that they may be involved in asthmatic inflammation (Joseph et al, 1983a). Macrophages from asthmatics release increased amounts of mediators, such as thromboxane, prostaglandins and platelet-activating factor (PAF).

Eosinophils

Histological studies suggest that eosinophil infiltration is a feature of asthmatic airways and differentiates asthma from other inflammatory conditions. Allergen inhalation results in a marked increase in eosinophils in bronchoalveolar lavage fluid at the time of the late reaction (de Monchy et al, 1985), and there is a relationship between peripheral eosinophilia and bronchial hyperresponsiveness (Frigas and Gleich, 1986).

Eosinophils release a variety of mediators, including leukotriene C4 and PAF, and basic proteins such as major basic protein, eosinophil cationic protein and eosinophil-derived neurotoxin, which are toxic to airway epithelium. Activated eosinophils in the airway lumen may thus lead to the epithelial damage, which is so characteristic of asthma.

Neutrophils

While neutrophil infiltration is characteristic of some animal models of asthma (O'Byrne et al, 1985), the role of neutrophils in human asthma is less certain. In some animal models neutrophil infiltration apparently follows the development of increased responsiveness, and neutrophil depletion with cyclophosphamide does not affect its development (Murlas and Roum, 1985).

Epithelial cells

Airway epithelial damage may be a critical feature of airway hyperesponsiveness and may explain how several different mechanisms, such as ozone exposure, virus infection and allergen exposure, can lead to its development, since all these stimuli may lead to epithelial disruption. Epithelial disruption may contribute to bronchial hyperresponsiveness in a number of ways.

Recent studies have demonstrated that mechanical removal of epithelial cells *in vitro* results in increased responsiveness of airway smooth muscle to spasmogens (Barnes et al, 1985; Flavahan et al, 1985), and suggests that epithelial cells may release a relaxant factor by analogy with endothelial-derived relaxant factor in vessels. Damage of epithelium would thus remove the protective effect of this relaxant factor, leading to exaggerated bronchoconstrictor responses.

Epithelial damage will also expose sensory nerve endings, which may be activated by inflammatory mediators, leading to inflammation via an axon reflex mechanism (Barnes, 1986a). Epithelial cells themselves may release inflammatory mediators, such as leukotriene B4 and 15-HETE, which is chemotactic for inflammatory cells (Hunter et al, 1985).

Platelets

Abnormalities of platelet function have been found in asthma, and animal studies suggest that platelets may be implicated in certain types of bronchial hyperresponsiveness (Morley et al, 1984). Platelets may release a variety of mediators, such as serotonin, thromboxane and 5- and 12-lipoxygenase products, and may be activated by IgE-dependent mechanisms (Joseph et al, 1983b).

Inflammatory mediators

Many different mediators have been implicated in asthma and they may have a variety of affects on the airways which account for many of the pathological features of asthma (Barnes, 1987b). Thus, mediators such as histamine, prostaglandins and leukotrienes contract airway smooth muscle, increase microvascular leakage, increase mucus secretion and attract other inflammatory cells. It is therefore possible that interaction between inflammatory mediators might account for bronchial hyperresponsiveness. Guinea-pig airway smooth muscle contraction *in vitro* may be potentiated by mediators such as 15-HETE (Copas et al, 1982) and leukotrienes C4 and D4 (Crease and Bach, 1983). Inhaled leukotriene D4 does not increase bronchial responsiveness to histamine in humans, however (Barnes et al, 1984). *In vivo*, prostaglandin D2 potentiates the bronchoconstrictor response to histamine and cholinergic agonist in asthmatic subjects (Fuller et al, 1985). These effects are transient and therefore unlikely to account for the sustained bronchial hyperresponsiveness of asthma. Only one mediator, PAF, is able to cause consistent prolonged increase in non-specific bronchial responsiveness.

Platelet-activating factor

PAF may be produced by several of the inflammatory cells involved in asthma, such as macrophages, eosinophils and neutrophils, but not from mast cells. In animals, PAF may cause a prolonged increase to bronchial responsiveness (Mazzoni et al, 1985; Chung et al, 1986) and our recent studies have demonstrated that inhaled PAF causes an increased brochial response to methacholine in normal subjects, whereas lyso-PAF is without effect (Cuss et al, 1986). The maximal effect is observed 3 days after inhalation and may persist for up to 4 weeks. Similar changes have also been observed in asthmatic subjects (Chung et al, 1987). Because PAF is rapidly inactivated *in vivo*, this suggests that it must trigger a series of inflammatory events which can account for the very prolonged increase in bronchial responsiveness.

PAF-induced bronchial hyperresponsiveness is platelet-dependent in guinea-pigs, since it may be prevented by prior depletion of platelets but not neutrophils by a cytotoxic antibody (Mazzoni et al, 1985), but whether this is so in humans is not certain. Inhaled PAF has no effect on circulating platelets in man, but causes a profound fall in circulating neutrophils and eosinophils (Chung et al, 1987). PAF, like antigen, stimulates accumulation of eosinophils in lung (Lellouch-Tubiana et al, 1985) and in the skin of atopic subjects (Henocq and Vargaftig, 1986). This selective attraction of eosinophils might explain how PAF can produce such a prolonged increase in responsiveness, since eosinophils may lead to damage and shedding of airway epithelium as discussed above. Since eosinophils themselves are a rich source of PAF (Lee et al, 1984), they can attract further eosinophils and there is the potential for a continued inflammation (Fig 1).

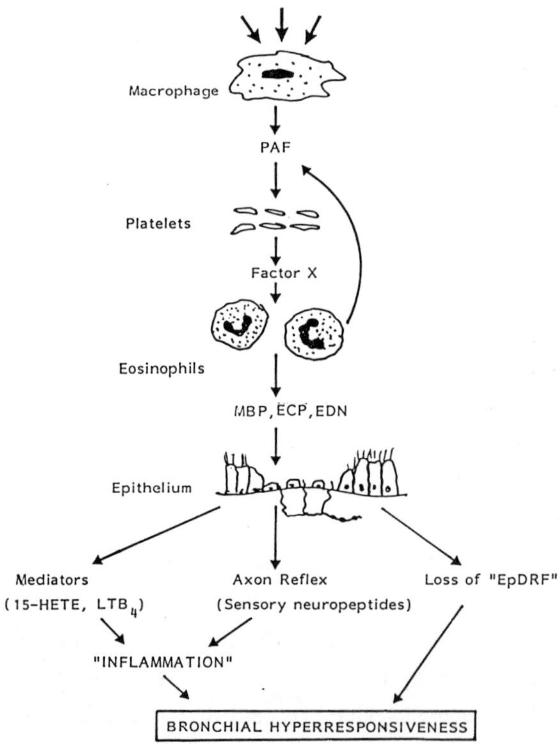

Fig 1

Possilbe mechanism for PAF-induced airway hyperresponsiveness

MBP = major basic protein,
ECP = eosinophil cationic protein
EDN = eosinophil derived neurotoxin
"Ep DRF" = putative epithelial derived relaxant factor

PAF has other properties which may be relevant in asthma. In animals, PAF is a potent inducer of airway microvascular leak, being the most potent agent so far described (Evans et al, 1986). This may lead to airway oedema and plasma extravasation which may be involved in the creation of hyperresponsiveness (Persson, 1986).

Several specific antagonists of PAF are available and their use in models of disease should make it possible to evaluate the role of endogenous PAF. One such antagonist is derived from the leaf of Ginkgo biloba, an ancient Chinese herbal remedy for chest disease. Ginkgolides (BN 52063) inhibit PAF-induced microvascular leakage in guinea-pigs (Barnes et al, 1986a), and, when given orally to man, inhibit PAF-induced platelet aggregation and wheal and flare response in the skin (Barnes et al, 1986b). Whether PAF-antagonists have a role in human asthma is not yet determined, but in animals these drugs have some effect on the acute bronchoconstrictor response to allergens (Braquet et al, 1985; Darius et al, 1986). Considerable caution must be exerted in proposing a role for PAF in bronchial hyperresponsiveness, since previous claims for various mediators in asthma have proved incorrect. The use of specific antagonists should answer these questions and it is possible that PAF is involved in certain forms of asthma. In any case, PAF-induced hyperresponsiveness may be a useful model in understanding mechanisms and in investigation of therapeutic strategies.

Neural mechanisms

Autonomic nervous control of the airways is complex (Nadel and Barnes, 1984; Barnes, 1986b) and several studies have investigated the possibility that defects in autonomic control may contribute to bronchial hyperresponsiveness and the pathology of asthma. Several abnormalities of autonomic function, such as enhanced cholinergic and α-adrenergic responses or reduced β-adrenergic responses, have been proposed. Current thinking suggests that these abnormalities are likely to be secondary to the disease, rather than primary defects (Barnes, 1986b). It is possible that airway inflammation may interfere with autonomic control by several mechanisms (Barnes, 1986c). Inflammatory mediators may stimulate cholinergic reflex bronchoconstriction by activation of afferent nerve endings, and may also facilitate release of acetylcholine from motor nerve endings in the airway. Inflammatory mediators also enhance airway α-adrenergic receptor function (Kneussl and Richardson, 1978; Barnes et al, 1983), although whether this is relevant in asthma is doubtful.

Mediators could also have an effect on β-receptor function. PAF appears to reduce the bronchodilator effect of isoprenaline in guinea-pigs *in vivo*, although it has no effect on the relaxant effect of isoprenaline *in vitro* or on the density or affinity of airway β-receptors (Barnes et al, 1986c).

Airway neuropeptides

Many different neuropeptides have now been identified in human airways which have potent effects on airway function (Barnes, 1987a). It is possible that these peptides might be implicated in asthma. Vasoactive intestinal peptide is a potent relaxant of human airway smooth muscle *in vitro* (Palmer et al, 1986) and is a cotransmitter in cholinergic nerves. If this peptide is degraded more rapidly in asthma by enzymes released from inflammatory cells, this could reduce its putative "braking" effect on cholinergic nerves, leading to exaggerated bronchoconstrictor responses (Barnes, 1986d).

Axon Reflexes

Sensory neuropeptides, substance P, neurokinin A and calcitonin gene-related peptide, may also be involved in asthma, since these peptides could be released by a local axon reflex (Barnes, 1986a). Damage to airway epithelium may expose unmyelinated C-fibre afferent nerves (Laitinen et al, 1985), which may then be triggered by inflammatory mediators such as bradykinin (Fuller et al, 1986). This might release sensory neuropeptides from collaterals of these nerves, with resultant bronchoconstriction, microvascular leakage and mucus secretion. Substance P may also degranulate mast cells (Barnes et al, 1986d) and have chemotactic activity (Payan et al, 1984). Axon reflexes, as in the skin and gut, may thus spread the inflammatory changes from areas of localised epithelial damage up and down the airway and may, therefore, contribute to bronchial hyperresponsiveness.

Conclusions

Asthma is a complex inflammatory disease of the airways. Several different inflammatory cells, such as eosinophils, macrophages, neutrophils, epithelial cells and platelets, may be involved, with release of many mediators which result in bronchial hyperresponsiveness. The role of mast cells in asthma has previously been over-emphasised and, while these cells may be involved in immediate bronchoconstrictor responses to allergen, they are unlikely to play a major role in the pathogenesis of bronchial hyperresponsiveness. Although inflammatory mediators, such as histamine, prostaglandins, leukotrienes and bradykinin may produce many of the pathological features of asthma, they cannot easily account for bronchial hyperresponsiveness. Only PAF causes a prolonged increase in bronchial responsiveness, although its role in asthma will only be revealed by the use of specific antagonists. Neural mechanisms, such as axon reflexes, may also be involved in the pathogenesis of bronchial asthma. These inflammatory mechanisms may lead to an increase in bronchial responsiveness, which is associated with increased asthma symptoms. Corticosteroids, which inhibit virtually every step in the inflammatory response, are able to reduce bronchial responsiveness, and are effective in controlling asthmatic symptoms. However, steroids are often unable to reduce bronchial responsiveness in asthmatics to normal. This suggests that there is an irreversible component of bronchial hyperresposiveness, which may be structural - such as hypertrophy of airway smooth muscle or chronic induration of the submucosa. These changes cannot be reversed by therapy, but presumably can be prevented by effective suppression of the inflamed airway. This may mean chronic therapy with anti-inflammatory drugs, such as inhaled corticosteroids, rather than over-reliance on bronchodilators, such as β-adrenergic agonists.

REFERENCES

Barnes, N.C., Piper, P.J. and Costello, J.F. (1984). Actions of inhaled leukotrienes and their interactions with other allergic mediators. Prostaglandins. 28, 629-631.

Barnes, P.J. (1985). Clinical studies with calcium antagonists in asthma. Br J Clin Pharmacol. 20, S895-S995.

Barnes, P.J. (1986a). Asthma as an axon reflex. Lancet. 1, 242-245.

Barnes, P.J. (1986b). Neural control of human airways in health and disease. Am Rev Respir Dis. 134, 1289-1314.

Barnes, P.J. (1986c). Airway inflammation and autonomic control. Eur J Respir Dis. 69 (Suppl 147), 80-87.

Barnes, P.J. (1986d). Non-adrenergic non-cholinergic neural control of human airways. Arch int Pharmacodyn. 280, 208-228.

Barnes, P.J. (1987a). Airway neuropeptides and asthma. Trends Pharm Sci. 8, 24-27.

Barnes, P.J. (1987b). Inflammatory mediator receptors and asthma. Am Rev Respir Dis. In press.

Barnes, P.J., Skoogh, B.-.E., Brown, J.K. and Nadel, J.A. (1983). Activation of alpha-adrenergic responses in tracheal smooth muscle: a post-receptor mechanism. J Appl Physiol. 54, 1469-1476.

Barnes, P.J., Cuss, F.M.C. and Palmer, J.B.D. (1985). The effect of airway epithelium on smooth muscle contractility in bovine trachea. Br J Pharmacol. 86, 685-691.

Barnes, P.J., Chung, K.F., Rogers, D.F. and Evans, T.W. (1986a). Increased airway vascular permeability induced by platelet activating factor: effect of specific antagonism and platelet depletion. Br J Pharmacol. 89, 764P.

Barnes, P.J., Chung, K.F., Dent, G., Guinot, Ph., McCusker, M. and Page, C.P. (1986b). Effectiveness of a specific antagonist of platelet-activating factor, BN 52063, in man. Br J Pharmacol. In press.

Barnes, P.J., Grandordy, B., Page, C.P., Rhoden, K.J. and Robertson, D.N. (1986c). The effect of PAF induced bronchial hyperreactivity on beta-adrenoceptor function. Br J Pharmacol. 89, 742P.

Barnes, P.J., Brown, M.J., Dollery, C.T., Fuller, R.W., Heavey, D.J. and Ind, P.W. (1986d). Histamine is released from skin by substance P but does not act as the final vasodilator in the axon reflex. Br J Pharmacol. 88, 741-745.

Boushey, H.A., Holtzman, M.J., Sheller, J.R. and Nadel, J.A. (1980).

Bronchial hyperreactivity. Am Rev Respir Dis. 121, 389-413.

Braquet, P., Etienne, A., Touvay, C., Bourgain, R., Lefort, J. and Vargaftig, B.B. (1985). Involvement of platelet activating factor in respiratory anaphylaxis, demonstrated by Paf-acether inhibitor BN 52021. Lancet. 1, 1501.

Chung, K.F. (1986). Role of inflammation in the hyperreactivity of the airways in asthma. Thorax. 41, 657-662.

Chung, K.F., Aizawa, H., Leikauf, G.D., Ueki, I.F., Evans, T.W. and Nadel, J.A. (1986). Airway hyperresponsiveness induced by platelet-activating factor: role of thromboxane generation. J Pharmacol Exp Ther. 236, 580-584.

Chung, K.F., Cuss, F.M., Evans, T.W. and Barnes, P.J. (1987). Platelet-activating factor: relevance to asthma. In: PAF, Pulmonary Hyperreactivty and Asthma. Holme G, Morley J, eds. Academic Press. In press.

Copas, J.L., Borgeat, P. and Gardiner, P.J. (1982). The actions of 5-,12- and 15-HETE on tracheobronchial smooth muscle. Prostagland Leuk Med. 8, 105-114.

Creese, B.R. and Bach, M.K. (1983). Hyperreactivity of airways smooth muscle produced in vitro by leukotrienes. Prostagland Leuk Med. 11, 161-169.

Cuss, F.M., Dixon, C.M.S. and Barnes, P.J. (1986). Effects of inhaled platelet activating factor on pulmonary function and bronchial responiveness in man. Lancet. 2, 189-192.

Darius, H., Lefer, D.J., Smith, B. and Lefer, A.M. (1986). Role of platelet-activating factor - acether in mediating guinea pig anaphylaxis. Science. 232, 58-60.

De Monchy, J.G.R., Kauffman, H.F., Venge, P., Koeter, G.H., Jansen, H.M., Sluiter, H.J. and de Vries, K. (1985). Bronchoalveolar eosinophils during allergen-induced late asthmatic reactions. Am Rev Respir Dis. 131, 373-376.

Dunnill, M.S. (1960). The pathology of asthma with special reference to changes in the bronchial mucosa. J Clin Path. 13, 27-33.

Evans, T.W., Chung, K.F. and Barnes, P.J. (1986). Platelet activating factor increases vascular permeability in guinea-pig airways. Clin Sci. 71, 1P.

Flavahan, N.A., Aarhus, L.L., Rimele, T.J. and Vanhoutte, P.M. (1985). Respiratory epithelium inhibits bronchial smooth muscle tone. J Appl Physiol. 58, 834-838.

Frigas, E. and Gleich, G.J. (1986). The eosinophil and the pathology of asthma. J Allergy Clin Immunol. 77, 527-537.

Fuller, R.W., Dixon, C.M.S., Dollery, C.T. and Barnes, P.J. (1986). Prostaglandin D2 potentiates airway responses to histamine and methacholine. Am Rev Respir Dis. 133, 252-254.

Fuller, R.W., Dixon, C.M.S., Cuss, F.M.C. and Barnes, P.J. (1987). Bradykinin-induced bronchoconstriction in man: mode of action. Am Rev Respir Dis. 135, 176-180.

Grandordy, B.M., Cuss, F.M., Sampson, A.S., Palmer, J.B. and Barnes, P.J. (1986). Phosphatidylinositol response to cholinergic agonists in airway smooth muscle: relationship to contraction and muscarinic receptor occupancy. J Pharmacol Exp Ther. 238, 273-279.

Henocq, E. and Vargaftig, B.B. (1986). Accumulation of eosinophils in response to intracutaneous PAF-acether and allergens in man. Lancet. 1, 1378-1379.

Hunter, J.A., Finkbeiner, W.E., Nadel, J.A., Goetzl, E.J. and Holtzman, M.J. (1985). Predominant generation of 15-lipoxygenase metabolites of arachidonic acid by epithelial cells from human trachea. Proc Natl Acad Sci USA. 82, 4633-4637.

Joseph, M., Tonnel, A.B., Tarpier, G. and Capron, A. (1983). Involvement of immunoglobulin E in the secretory process of alveolar macrophages from asthmatic patients. J Clin Invest. 71, 221-230.

Joseph, M., Auriault, C., Capron, A., Vorng, H. and Viens, P. (1983). A new function for platelets: IgE-dependent killing of schistozomes. Nature. 303, 310-312.

Juniper, E.F., Frith, P.A. and Hargreave, F.E. (1981). Airway responsiveness to histamine and methacholine: relationship to minimum treatment to control symptoms of asthma. Thorax. 36, 575-579.

Kerrebijn, K.F., von Essen-Zandvliet, E.E.M. and Neijens, H.J. (1987). Effect of long-term treatment with inhaled corticosteroids and beta-agonists on bronchial responsiveness in asthmatic children. J Allergy Clin Immunol. In press.

Kneussl, M.P. and Richardson, J.B. (1978). Alpha-adrenergic receptors in human and canine tracheal and bronchial smooth muscle. J Appl Physiol. 45, 307-311.

Kraan, J., Koeter, G.H., V.d. Mark, T.W., Sluiter, H.J. and de Vries, K. (1985). Changes in bronchial hyperreactivity induced by 4 weeks of treatment with antiasthma drugs in patients with allergic asthma: a comparison between budesonide and terbutaline. J Allergy Clin Immunol. 76, 628-636.

Laitinen, L.A., Heino, M., Laitinen, A., Kava, T. and Haahtela, T. (1985). Damage of the airway epithelium and bronchial reactivity in patients with asthma. Am Rev Respir Dis. 131, 599-606.

Lee, T.C., Lenihan, D.J., Malone, B., Roddy, L.L. and Wasserman, S.I. (1984). Increased biosynthesis of platelet activating factor in activated human eosinophils. J Biol Chem. 259, 5526-5530.

Lellouch-Tubiana, A., Lefort, J., Pirotzky, E., Vargaftig, B.B. and Pfister, A. (1985). Ultrastructural evidence for extravascular platelet recruitment in the lung upon intravenous injection of platelet activating factor (Paf-acether) to guinea-pigs. Br J Exp Pathol. 66, 345-355.

Mazzoni, L., Morley, J., Page, C.P. and Sanjar, S. (1985). Induction of airway hyper-reactivity by platelet activating factor in the guinea-pig. J Physiol. 365, 107.

Morley, J., Sanjar, S. and Page, C.P. (1984). Platelet activation as a basis for asthma exacerbation. Lancet. 2, 1142-1144.

Murlas, C.G. and Roum, J.H. (1985). Sequence of pathologic changes in the airway mucosa of guinea pigs during ozone-induced bronchial hyperreactivity. Am Rev Respir Dis. 131, 314-320.

O'Byrne, P.M., Walters, E.H., Gold, B.D. et. al. (1985). Neutrophil depletion inhibits airway hyperresponsiveness induced by ozone exposure in dogs. Am Rev Respir Dis. 130, 214-219.

Palmer, J.B., Cuss, F.M.C. and Barnes, P.J. (1986). VIP and PHM and their role in non-adrenergic inhibitory responses in isolated human airways. J Appl Physiol. 61, 1322-1328.

Payan, G.P., Levine, J.D. and Goetzl, E.J. (1984). Modulation of immunity and hypersensitivity by sensory neuropeptides. J Immunol. 132, 1601-1604.

Persson, C.G.A. (1986). The role of microvascular permeability in the pathogenesis of asthma. Eur J Respir Dis. 68 (Suppl 144), 190-216.

Vincenc, K.S., Black, J.L., Yan, K., Armour, C.L., Donnelly, P.D. and Woolcock, A.J. (1983). Comparison of in vivo and in vitro responses to histamine in human airways. Am Rev Respir Dis. 128, 875-879.

EFFECTS OF BN 52066 ON PAF-ACETHER INDUCED WEAL AND FLARE IN MAN

Ph. Guinot(1), P.Braquet(1), J. Duchier(2), A. Cournot(2)

1 - I.H.B. Research Labs, 17 avenue Descartes, F-92350 Le Plessis Robinson, France

2 - Therapharm Recherches, F-75016 Paris, France

Introduction

It has been suggested that PAF-acether may be an important mediator in asthma (5) and a PAF-acether antagonist may therefore have a potentially important role (3). PAF-acether has been shown to induce a dual inflammatory response in the skin of man (1) and we investigated the effect of BN 52063, a PAF-acether antagonist (2) on this response. BN 52063 orally inhibited the inflammatory response to a sub-cutaneous injection of PAF-acether. This effect proved to be dependent: on the dose of injected PAF-acether, on the dose of BN 52063, and on the time of challenge after the intake of the drug.

A late cutaneous response was not observed in any of the subjects. BN 52063 was also demonstrated to be tolerated at doses of 20, 40, 80 and 120 mg with no significant side effects.

A - First Experiment

Method

Five healthy male volunteers (age range 21-27) gave their informed consent to enter this single-blind cross-over trial. The protocol for the study was approved by the local Ethical Committee.

Before inclusion, the blood pressure, pulse, ECG and laboratory parameters for each volunteer were confirmed to be within normal limits. Subjects were excluded if there was evidence of renal, hepatic, cardiac, haematological and gastro-intestinal disorders, or drug abuse. Concomitant medication was not permitted for two weeks prior to or during the study.

Subjects were randomised to receive increasing single doses of BN

52063 (20 mg, 40 mg, 80 mg, 120 mg) and placebo separated by at least one week. Clinical and laboratory parameters were closely monitored for 24 hours following each dose.

Ninety minutes after taking BN 52063 (80 mg) or placebo, each subject received sub-cutaneous injections of PAF-acether in the forearm (400 ng in 0.1 ml of 4% human albumin, 50 ng in 0.1 ml of saline and 100 ng in 0.2 ng of saline solution) in order to compare several methods and dose dependent effects of PAF-acether injection.

Saline and albumin solutions were injected separately to act as negative controls. All the injections were given and the responses measured by the same investigator. The cutaneous weal and flare responses were assessed at 15, 30, 60, 120 minutes and 6 hours after injection. The surface area in mm^2 was measured using sellotape and a planimeter (COMSA/Prorobot Instrument) coupled to an Apple MacIntosh computer. Results were recorded as means + SEM.

Results

There were no significant effects of BN 52063 on the blood pressure, pulse, ECG and laboratory parameters at each dosage given. No serious side effects were reported: four subjects reported headaches, three subjects complained of tiredness and one of frequency of micturition, but these did not necessitate stopping treatment and were not dose-related.

The effect of BN 52063 80 ng on PAF-acether induced flare and weal reaction are shown in Figures 1, 2 and 3.

B - Second Experiment (preliminary results)

Method

In a double-blind cross-over trial a single volunteer received a single dose of BN 52063 (80 mg) or placebo and the cutaneous reaction to repeated injection of PAF-acether (400 ng- S.C.HSA) was monitored before intake of the drug and 1, 2, 4, 6, and 8 hours after intake of the drug.

The same study design was used in three other volunteers with a single dose of 120 mg or Placebo.

Results

The results on flare reaction are shown in Figures 4 and 5.

Conclusion

These experiments demonstrate an inhibition of the acute

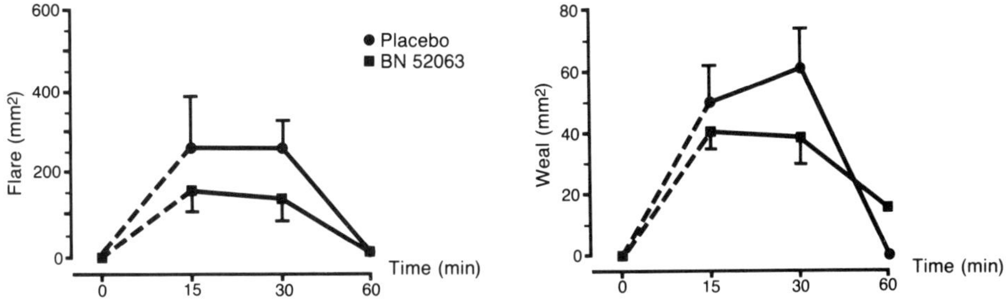

Fig. 1 : Effect of BN 52063 (80 mg, single dose, po, 90 min before challenge) on PAF-acether (50 ng, sc, saline)-induced flare and weal reactions in human.

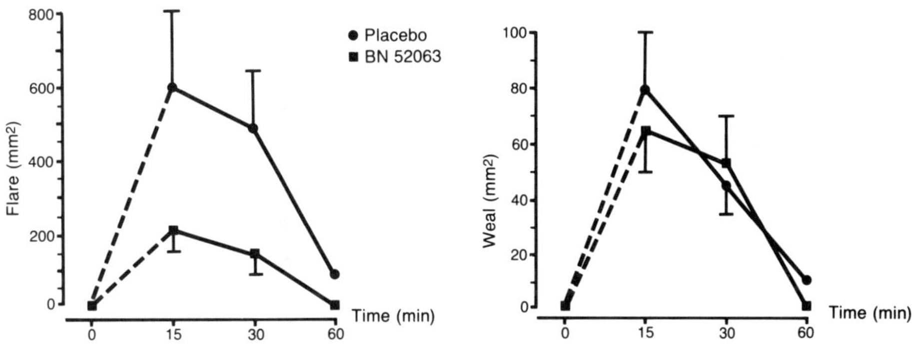

Fig. 2 : Effect of BN 52063 (80 mg, single dose, po, 90 min before challenge) on PAF-acether (100 ng, sc, saline)-induced flare and weal reactions in human.

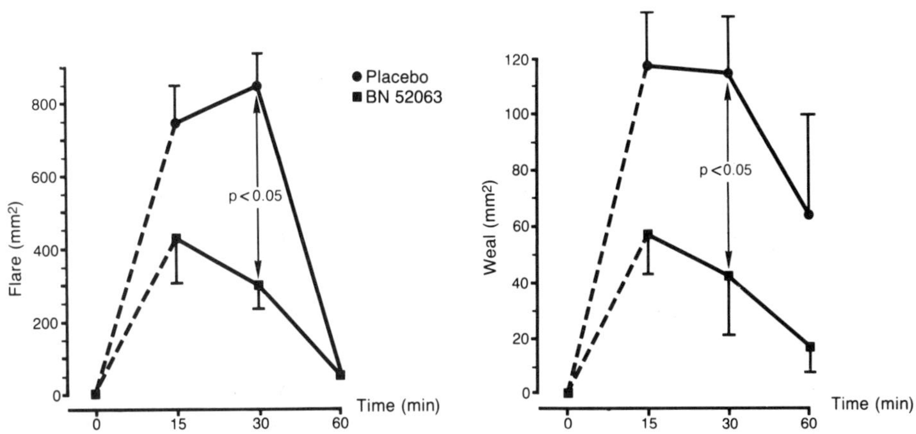

Fig. 3 : Effect of BN 52063 (80 mg, single dose, po, 90 min before challenge) on PAF-acether (400 ng, sc, HSA)-induced flare and weal reactions in human.

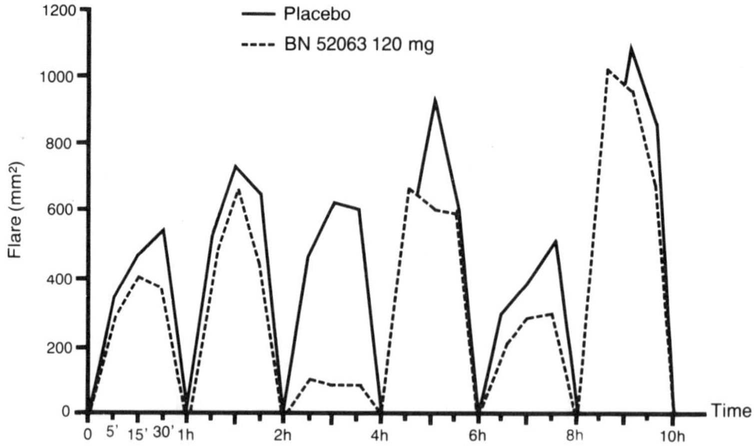

Fig. 4 : Effect of BN 52063 (80 mg, single dose, po) and placebo on PAF-acether (400 ng, sc, HSA)-induced flare reaction in humans (mean of three subjects)

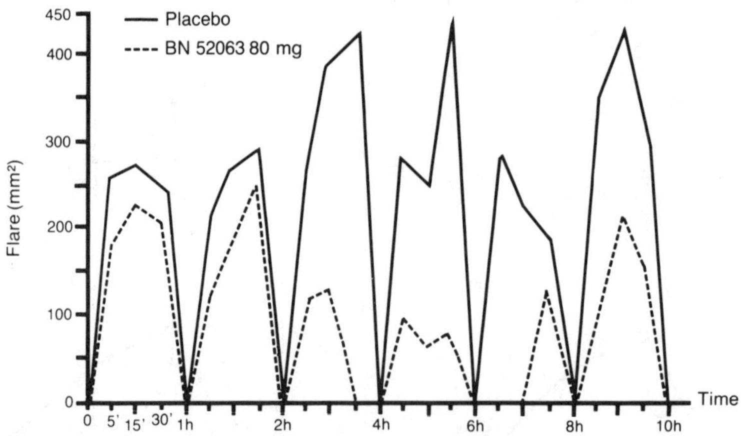

Fig. 5 : Effect of BN 52063 (120 mg, single dose, po) and placebo on PAF-acether-induced flare reaction in humans (mean of three subjects)

PAF-acether induced cutaneous reaction in man by BN 52063. Furthermore, our recent trials confirmed our first findings (4) and also indicate that the effect of BN 52063 an this models depends on the quantity of PAF-acether injected, on the dosage of BN 52021, and on the time of challenge after drug intake.

References

1. *Archer, C.B., Page, C.P., Paul, W., Morley, J. and Mac Donald, D.M. (1985). Actions of disodium cromaglycate (DSCG) on human skin responses to histamine, codenic and PAF-acether. Agents Actions 16 : 6-8*

2. *Braquet, P. (1984). Treatment or prevention of PAF-acether-induced disorders by a new series of highly specific inhibitors. Belg. BE 901, 915 (July 19, 1984 - see CA 103 : 189808d, 1985)*

3. *Braquet, P., Etienne, A., Touvay, C., Bourgain, R.H., Lefort, J. and Vargaftig, B.B. (1985). Involvement of platelet activating factor in respiratory anaphylaxis demonstrated by PAF-acether inhibitor BN 52021, Lancet i: 1501*

4. *Guinot, Ph., Braquet, P., Duchier, J. and Cournot, A. (1986). Inhibition of PAF-acether-induced weal and flare reaction in man by a specific PAF antagonist. Prostaglandins 32 : 160-163.*

5. *Vargaftig, B.B., Chignard, M., Benveniste, J. Lefort, J. and Wal, F. (1981). Background and present status of research on platelet-activating factor (PAF-acether). Ann. NY Acad. Sci. 370 : 119-137*

EFFECTS OF THE PAF-ANTAGONIST CV-3988 ON PAF-INDUCED CHANGES IN MUCUS SECRETION AND IN RESPIRATORY AND CIRCULATORY VARIABLES IN FERRETS.

M. Lang, D. Hansen and H.-L. Hahn.

Medizinische Poliklinik, University of Würzburg, 8700 Würzburg

Introduction

Platelet activating factor (PAF) is released from polymorphonuclear leukocytes (9), eosinophils (10), macrophages (1,2) and other cells following activation by IgE-mediated mechanisms. PAF in turn activates platelets and leads to their accumulation in lung tissue (15). Many, but not all of the effects of exogenously applied PAF resemble symptoms seen in bronchial asthma, thus the rôle of PAF in asthma is unclear. Symptoms typical of asthma are bronchoconstriction (6,23), mucus secretion (6), tissue eosinophilia (4) and long lasting hyperreactivity (14). Symtoms not typical of asthma are leukopenia, hypotension and a dramatic increase in vascular permeability with subsequent haemoconcentration, pulmonary oedema and shock (6,3). Some of these effects are mediated by platelets, others appear to be direct because they are not changed by platelet depletion. Platelet-mediated effects include bronchoconstriction and bronchial hyperreactivity (14,19,23) although there is no universal agreement on this (21). Direct effects include increased vascular permeability, oedema, and hypotension (7,16). Competitive receptor antagonists of PAF have been developed and selection has been based on their potency to displace PAF from the specific receptor on platelets.

The question whether PAF is a major mediator of asthma will ultimately be answered by studies in which antagonists are used to prevent IgE-mediated allergic reactions. However, before these compounds can be used as tools for identifying the rôle of PAF in asthma it has to be shown that they are reliable blockers of the effects of PAF. Compounds engineered to antagonize the PAF receptor on platelets may only antagonize platelet-mediated, but not direct effects of PAF. If they do not antagonize direct effects of PAF this may be because such effects are mediated by receptor subtypes different from those on platelets (8,9) or because they are not receptor mediated. As a phospholipid PAF can be expected to have nonspecific effects on cell membranes which might be unaffected by receptor antagonists. Only if a specific receptor antagonist blocks all effects of PAF can it be expected to prevent asthma if asthma is PAF mediated.

Takeda compound CV-3988 inhibits or blocks a variety of PAF-induced changes, e.g. platelet aggregation and hypotension (22). We wanted to know to what extent this compound blocked other effects of PAF, especially the PAF-induced increase in mucus secretion which we have described previously (6).

Methods

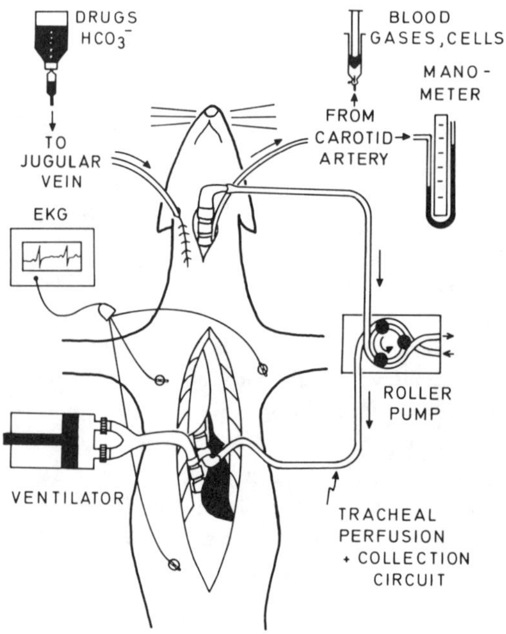

Fig. 1: Experimental setup: isolated perfused segment of trachea with intact nerve and blood supply.

We anaesthetized 28 female ferrets, mean weight 760 g (SD 98 g) with pentobarbital (Nembutal[R]) at an initial dose of 46 ± 6 mg/kg (mean ± SD) given intraperitoneally. During surgery, the animals inhaled an oxygen-enriched gas mixture. We dissected the jugular vein under a stereo-microscope (OPMI I, Zeiss) and inserted a polyethylene catheter (PE 60 to PE 100) through which we infused a modified Ringer's lactate solution (Sterofundin[R],

Braun Melsungen). We added 50 meq $NaHCO_3$/litre to prevent metabolic acidosis. Supplemental doses of anaesthetic (total dose 93 ± 20 mg/kg, mean ± SD) and drugs were also applied through this catheter. We cannulated the carotid artery to measure blood pressure and to obtain blood samples for gas analysis and cell counts. We cannulated the trachea just below the larynx and ventilated the animals with a Harvard respirator (model 661). We opened the thorax by median sternotomy starting from the xiphisternum upwards. End-expiratory pressure was set at 5 cm H_2O to prevent collapse of the lungs during expiration. We carefully separated the trachea from the superior vena cava and opened the trachea 1 cm above the bifurcation. We inserted a cannula into the caudad opening and ventilated the animal with a volume of 20 ± 2 ml (mean ± SD) at 31 ± 2 strokes per minute. Another cannula was inserted into the cephalad opening for perfusion of the upper trachea (fig. 1). We closed the thorax and inserted a chest tube to maintain negative pleural pressure (-5 cm H_2O). The two cannulae inserted into the upper trachea (top and bottom) were connected through silicone tubing to a roller pump (Harvard peristaltic pump, model 1201) and thence to a reservoir containing 7 ml medium M-199 in Earle's balanced salt solution, so the isolated segment could be perfused continuously with medium and the perfusate could be changed without stopping the roller pump.

We inserted 3 needle electrodes into the animals' skin for continuous monitoring of the ECG (Hellige Servomed compact monitor) which was also recorded briefly at 5-min-intervals on a single channel recorder (Allco model ED 142 B thermal writer) during collection periods. Mean blood pressure was measured with a Hg-manometer through the cannula in the carotid artery. Blood samples were taken from the same artery. pO_2, pCO_2 and pH were measured with a Corning 178 pH/blood gas analyzer (Corning Medical Corp., Medfield, Mass., USA). 125 µl were needed to fill the capillary. Another 500 µl were collected in an EDTA-coated tube and leucocytes, erythrocytes and thrombocytes were counted in a haematology laser counter (ELT-8, Moltronic, Heidelberg). At the end of the experiment (approx. 1 hour after the application of PAF) we excised the lungs, weighed them before and after freeze-drying and obtained a wet:dry ratio.

PAF (L-α-lecithin, molecular weight 523.7, Serva, Heidelberg) was dissolved in 100% ethanol to a 10^{-2} molar solution which was stored at -20°. Further dilutions were made with Ringer's lactate solution. A dose of 10^{-6} M kg^{-1} was injected in all of these experiments. The antagonist CV-3988 (molecular weight 619.79) was made up in 0.9% NaCl under gentle warming and a solution of 3-4 mg/ml was injected to give a total dose of 12 mg/kg ($2x10^{-5}$ M kg^{-1}).

Samples of perfusate were emptied into dialysis bags (molecular weight cutoff, 12000 to 14000, Servapor, Serva, Heidelberg) and dialyzed for 48 hours against distilled water to remove unbound sulfate. We added nonradioactive $NaSO_4$ to displace $Na^{35}SO_4$ molecules bound covalently and we added sodium azide to prevent bacterial growth. When the radioactivity in the dialysis water had dropped to background levels we emptied each dialysis bag into a 20 ml scintillation vial, added 10 ml scintillation fluid (Lumagel, Baker Chemicals) and counted radioactivity in a beta-counter (Betamatic I, Kontron).

Time course of experiments:

After connecting the tracheal segment to the perfusion circuit we added 200 µCi $Na^{35}SO_4$ to the perfusion volume of 7 ml and injected 100 µCi $Na^{35}SO_4$ in 1 ml Ringer's solution i.v. Radioactivity was drained from the segment 2 h later at the start of the collecting periods. After 3 control samples we slowly injected the antagonist CV-3988 through the jugular catheter over 15 minutes while continuing to sample the perfusate every 5 minutes. At the end of each sampling period, when perfusate was being drained from the circuit, we recorded ECG and blood pressure and collected arterial samples for blood gases and cell counts. In experiments without antagonist we collected 6 control samples. From the 3 values obtained during the slow injection of the antagonist we calculated a mean control value. At time 0 we applied PAF 10^{-6} M kg^{-1} as a bolus dose. Heart rate and blood pressure were measured every minute up to 15 min, then at 5 min-intervals until the end of the experiment. Arterial samples were taken at 2.5, 5, 10, 15, 20 and 30 min after PAF. To ascertain viability of glands, we applied acetylcholine (ACh) 10^{-4} M at 30 minutes and measured the response over three 5-min collecting periods. Results of experiments were considered valid only if ACH caused at least a doubling of secretion.

Statistical evaluation:

Differences obtained between treatments (antagonist vs. no antagonist) were analyzed statistically using the unpaired t-test. Differences within animals (e.g. before and after PAF) were analyzed using Student's paired t-test. We considered differences as significant if the probability of the null hypothesis (p) was 5% or less ($p \leq 0.05$). Data are presented as mean ± standard error ($\bar{x}$ ± SE) unless otherwise stated.

Results

Mucus secretion:

CV-3988 approximately halved the PAF-induced increase in the release of non-dialyzable $Na^{35}SO_4$ from tracheal submucosal glands. $Na^{35}SO_4$ secretion increased 84 ± 23 % without and 41 ± 7 % with the antagonist ($p<0.1$). The secretory effect of ACh 10^{-4} M, given at the end of an experiment to assess gland viability was the same in CV-3988-treated as in control animals (mean increase, 126 ± 24 % vs. 133 ± 18 %, control vs. CV-3988).

Blood cells (fig. 2):

There was a steep fall in leukocyte counts 2.5 min after PAF application which was unchanged by the antagonist. Only slight recovery was seen over the following 30 minutes. Thus CV-3988 was ineffective in reducing PAF-induced leukopenia. Control cell counts for erythrocytes were the same for both groups. PAF-induced haemoconcentration was more severe in CV-3988-treated than in control animals. Differences in erythrocyte counts were significant at 10 and at 15 minutes. Thrombopenia after PAF was less in CV-3988 treated than in control animals. Differences in platelet counts were significant at 10 minutes.

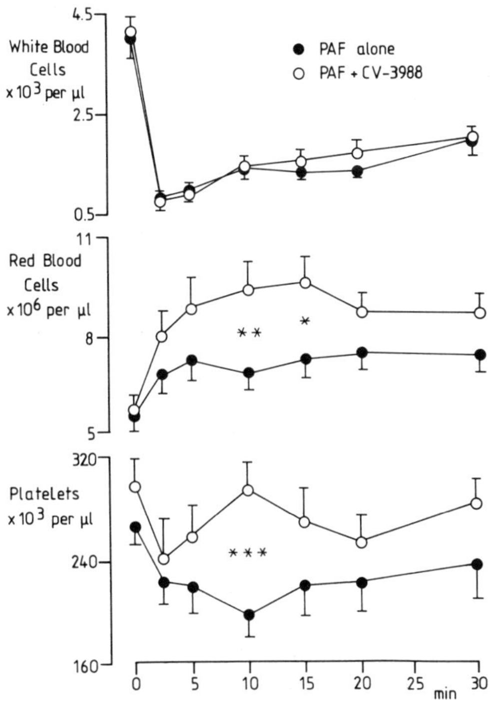

Fig. 2: Effect of PAF alone and of PAF + CV-3988 on blood cells. Mean data ± SE. * $p < 0.05$ ** $p < 0.01$ *** $p < 0.001$

Blood gases, circulatory variables and lung weights:

PAF-induced hypoxaemia, hypercarbia and acidosis were not changed significantly by CV-3988 although there was a tendency for pO_2 to be lower and for pCO_2 to be higher in CV-3988-treated than in untreated animals. Likewise CV-3988 had no effect on PAF-induced hypotension and on changes in heart rate (tachycardia followed by bradycardia). Wet lung weights were significantly higher in CV-3988-treated than in control animals (7.9 ± 0.6 vs. 9.6 ± 0.6 g, $p<0.05$, control vs. CV-3988), although animal weights were the same. The wet:dry ratio was also higher in CV-3988-treated animals (6.6 ± 0.2 vs. 7.4 ± 0.5. con vs. CV-3988), but this difference was not statistically significant.

Discussion:

CV-3988 at a molar dose 20 times higher than the dose of PAF had two beneficial effects: prevention of PAF-induced thrombopenia and 50% inhibition of PAF-induced mucus secretion although the latter did not quite reach statistical significance. This may indicate that PAF-induced hypersecretion and thrombopenia are interrelated. Platelets accumulating in the lungs following PAF injection may release mediators which cause mucus hypersecretion. Blood levels of thromboxane B_2 and prostaglandins are elevated after application of PAF (3) and leukotrienes are released from leukocytes following administration of PAF (11). Prostaglandins E_1 and $F_{2\alpha}$ and leukotrienes C_4 and D_4 are known to increase mucus secretion (12,13,17,18,20), so they could have been responsible for the increase in mucus secretion seen after PAF. A direct effect of PAF on mucus secretion had been ruled out in earlier experiments from our own laboratory (5,24). The residual effect of PAF on mucus secretion seen despite application of CV-3988 was probably due to the continued secretion of mediators from leukocytes whose fall was completely unaffected by the antagonist. In contrast to these beneficial effects was the significant augmentation by CV-3988 of PAF-induced haemoconcentration indicating an increase in plasma extravasation. At the same time lung wet weights were increased, thus preferential extravasation may have been in the lungs. This could explain the tendency of CV-3988 to worsen blood gases.

Summarizing, CV-3988 antagonized some effects of PAF, augmented others and left yet other effects (leukopenia) unchanged. Antagonism to the PAF receptor on platelets did not appear to correlate with overall effectiveness of this specific PAf antagonist, which would lead us to predict that platelet receptor antagonism will not correlate well with the clinical efficacy of a compound. Our results further imply that CV-3988 would not be a good probe for studying mechanisms of asthma. If CV-3988 were shown to cause significant inhibition of asthma symptoms this would, of course, indicate PAF and platelet involvement in the asthmatic reaction. However, a negative result (lack of an effect against asthma) would not allow us to conclude that PAF is not involved in the asthmatic reaction because we know from these experiments that the antagonist does not block all effects of PAF. Possible reasons for partial effectiveness of a highly specific receptor antagonist are [1] that CV-3988 is a partial agonist. This appears to have been the case with CV-3988 which augmented PAF-induced plasma extravasation. [2] that CV-3988 antagonizes the "wrong" receptor. This is possible because receptor heterogeneity has recently been demonstrated (9,8). [3] that not all effects of PAF are receptor mediated. In view of the membrane perturbing properties and detergent-like effects of many phospholipids we consider this a likely possibility in view of the fact that relatively high doses of PAF had to be used in these experiments in order to study the effects of agonist and antagonist on mucus secretion. Previous experiments from our laboratory have shown that PAF has weaker (though still significant) effects on mucus secretion at 10^{-7}M kg^{-1} and is ineffective at 10^{-8}M kg^{-1}. We used 10^{-6}M kg^{-1} PAF to make sure we were operating well above the noise level. Experiments using lower doses of PAF are under way in our laboratory.

References

1. Arnoux, B., D. Duval, J. Benveniste (1980) Release of platelet-activating-factor (PAF-acether) from alveolar macrophages by the calcium ionophore A23178 and phagocytosis. Eur. J. Clin. Invest. 10, 437-441.
2. Arnoux, B., M.H. Simoès-Caeiro, A. Landes, M. Mathieu, P. Duroux, J. Benveniste (1982) Alveolar macrophages from asthmatic patients release platelet activating factor (PAF-acether) and lyso-PAF-acether when stimulated with the specific allergen. Am. Rev. Respir. Dis. 125 (4, part 2) 70.
3. Bessin P., J. Bonnet, D. Apffel, C. Soulard, L. Desgroux, I. Pelas, J. Benveniste (1983) Acute circulatory collapse caused by platelet-activating factor (PAF-acether) in dogs. Eur. J. Pharmacol. 86, 403-413.
4. Denjean, A., B. Arnoux, A. Lockhart, R. Masse, J. Benveniste (1984) Modification of alveolar cell population after PAF-acether-induced bronchoconstriction in baboons. Am. Rev. Respir. Dis. 129 Suppl., A 3.
5. Hahn, H.L., I. Purnama, M. Lang, U. Sannwald, H. Stenzel (1985) Effects of platelet activating factor on release of mucus secretion from tracheal submucosal glands in the ferret. Am. Rev. Respir. Dis. 131, A 27.
6. Hahn, H.L., I. Purnama, M. Lang, U. Sannwald (1986) Effects of platelet activating factor on tracheal mucus secretion, on airway mechanics and on circulating blood cells in live ferrets. Prog. Respir. Res., in press.
7. Halonen, M., J.D. Palmer, I.C. Lohman, L.M. McManus, R.N. Pinckard (1981) Differential effects of platelet depletion on the physiologic alterations of IgE anaphylaxis and acetyl glyceryl ether phosphorylcholine infusion in the rabbit. Am. Rev. Respir. Dis. 124, 416-421.
8. Hwang, S.B., C.S. Lee, M.J. Cheah, T.Y.Shen (1983) Specifific receptor sites for 1-O-alkyl-2-O-acetyl-sn-glycero-3-phosphocholine (patelet activating factor) on rabbit platelet and guinea pig smooth muscle membranes. Biochemistry 22, 4756-4763.

9. Lambrecht, G., M.J. Parnham (1986) Kadsurenone distinguishes between different platelet activating factor subtypes on macrophages and polymorphonuclear leucocytes. Br. J. Pharmac. 87, 287-289.
10. Lee, T.C., D.J. Lenihan, B. Malone, L.L. Roddy, S.I. Wasserman (1984) Increased biosynthesis of platelet-activating factor in activated human eosinophils. J. Biol. Chem. 259, 5526-5530.
11. Lin, A.H., D.R. Morton, R.R. Gorman (1982) Acetyl glyceryl ether phosphorylcholine stimulates leukotrienes B_4 synthesis in human polymorphonuclear leukocytes. J. Clin. Invest. 70, 1058-1065.
12. Marom, Z., J.H. Shelhamer, M.A. Bach, D.R. Morton, M. Kaliner (1982) Slow-reacting substances, leukotrienes C_4 and D_4 increase the release of mucus from human airways in vitro. Am. Rev. Resp. Dis. 126, 449-451.
13. Marom, Z., J.H. Shelhamer, M Kaliner (1981) Effects of arachidonic acid, monohydroxyeicosatetraenoic acid, and prostaglandins on the release of mucous glycoproteins from human airways in vitro. J. Clin. Invest. 67, 1695-1702.
14. Mazzoni, L., J. Morley, C.P. Page, S. Sanjar (1985) Induction of airway hyper-reactivity by platelet activating factor in the guinea-pig. J. Physiol. 365, 107 P.
15. Morley, J., C.P. Page, S. Sanjar (1985) Platelets in asthma. Lancet 2, 726-727.
16. Namm, D.H., A.S. Tadepalli, J.A. High (1982) Species specifity of the platelet responses to 1-O-alkyl-sn-glycero-3-phosphocholine. Thromb. Res. 25, 341-350.
17. Peatfield, A.C., P.J. Piper, P.S. Richardson (1982) The effect of leukotriene C_4 on mucin release into the cat trachea in vivo and in vitro. Br. J. Pharmacol. 77, 391-393.
18. Richardson, P.S., R.J. Phipps, K. Balfre, R.L. Hall (1978) The roles of mediators, irritants and allergens in causing mucin secretion from the trachea. In: Respiratory tract mucus. Ciba Foundation Symposium 54. Amsterdam, Elsevier, p.111-131.
19. Schellenberg, R.R., B. Walker, F. Snyder (1983) Platelet-dependant contraction of human bronchus by platelet-activating factor. J. Allery Clin. Immunol. 71, 145.
20. Shelhamer, J.H., Z. Marom, M. Kaliner (1980) Immunologic and neuropharmacologic stimulation of mucous glycoprotein release from human airways in vitro. J. Clin. Invest. 66, 1400-1408.
21. Stimler, N.P., J.T. O'Flaherty (1983) Spasmogenic properties of platelet activating factor: evidence for a direct mechanism in the contractile response of pulmonary tissues. Am J. Pathol. 113, 75-84.
22. Terashita, Z., S. Tsushima, Y. Yoshioka, H. Nomura, Y. Inada, K. Nishikawa (1983) CV-3988 - a specific antagonist of platelet activating factor (PAF). Life Sci. 32, 1975-1982.
23. Vargaftig B.B., J. Lefort, M. Chignard, J. Benveniste (1980) Platelet-activating factor induces a platelet-dependent bronchoconstriction unrelated to the formation of prostaglandin derivatives. Eur. J. Pharmacol. 65, 185-192.
24. Wirtz, H., M. Lang, U. Sannwald, H.L. Hahn (1986) Mechanism of platelet activating factor (PAF)- induced secretion of mucus from tracheal submucosal glands in the ferret. Fed. Proc. 45, 226.

Hans-L. Hahn, MD, PhD, Medizinische Poliklinik, University of Würzburg, Klinikstraße 8, 8700 Würzburg - West Germany

EFFECT OF THE PAF-ANTAGONIST SRI 63-441 ON THE ALLERGIC REACTION IN AWAKE DOGS WITH NATURAL ASTHMA.

H. Stenzel, B. Hümmer and H.-L. Hahn.

Medizinische Poliklinik, University of Würzburg, West Germany.

Introduction:

Platelet activating factor (PAF) is released by macrophages (1,2), polymorphonuclear leukocytes (13), eosinophils (14) and other cells. PAF imitates many symptoms of anaphylaxis and is believed by some authors to be an important mediator of bronchial asthma. PAF causes an increase in mucus secretion (6), bronchoconstriction (3,5), an accumulation of eosinophils in lung tissue (4) and increased bronchial reactivity (3,17). However, other effects of PAF, i.e. PAF-induced leukopenia, hypotension and haemoconcentration are not typical of bronchial asthma.

If PAF is an important mediator in bronchial asthma, antagonists of PAF should inhibit or block the allergic reaction. SRI 63-441 (Sandoz Research Institute, East Hanover, N.J., USA) is a competitive antagonist of PAF receptors on the platelets of several species. SRI 63-441 inhibits one or more of the following PAF-induced reactions: hypotension, extravasation and bronchoconstriction in guinea pig, dog and cebus monkey (7). We decided to test the efficacy of SRI 63-441 in blocking or inhibiting allergen-induced reactions in a colony of 5 dogs allergic to Ascaris suum antigen. This model of asthma has been described previously (8,10,11,16). The allergic reaction in the Ascaris suum sensitive dog is mediated predominantly by antibodies of the IgE type (10,12,16) and closely resembles human asthma.

Methods:

We trained 5 dogs (24-31 kg) allergic to Ascaris suum antigen to walk on a treadmill (Jaeger, Würzburg, W.-Germany) to divert their attention and to induce an even breathing pattern. During this training period, the dogs became familiar with the personnel, equipment and procedures in the laboratory. Subsequently we surgically exteriorized the cervical vagus nerves and placed them in skin loops. This was required for other experiments. 3 weeks later we created a chronic tracheostomy. Training on the treadmill was resumed within 2 days after each operation. At the beginning of each experiment the animals were intubated with a cuffed endotracheal tube (Rüsch, 8 - 11 mm ID). We measured inspired and expired airflow using pneumotachometers (Fleisch No.3) connected to differential pressure transducers (Validyne DP45). An ultrasonic nebulizer (DeVilbiss No. 65) was placed between the inspiratory pneumotachograph and the non-rebreathing valve (Fig. 1). The dogs learned to swallow an oesophageal balloon catheter for measurement of transpulmonary pressure. The balloon was advanced to a position 5 cm above the stomach and pressure was recorded by a pressure transducer (Validyne DP45). Tracheal gas was sampled at the outlet of the endotracheal tube and analyzed continuously for CO_2 and O_2. CO_2 was analyzed with an infrared absorption device (CO_2-Test, Jaeger), which had a 90 % response time of 100 ms. O_2 was analyzed with a zirconium oxide chamber (O_2-Test, Jaeger) with the same response time. The lag between injection of a pulse of gas into the endotracheal tube and the response of the gas analyzers was 1820 ms for O_2 and 1070 ms for CO_2. Heart rate was monitored with a three-lead electrocardiogram from leads attached to the chest wall and back. Primary signals were fed into a pulmonary mechanics analyzer (Model 6, Buxco Electronics, Sharon, Conn., U.S.A.) We derived tidal volume by electronic integration of inspired and expired air flow, pulmonary resistance (R_L) and compliance (C_L) by a method of electrical subtraction. From the volume-time trace we calculated respiratory rate, minute volume (V_E), time of inspiration (T_i), time of expiration (T_e), and total breath duration (T_t). In addition we measured end tidal CO_2 and O_2. We delayed flow, pressure and CO_2 using a digital delay (Buxco Electronics) to synchronize the signals for gases, flow and pressure. Analog signals from the pulmonary mechanics analyzer went into an ink jet recorder (Siemens-Elema) for analog recording of up to 8 signals. Simultaneously, all signals were fed into a data logger (DL 24, Buxco Electronics) for analog-to-digital conversion and from there into a computer system (IBM PC XT). Data were averaged for each breath and printed out by an ink jet printer (Model PT 89, Siemens). Results analyzed by the computer were compared routinely with those obtained from tracings of the analog recorder for accuracy. On days without experiments we trained dogs on the treadmill for at least one hour to keep them conditioned to all procedures.

Single experiment:

We intubated the dog, advanced an oesophageal balloon catheter through a bite block into the oesophagus, attached ECG leads and connected the endotracheal tube to a non-rebreathing valve. The experiment was preceded by a warm up period of at least 30 min to achieve a steady breathing pattern and a constant heart rate. The experiment itself began with a 5 min control period, after which the dogs inhaled a 1:10 or 1:100 dilution in NaCl of the Ascaris suum antigen (Greer Laboratories, Lenoir, N.J., U.S.A.) for 20-45 sec. The response to the antigen was measured for 15 min.

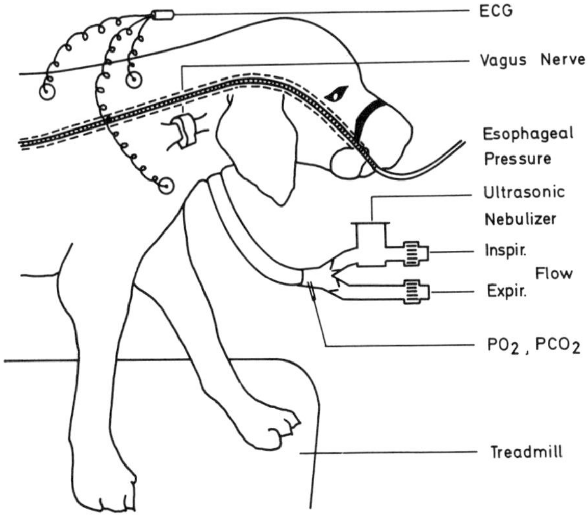

Fig. 1. Schematic diagram of dog model: the Ascaris-sensitive dog studied awake. Chronic tracheostomy, inspired and expired air flow measured through pneumotachometers, transpulmonary pressure by oesophageal catheter, heart rate from a 3 lead ECG. Exteriorized vagus nerves (skin loops) not used in these experiments.

Study design:

One crossover consisted of 2 experiments 14 days apart: the first allergen challenge was performed after treatment with placebo (0.9 % NaCl, solvent for SRI 63-441), the second after treatment with the PAF-antagonist SRI 63-441. Another crossover was started 2 weeks later. Each animal underwent two such crossovers.

Treatment:

Intravenous injection of 5 mg kg^{-1} SRI 63-441 was followed by inhalation of 10 mg SRI 63-441 in 10 ml 0.9 % NaCl from a DeVilbiss No. 65 nebulizer starting one hour before exposure to Ascaris suum antigen. The dog was placed on the treadmill immediately after the end of the inhalation from the nebulizer which took approximately 20 minutes. In placebo experiments the same protocol was followed, but 0.9 % NaCl was substituted for SRI 63-441.

Statistical analysis:

Averages were calculated every 30 sec during the experiment. Markers could be inserted by computer after the experiment and 30 sec averages could be recalculated starting from those markers. In this series of experiments we placed a marker at the start of the allergic reaction because the interval between the inhalation of allergen and the start of the reaction, though highly reproducible for a given dog, differed between dogs. Average results for each treatment were derived by averaging data first within and then between animals (n=5). Statistical evaluation of differences within placebo and within treatment experiments was by one way analysis of variance. The significance of differences between baseline and response to Ascaris suum antigen was assessed by Dunnett's Test. Differences between placebo and drug were evaluated by paired T-test (N=5).

Results:

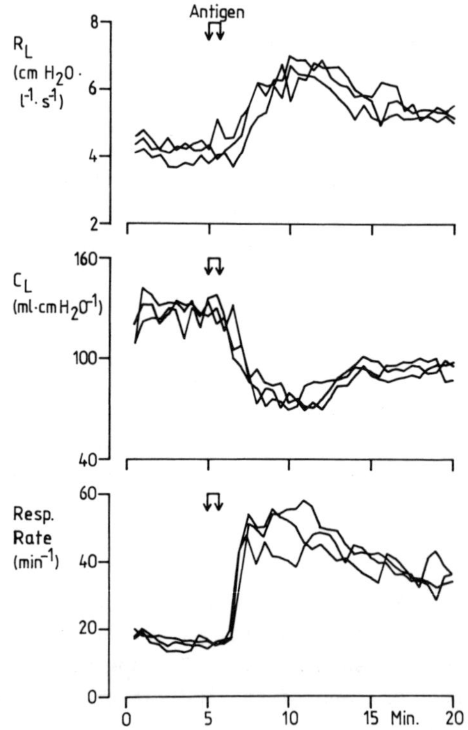

Fig. 2. Reproducibility of experiments: 3 experiments performed in the same dog at intervals of 4 weeks. Highly reproducible reactions to Ascaris suum antigen: increases in lung resistance (R_L, top), respiratory rate (bottom) and decreases in compliance (C_L, middle).

Experiments within animals were highly reproducible (Fig. 2). The lag from the start of antigen inhalation to the start of the allergic reaction varied between 0.5 and 3.5 min between animals. We normalized the start of the time axis to the start of the allergic reaction (fig. 3). Inhalation of Ascaris suum antigen caused significant increases in R_L, resp. rate, V_E, V_{Ti}/T_i and V_{Te}/T_e, and significant decreases in C_L, V_{Ti}, V_{Te}, T_i, T_e and T_t. Most of these changes were significant even when absolute data were used; all of them were significant when we smoothed data by expressing them as percent of baseline. Treatment with SRI 63-441 induced significant changes in baseline variables before application of Ascaris suum antigen: for instance, the PAF-antagonist increased baseline resistance 29 %, increased respiratory rate 41 % and reduced tidal volume 16 % (Fig. 3).

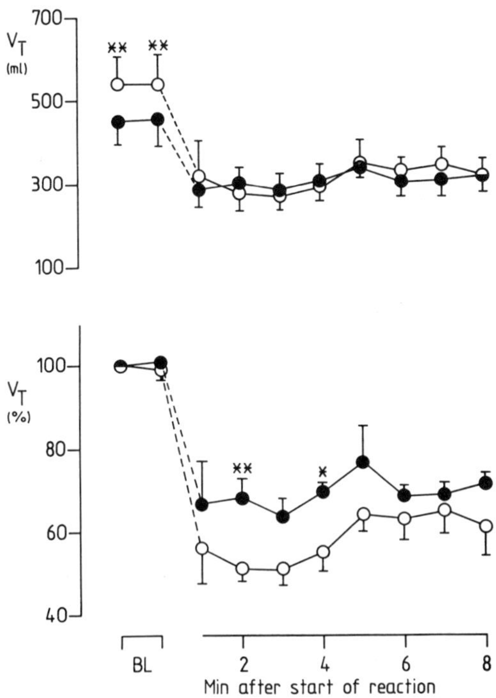

Fig. 3. Tidal volume (V_T) in awake dogs before and after inhalation challenge with Ascaris suum antigen. Data expressed in absolute units (top) and as per cent of baseline (bottom). Each curve represents average data from 2 experiments in each of 5 dogs. Data plotted as mean values ± standard error (x±SE) with n=5. Asterisks (*) indicate significance of difference between placebo (open symbols) and SRI 63-441 (closed symbols).

When absolute data were used, significant differences between placebo and SRI 63-441 were found only for baseline variables (C_L, resp. rate and V_T), not for variables measured after antigen inhalation (Fig. 3, top panel). When data were normalized to their new baselines after the antagonist, i.e., were expressed as % of baseline, SRI 63-441 significantly inhibited allergen-induced changes in R_L, (2 and 6 min after start of reaction), V_T (2 and 4 min, see fig. 3, bottom panel) and respiratory rate (2 min). C_L was not affected significantly, but there was a tendency for C_L to be increased.

Discussion:

Compound SRI 63-441 appears to be a partial agonist, causing moderate bronchoconstriction and significant changes in the control of respiration by itself. Subsequent peaks of the reaction were the same as without treatment so the difference to baseline and % changes were reduced. Clinically this would mean a patient exposed to allergen would still deteriorate to the same level as before and the difference to baseline would be less only because baseline values had deteriorated after treatment. This could hardly be interpreted as clinical improvement and partial agonism of SRI 63-441 would seriously limit the clinical usefulness of the compound. More important in this context, interpretation concerning involvement of PAF in the allergic reaction becomes very complicated. Possible interpretations of our results are as follows. [1] Since, in principle, deterioration of baseline variables predisposes to a more severe asthmatic reaction, the fact that the allergic reaction was unchanged after treatment indicates a protective effect of SRI 63-441. [2] Partial agonism of SRI 63-441 or a nonspecific membrane effect of SRI 63-441 (based on its phospholipid character) caused release of mediators from cells involved in the allergic reaction. Partially depleted cells released fewer mediators during the allergic reaction. No PAF involvement. [3] Partial agonism of SRI 63-441 leading to elevated baseline values caused tachyphylaxis of the PAF receptor - specific tachyphylaxis to PAF is known to occur rapidly. PAF released during the subsequent allergic reaction was less effective because it found receptors desensitized. Apparent protection was, in fact, tachyphylaxis. This possibility would imply a rôle for PAF in the allergic reaction although for reasons unrelated to receptor antagonism. [4] Elevated baseline values and reduced % changes after treatment were due to toxic effects of SRI 63-441 and were unrelated to PAF antagonism. [5] Mechanisms leading to baseline elevation were entirely different from those involved in the allergic reaction. The allergic reaction proceeded as before, there was no protection by SRI 63-441 and it would be incorrect to express data after allergen as per cent of (new) baseline because this would imply a relationship between the two which did not exist. [6] There could have been a mixture of mechanisms 1-5. In summary we cannot totally exclude the possibility that PAF was involved in the allergic reaction, but since allergen-induced changes (calculated from new baseline values) were only moderately reduced and since variables expressed in absolute units were totally unchanged (see table) PAF would not seem to be the only or the major mediator of the allergic reaction.

Table I. Respiratory variables before and after allergen following pretreatment with placebo and with SRI 63-441. Data in each column are expressed in absolute units (left) and as % of control (right).

Before/after Allergen	Resistance ($cm\ H_2O \cdot l^{-1} \cdot s^{-1}$)		Compliance ($ml \cdot cm\ H_2O^{-1}$)		Resp. rate (min^{-1})		Tidal vol. (ml)	
Placebo								
Before	3.48	100%	111.9	100%	18.6	100%	538.2	100%
After	5.67	163%	61.5	56%	59.6	305%	274.2	51%
SRI 63-441								
Before	4.48	100%	117.3	100%	26.3	100%	452.4	100%
After	6.55	151%	69.4	60%	55.9	207%	286.4	64%

Although our results suggest that PAF might not be an important mediator in bronchial asthma receptor heterogeneity may be an alternative explanation. Recent results show substantial heterogeneity of PAF receptors. Receptors on thrombocytes and leucocytes differ from those on macrophages (PAF_1 vs. PAF_2) (13). It is possible that antagonists "constructed" against one receptor are ineffective against another. The usual way of screening prospective PAF antagonists, i.e., testing their efficacy in displacing PAF from the PAF-receptor on platelets selects compounds antagonizing the platelet receptor. This receptor may not be as important for reactions in the respiratory system as the PAF-receptor on macrophages (1,2), on eosinophils (14) or on bronchial smooth muscle (9).

References:

1 Arnoux, B., D. Duval, J. Benveniste (1980) Release of platelet activating factor (PAF-acether) from alveolar macrophages by the calcium ionophore A 23187 and phagocytosis. Eur. J. Clin. Invest. 10, 437-441.

2 Arnoux, B., M.H. Simoès-Caeiro, A. Landes, M. Mathieu, P. Duroux, J. Benveniste (1982) Alveolar macrophages from asthmatic patients release platelet activating factor (PAF-acether) and lyso-PAF-acether when stimulated with the specific allergen. Am. Rev. Respir. Dis. 125 (4, part 2) 70.

3 Cuss, F.M., C.M. Dixon, P.J. Barnes (1986) Inhaled platelet activating factor causes bronchoconstriction and increased bronchial reactivity in

man. Am. Rev. Respir. Dis. 133 Suppl., A 212.
4 Denjean, A., B. Arnoux, A. Lockhart, R. Masse, J. Benveniste (1984) Modification of alveolar cell population after PAF-acether-induced bronchoconstriction in baboons. Am. Rev. Respir. Dis. 129 Suppl., A 3.
5 Denjean, A., B. Arnoux, R. Masse, A. Lockhart, J. Benveniste (1983) Acute effects of intratracheal administration of platelet activating factor in baboons. J. Appl. Physiol.: Respirat. Environ. Exercise Physiol. 55 (3), 799-804.
6 Hahn, H.-L., I. Purnama, M. Lang, U. Sannwald, H. Stenzel (1985) Effects of platelet activating factor on release of mucus from tracheal submucosal glands in the ferret. Am. Rev. Respir. Dis. 131 (4), A 27.
7 Handley, D.A., J.C. Tomesch, R.N. Saunders (1986) pers. comm. and Thromb. Haemostas. (in press).
8 Hirshman, C.A., D.A. Leon, N.A. Bergman (1981) The basenji-greyhound dog: antigen-induced changes in lung volumes. Respir. Physiol. 43, 377-388.
9 Hwang, S.B., C.S. Lee, M.J. Cheah, T.Y.Shen (1983) Specifific receptor sites for 1-O-alkyl-2-O-acetyl-sn-glycero-3-phosphocholine (patelet activating factor) on rabbit platelet and guinea pig smooth muscle membranes. Biochemistry 22, 4756-4763.
10 Kessler, G.-F., O.L. Frick, W.M. Gold (1974) Immunologic and physiologic characterization of the rôle of reaginic antibodies in experimental asthma in dogs. Int. Archs. Allergy Appl. Immunol. 47, 313-328.
11 Krell, R.D. (1978) Investigation of the rôle of histamine in antigen-induced bronchoconstriction in the ascaris-hypersensitive dog. Br. J. Pharmac. 62, 519-528.
12 Krell, R.D., L.W. Chakrin (1976) An in vitro model of canine immediate-type hypersensitivity reactions. Int. Archs. Allergy Appl. Immunol. 51, 641-655.
13 Lambrecht, G., M.J. Parnham (1986) Kadsurenone distinguishes between different platelet activating factor subtypes on macrophages and polymorphonuclear leucocytes. Br. J. Pharmac. 87, 287-289.
14 Lee, T.C., D.J. Lenihan, B. Malone, L.L. Roddy, S.I. Wasserman (1984) Increased biosynthesis of platelet-activating factor in activated human eosinophils. J. Biol. Chem. 259, 5526-5530.
15 Page, C.P., J. Morley (1984) Platelet activating factor. Sandoz asthma series 10, 17-22.
16 Patterson, R., J.F. Kelly (1974) Animal models of the asthmatic state. Ann. Rev. Med. 25, 53-68.
17 Rubin, A.E., L.J. Smith, R. Patterson (1986) Effect of platelet activating factor (PAF) on normal human airways. Am Rev. Respir. Dis. 133 Suppl., A 91.

Hans-L. Hahn, MD, PhD, Medizinische Poliklinik, University of Würzburg, Klinikstr. 8, 8700 WÜRZBURG - West Germany